METHODS IN MOLECULAR BIOLOGY™

For further volumes:
http://www.springer.com/series/7651

Mouse Models of Allergic Disease

Methods and Protocols

Edited by

Irving C. Allen

Department of Biomedical Sciences and Pathobiology, Virginia-Maryland Regional College of Veterinary Medicine, Virginia Polytechnic Institute and State University, Blacksburg, VA, USA

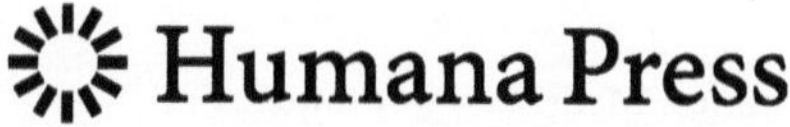

Editor
Irving C. Allen
Department of Biomedical Sciences and Pathobiology
Virginia-Maryland Regional College of Veterinary Medicine
Virginia Polytechnic Institute and State University
Blacksburg, VA, USA

ISSN 1064-3745 ISSN 1940-6029 (electronic)
ISBN 978-1-62703-495-1 ISBN 978-1-62703-496-8 (eBook)
DOI 10.1007/978-1-62703-496-8
Springer New York Heidelberg Dordrecht London

Library of Congress Control Number: 2013941724

Printed on acid-free paper

Humana Press is a brand of Springer
Springer is part of Springer Science+Business Media (www.springer.com)

Preface

A diverse spectrum of human disorders can be classified as allergic diseases, including asthma, anaphylaxis, and atopic dermatitis. In general, each of these disorders can be characterized as a complex genetic disease or syndrome, with specific environmental cofactors that contribute to exacerbations. Allergic diseases typically result in significant quality-of-life issues for the patient due to the sudden and acute nature of the exacerbations. Over the last half century, a dramatic increase in allergic diseases has been observed throughout industrialized nations, which has resulted in significant worldwide socioeconomic challenges.

The first complete draft sequences of the human genome were published over a decade ago. Since the publication of this scientific milestone, researchers have been expanding their focus towards increasing our understanding of the normal biological functions of our genes and associating genetic mutations with disease states. While the ultimate goal of biomedical research is to improve the health and welfare of the human population, there are significant limitations and restrictions associated with human research. For example, in addition to ethical and cost limitations, human studies of allergic diseases have been limited by the complex genetic and environmental interactions that result in significant pathogenic heterogeneity among individual patients. To circumvent these limitations, mouse models have been developed that serve as effective surrogates for many of the most prevalent human diseases. Indeed, allergy research has been significantly enhanced by the ability to manipulate gene expression in mice. It is now considered routine to generate mice that either lack or overexpress specific genes of interest. Likewise, novel technological approaches have provided researchers with the ability to conditionally alter gene expression in a cell type- and temporal-specific manner. These advances in mouse genetics have occurred in parallel with human clinical studies and have greatly complemented our understanding of the mechanisms associated with allergic diseases.

Mouse Models of Allergic Disease. Methods and Protocols has assembled a highly acclaimed group of contributors with extensive experience in genetics, allergy research, immunology, and in vivo model systems. Similar to the other volumes in the *Methods in Molecular Biology* series, these contributors have provided step-by-step protocols for the design and execution of experiments to thoroughly analyze critical elements associated with a diverse range of allergic diseases. Emphasis has been placed on mouse models that accurately recapitulate clinically relevant aspects of the respective human disease. The first section of this volume outlines protocols that are essential for effective ex vivo cell isolation and evaluation of specific cell types that are highly relevant to a diverse range of allergic diseases. While the greatest advantage of mouse research is the ability to model disease processes in vivo, the complexity of the whole animal often creates barriers to fully elucidate the mechanism underlying the disease state. Thus, it is often necessary to simplify the system through focused mechanistic studies on individual cell types. In the second section, we discuss in vivo protocols commonly used to evaluate prevalent mouse models of human allergic diseases, including mouse models of systemic anaphylaxis, contact hypersensitivity, allergic rhinitis, and asthma. We have devoted the third section to an overview of in vivo and ex vivo protocols that are commonly used to assess indirect mediators of allergic diseases, such as the nervous system, non-hematopoietic cells, and the composition of the gut microbiome. It is my sincere hope that *Mouse Models of Allergic Disease* will be considered an essential collection of protocols that allow both novice and expert researchers the ability to accurately develop, evaluate, and characterize the mechanisms associated with these disorders.

Blacksburg, VA, USA ***Irving C. Allen***

Contents

Contributors

IRVING C. ALLEN • *Department of Biomedical Sciences and Pathobiology, Virginia-Maryland Regional College of Veterinary Medicine, Virginia Polytechnic Institute and State University, Blacksburg, VA, USA*
BRIANNE R. BARKER • *Department of Biology, Drew university, Madison, NJ, USA*
ROBERT BRENNER • *Department of Physiology, University of Texas Health Science Center at San Antonio, San Antonio, TX, USA*
WILLIE JUNE BRICKEY • *Department of Microbiology and Immunology, University of North Carolina at Chapel Hill, Chapel Hill, NC, USA*
STEVEN L. BRODY • *Department of Internal Medicine, Pulmonary and Critical Care Division, Washington University in St. Louis, Saint Louis, MO, USA*
VIRGINIA MCMILLAN CARR • *Department of Otolaryngology, Head & Neck Surgery, Feinberg School of Medicine, Northwestern University, Chicago, IL, USA*
RITA CARSETTI • *Unit of B Cell Development, Research Center Ospedale Pediatrico Bambino Gesù (IRCSS), Rome, Italy*
SIMONA CASCIOLI • *Unit of B Cell Development, Research Center Ospedale Pediatrico Bambino Gesù (IRCSS), Rome, Italy*
DANIEL H. CONRAD • *Department of Microbiology and Immunology, Virginia Commonwealth University School of Medicine, Richmond, VA, USA*
DONALD N. COOK • *Laboratory of Respiratory Biology, National Institute of Environmental Health Sciences, National Institutes of Health, Research Triangle Park, NC, USA*
JAIME M. CYPHERT • *Matrix Biology Branch, Laboratory of Respiratory Biology, National Institute of Environmental Health Sciences, National Institutes of Health, Research Triangle Park, NC, USA*
BECKLEY K. DAVIS • *Department of Biology, Franklin & Marshall College, Lancaster, PA, USA*
JOHN D. DICKINSON • *Department of Internal Medicine, Pulmonary and Critical Care Division, Washington University in St. Louis, Saint Louis, MO, USA*
ELIZABETH DOYLE • *Department of Dermatology and Allergy, Allergie-Centrum-Charité,, Charité - Universitätsmedizin, Berlin, Germany*
JAN C. DUDDA • *Ludwig Institute for Cancer Research, The University of Lausanne, Lausanne, Switzerland*
CAROLYN G. DURHAM • *Department of Medicine, University of North Carolina, Chapel Hill, NC, USA*
KIMBERLY D. DYER • *Inflammation Immunobiology Section, Laboratory of Allergic Diseases, National Institutes of Allergy and Infectious Diseases, National Institutes of Health, Bethesda, MD, USA*
KATIA E. GARCIA-CRESPO • *Inflammation Immunobiology Section, Laboratory of Allergic Diseases, National Institutes of Allergy and Infectious Diseases, National Institutes of Health, Bethesda, MD, USA*

EZIO GIORDA • *Unit of B Cell Development, Research Center Ospedale Pediatrico Bambino Gesù (IRCSS), Rome, Italy*
LINDA H. GOWER • *Center for Stem Cell Biology, Vanderbilt University Medical Center, Nashville, TN, USA*
JOHN M. HARTNEY • *Integrated Department of Immunology, University of Colorado Denver and National Jewish Health, Denver, CO, USA*
JEREMIAH T. HERLIHY • *Department of Physiology, University of Texas Health Science Center at San Antonio, San Antonio, TX, USA*
EDA K. HOLL • *Department of Surgery, Duke University, Durham, NC, USA*
AMJAD HORANI • *Department of Pediatrics, Division of Pediatric Allergy, Immunology, and Pulmonary Medicine, Washington University in St. Louis, Saint Louis, MO, USA*
SCOTT A. HOSELTON • *Department of Veterinary and Microbiological Sciences, North Dakota State University, Fargo, ND, USA*
MIRJAM KOOL • *Department of Pulmonary Medicine, Erasmus Medical Center University Rotterdam, The Netherlands*
MARTINA KOVAROVA • *Pulmonary Division, Department of Medicine, University of North Carolina, Chapel Hill, NC, USA*
PATRICIA A. LABOSKY • *Office of Strategic Coordination, Division of Program Coordination, Planning, and Strategic Initiatives, Office of the Director, NIH, Bethesda, MD, USA*
BART N. LAMBRECHT • *Flemish Institute for Biotechnology Department for Molecular Biomedical Research Laboratory of Immunoregulation and Mucosal Immunology Ghent, Belgium; Erasmus Medical Center University Department of Pulmonary Medicine, Rotterdam, The Netherlands*
ROBIN G. LORENZ • *Department of Pathology, University of Alabama at Birmingham, Birmingham, AL, USA*
SABRINA MATTOLI • *Avail Biomedical Research Institute, Basel, Switzerland*
ANNE MCGOUGH • *Center for Stem Cell Biology, Vanderbilt University Medical Center, Nashville, TN, USA*
MARTIN METZ • *Department of Dermatology and Allergy, Charité - Universitätsmedizin, Berlin, Germany*
HIDEKI NAKANO • *Laboratory of Respiratory Biology, National Institute of Environmental Health Sciences, National Institutes of Health, Research Triangle Park, NC, USA*
CAROLINE M. PERCOPO • *Inflammation Immunobiology Section, Laboratory of Allergic Diseases, National Institutes of Allergy and Infectious Diseases, National Institutes of Health, Bethesda, MD, USA*
PHILIPPE POULLIOT • *Department for Molecular Biomedical Research, Laboratory of Immunoregulation and Mucosal Immunology, VIB, Ghent University, Ghent, Belgium*
ADEEB H. RAHMAN • *Division of Liver Diseases, Mount Sinai School of Medicine, New York, NY, USA*
ANNETTE ROBICHAUD • *SCIREQ Scientific Respiratory Equipment Inc., Montreal, QC, Canada*
ALAN M. ROBINSON • *Department of Otolaryngology, Head & Neck Surgery, Feinberg School of Medicine, Northwestern University, Chicago, IL, USA*
M. MANUELA ROSADO • *Research Center Ospedale Pediatrico Bambino Gesù (IRCCS), Rome, Italy*
HELENE F. ROSENBERG • *Inflammation Immunobiology Section, Laboratory of Allergic Diseases, National Institutes of Allergy and Infectious Diseases, National Institutes of Health, Bethesda, MD, USA*

MARCO SCARSELLA • *Unit of B Cell Development, Research Center Ospedale Pediatrico Bambino Gesù (IRCCS), Rome, Italy*
MATTHIAS SCHMIDT • *Avail Biomedical Research Institute, Basel, Switzerland*
JANE M. SCHUH • *Department of Veterinary and Microbiological Sciences, North Dakota State University, Fargo, ND, USA*
LISA M. SCHWIEBERT • *Department of Cell, Developmental, and Integrative Biology, University of Alabama at Birmingham, Birmingham, AL, USA*
IURII SEMENOV • *Frank Reidy Research Center for Bioelectrics, Old Dominion University, Norfolk, VA, USA*
JENNIFER SKELTON • *Center for Stem Cell Biology, Vanderbilt University Medical Center, Nashville, TN, USA*
SANCHAITA S. SONAR • *Institute for Molecular Health Sciences, ETH Zurich, Zurich, Switzerland*
JAMIE L. STURGILL • *Department of Microbiology and Immunology, Virginia Commonwealth University School of Medicine, Richmond, VA, USA*
EVA M. STURM • *Inflammation Immunobiology Section, Laboratory of Allergic Diseases, National Institutes of Allergy and Infectious Diseases, National Institutes of Health, Bethesda, MD, USA*
JULIA TROSIEN • *Department of Dermatology and Allergy, Allergie-Centrum-Charité, Charité - Universitätsmedizin, Berlin, Germany*
MONIQUE A.M. WILLART • *Department for Molecular Biomedical Research, Laboratory of Immunoregulation and Mucosal Immunology, VIB, Ghent University, Ghent, Belgium*

Chapter 1

Transgenic Mouse Models

Jennifer Skelton, Linda H. Gower, Anne McGough, and Patricia A. Labosky

Abstract

The generation of transgenic mouse models has been a powerful technique for several decades and is still widely used. There have been many manuals and general reviews of this technology. This chapter is designed to be a "how-to" resource with detailed specifics.

Key words Mice, Transgenics, Microinjection, Pronuclear injection, Animal models

1 Introduction

The first report of injection of foreign DNA into mouse embryos was in 1974 by Ruldolf Jaenisch and Beatrice Mintz at Fox Chase Cancer Center in Philadelphia [1]; these investigators were injecting viral DNA into mouse embryos. The first report of transgenic mice was published in late 1980 from Frank Ruddle's group at Yale [2] and this was followed up by several other groups publishing similar technical success: Ralph Brinster, Richard Palmiter, and colleagues at the University of Pennsylvania [3], Frank Costantini and Elizabeth Lacy at Oxford who also achieved germ line transmission [4], and Erin Wagner, Beatrice Mintz, and colleagues at Fox Chase Cancer Center [5]. This technology has led to the development of a plethora of applications reviewed elsewhere [6]. Transgenic mice have been used to conduct cell lineage ablation, overexpression of genes of interest, analysis of promoters and enhancers driving tissue-specific expression, and the production of animal models to address questions of human disease.

Here we will describe the procedures commonly used to generate transgenic mice through pronuclear injection of foreign DNA constructs. The DNA, either plasmid or BAC DNA, is introduced into the mouse zygote just after fertilization via injection. Injected embryos are placed into a foster mother and the resulting offspring examined for possession of the transgene. Those founder animals

Irving C. Allen (ed.), *Mouse Models of Allergic Disease: Methods and Protocols*, Methods in Molecular Biology, vol. 1032,
DOI 10.1007/978-1-62703-496-8_1, © Springer Science+Business Media, LLC 2013

are then bred to test for germ line transmission and offspring analyzed for transgene expression and subsequent phenotype.

We have divided this chapter into relevant units as follows: (1) Preparation of mice; (2) Harvesting of Embryos for Microinjection; (3) Preparation of DNA for Microinjection; (4) Microinjection of DNA; and (5) Surgical Transfer of Embryos to Foster Dams.

2 Materials

2.1 Preparation of Vasectomized Male Mice

1. 6–8-week-old CD-1 male mice (Charles Rivers 022) or similar strain.
2. Scale appropriate to weigh mice.
3. Anesthesia (*see* **Notes 1** and **2**).
4. Analgesic (*see* **Note 1**).
5. BD *Micro-Fine* IV Insulin Syringes.
6. Sterile surgical pack: Scissors, iris scissors, serrated forceps, fine forceps #5.
7. Disposable Cautery Unit.
8. Suture (5-0 Ethicon vicryl).
9. Surgical glue or Skin Staples/wound clips.

   If using staples: Staple/clip Applicator and Staple/clip remover.
10. 3M Tegaderm for surgical drapes.
11. 95 % Alcohol.
12. Chlorascrub swabstick.
13. Iodine swab.
14. Clippers with #40 clipper blade.
15. Puralube Eye ointment.
16. Sterile Gloves.
17. Warming pad.
18. Clean cage.

2.2 Preparation of Pseudopregnant Females (Fosters)

1. CD-1 female mice 25 g or larger (4–5 weeks) (Charles Rivers 022) (or similar strain).
2. CD-1 vasectomized male mice.
3. Clean cage.
4. Blunt forceps (Graefe extra fine serrated forceps).

2.3 Preparation of Donor Females

1. Female mice 3–5 weeks of age (the following mouse strains are the most common for this procedure: B6D2F1; C57Bl6; C57Bl6/J; Albino Bl6/J; FVB; or 129S6). The mice are typically acquired from Taconic Farms, Harlan or The Jackson Laboratory.

2. BD *Micro-Fine* IV Insulin Syringes.
3. 0.9 % NaCl or sterile water.
4. 1.5 ml microfuge tubes.
5. Pregnant Mare Serum Gonadotropin (PMS) (Harbor-UCLA Research; 2,000 IU per ampoule). Dissolve 2,000 IU (one ampoule) in 40 ml of 0.9 % saline or sterile water. Aliquot 1,000 μl of the PMS stock solution into labeled microfuge tubes and store in −80 °C freezer for up 4 months. Inject 0.1 ml per mouse (5 IU) via intraperitoneal route. Caution: wear gloves when preparing this solution.
6. Human chorionic gonadotropin (hCG) (Harbor-UCLA Research; 1,000 IU per ampoule). Dissolve 1,000 IU (one ampoule) in 2.0 ml of 0.9 % saline or sterile water. Aliquot 100 μl of the hCG stock solution into labeled microfuge tubes and store in −80 °C freezer for up 5 months. Add 0.9 ml 0.9 % saline or sterile water to the tube when ready to use. Inject 0.1 ml per mouse (5 IU) via intraperitoneal route. Caution: wear gloves when preparing this solution.

2.4 Harvesting of Embryos for Microinjection

1. Appropriately superovulated and mated female mice.
2. Dissection instruments (blunt scissors, blunt forceps, sharp scissors, sharp forceps).
3. Hyaluronidase aliquot (Sigma Aldrich). Dissolve lyophilized hyaluronidase in distilled water to make a 10mg/ml solution. Filter sterilize through a 0.2 μm syringe filter. Aliquot 20 μl into labeled microfuge tubes and store in −20 °C freezer for up to 3 months. Use one aliquot per dish of M2 medium.
4. 5–35 mm dishes.
5. Mouse Embryo Culture Medium (i.e., M2 medium from EMD Millipore Corporation).
6. Embryo Culture Medium (i.e., EmbryoMax® KSOM Embryo Culture (1×), Powder, w/o Phenol Red from EMD Millipore Corporation).
7. Transfer pipettes.
8. Mouth pipette.
9. Flat mouth pieces (Biotech Inc.).
10. Mineral oil.
11. Kimwipes.
12. 95 % Alcohol.

2.5 Preparation of DNA for Microinjection

1. Qiagen QIAquick PCR Purification Kit column kit.
2. DNA fragment for injection.
3. Fluorometer.

4. Microcentrifuge.
5. 1.5 ml microfuge tubes.
6. 0.5 ml microfuge tubes.
7. 0.5 M EDTA.
8. 1 M HCl.
9. 1 M Tris–HCl.
10. 0.22-μm filter.
11. ddH2O.
12. 1× TE Microinjection Buffer: Prepare a 5 mM Tris–HCl and 0.1 mM EDTA solution with ddH_2O. Adjust the pH to 7.4 with 1 M HCl. Filter the solution and store at 4 °C for up to 3 months.

2.6 Microinjection of DNA

1. Inverted microscope (i.e., Leica DMI3000B Leica Microsystems).
2. Micromanipulators.
3. Mouth pipette.
4. Transfer glass.
5. Mouse Embryo Culture Medium (i.e., M2 medium from EMD Millipore Corporation).
6. Embryo Culture Medium (i.e., EmbryoMax® KSOM Embryo Culture (1×), Powder, w/o Phenol Red from EMD Millipore Corporation).
7. Embryo tested Mineral oil.
8. Depression slide.
9. Holding pipette (i.e., Fisher/Eppendorf).
10. Injection needle (i.e., Capillary glass for Injection needles from World Precision Instruments).

2.7 Surgical Transfer of Embryos to Foster Dams

1. Scale appropriate for weighing a mouse.
2. Anesthetic (*see* **Notes 1** and **2**).
3. Analgesic (*see* **Note 1**).
4. BD *Micro-Fine* IV Insulin Syringes.
5. Sterile surgical pack: Scissors, iris scissors, serrated forceps, two pair of fine forceps #5, Schwartz Micro serraphine clips.
6. Suture.
7. Surgical glue or Skin Staples/wound clips If using staples: Staple/clip Applicator and Staple/clip remover.
8. 3M Tegaderm for surgical drapes.
9. 95 % Alcohol.
10. Chlorascrub swabstick.
11. Iodine swab.

12. Clippers (Oster A5) with #40 clipper blade.
13. Puralube Eye ointment.
14. Sterile Gloves.
15. Warming pad.
16. Mouth pipette.
17. Flat mouth pieces.
18. Clean cage.
19. Cage identification.

3 Methods

3.1 Preparation of Vasectomized Male Mice

1. Anesthetize one mouse.
2. Administer analgesia.
3. Once the mouse is anesthetized, shave lower abdomen to cover an area much larger than the expected incision area.
4. Apply eye ointment to eyes.
5. Wet the shaved area with 95 % alcohol, taking care not to wet the entire mouse as this will lower body temperature unnecessarily.
6. Using a Chlorascrub stick, start in the center of surgical field and draw concentric circles out from the incision site toward the outer edges of the shaved area (*see* Fig. 3b).
7. Rewet the area with 95 % alcohol, again being careful not to wet the entire mouse.
8. Repeat the Chlorascrub step three times.
9. Repeat the scrub with an iodine swab one time in the same manner.
10. Open a surgery pack and don sterile gloves.
11. Make a small side-to-side incision through the skin just above the penis with scissors.
12. Open the abdominal wall with iris scissors, locate left testis, and exteriorize.
13. Locate the epididymis/vas deferens and gently separate them from the surrounding fat and tissue using the serrated and fine forceps.
14. Cauterize both ends of about a 0.5–0.75 cm section of the vas deferens.
15. Replace that testis into the abdomen and exteriorize the right testis and cauterize both ends of a section of that vas deferens.
16. Replace second testis into the abdomen and close the abdominal wall with absorbable sutures, using one or two single interrupted sutures.

17. Close skin with staples, nonabsorbable sutures, or surgical glue and place in a prewarmed cage for recovery.
18. Observe the mouse until it is fully ambulatory.
19. Observe daily for 7–10 days post-surgery for infection, redness, swelling, pain, etc. Report any postsurgical complications to the Veterinarian or Veterinary Technician. If staples or sutures were used to close skin incision they are to be removed at the end of the 7–10-day observation period.
20. The males may be used for pseudopregnant matings after 10 days.

3.2 Pseudopregnant Females (Fosters)

1. Remove CD-1 females from the cage and check the vulva for signs of estrus. Appropriate females will have moist, swollen, pink mucus membranes.
2. Place one female with one vasectomized male.
3. Check for a copulation plug the following morning using the blunt forceps if necessary.
4. Identify females with ear punches if necessary and label each cage by date of plug.

3.3 Donor Females: Superovulation of Female Mice for Pronuclear DNA Microinjections (See Notes 3–7)

1. Female mice are ordered 2 weeks before the scheduled injection day.
2. PMSG is usually administered between 11 a.m. and 1 p.m. Wearing gloves, an appropriate amount of PMSG should be thawed immediately before use and used within 30 min. Withdraw an appropriate amount of PMSG from the microfuge tube using one insulin syringe per strain.
3. Using the prepared syringe, inject 0.1 ml (5 IU) of PMSG solution per mouse intraperitonealy (IP). Continue with remaining mice.
4. Note the date and time that PMSG was administered on the cage cards and place the cages back in their respective locations in the animal facility.
5. Two days following administration of PMSG, hCG is given to each mouse by IP injection. hCG is also administered between 11 a.m. and 1 p.m. Wearing gloves, thaw an appropriate amount of hCG immediately before use and use within 30 min. Add 0.9 ml of sterile 0.9 % NaCl to the thawed microfuge tube containing hCG and mix well.
6. Using the diluted hCG solution and prepared syringe, inject 0.1 ml (5 IU) of hCG solution per mouse IP.
7. Following the administration of hCG, place each female with a stud male mouse. Check each female mouse for copulation plugs the following morning (*see* **Note 8**).

3.4 Harvesting of Embryos for Microinjection

1. Prepare the following 35 mm culture dishes containing the appropriate medium: *Culture dish 1* should contain ~2.5–3 ml of M2 medium and add a hyaluronidase aliquot after oviduct collection; *Culture dish 2* should contain 1–10 μl dot of M2 medium covered with mineral oil for washing away hyaluronidase; *Culture dish 3* should contain ~100 μl of M2 for the microscope set up and for moving embryos from the wash dish to the microscope; *Culture dish 4* should contain ~2.5–3 ml of KSOM for washing off the M2 medium. *Culture dish 5* should contain multiple (5–10)–10 μl KSOM dots covered with mineral oil. The two KSOM dishes will be placed in a humidified 5 % CO_2 incubator at 37 °C to equilibrate while zygotes are harvested.
2. Following overnight mating, sacrifice superovulated female mice by CO_2 overdose. Follow CO_2 overdose by a secondary method to ensure death, such as cervical dislocation. Also, verify death by monitoring mice for breathing.
3. Lay females on their backs and wet their abdomens with alcohol.
4. Pick up the skin with the dull forceps. Using scissors, cut the skin at the lower part of the abdomen.
5. Grasp the opposite sides of the cut that was just made and pull apart the incision to open the abdomen.
6. With fine scissors, cut through the peritoneum to open the abdominal cavity (Fig. 1a).
7. With blunt forceps, move the viscera to the side so the uterine horns can be easily observed. Locate the uterus (Fig. 1b) and with fine forceps, grasp the top part of the uterus (Fig. 1c).
8. Using fine forceps or scissors, pull the connective tissue away from the ovary and oviduct (Fig. 1c). Make a cut between the ovary and oviduct using fine scissors (Fig. 1d).
9. Make a second cut at the top of the uterus while grasping the oviduct with fine forceps (Fig. 1e).
10. Place the isolated oviduct in a 35 mm culture dish containing about 3 ml of M2 medium (Culture dish 1) and repeat the process on the other side. Repeat this process for the other embryo donors.
11. Once all oviducts have been collected, add one aliquot of hyaluronidase solution to the M2 medium dish and move the dish to a dissection microscope.
12. Using fine forceps, grasp one oviduct and focus the stereomicroscope on the oviduct.
13. Locate the ampulla on the oviduct. The ampulla is the swollen area near the upper portion of the infundibulum of the oviduct that contains the freshly ovulated and fertilized embryos.

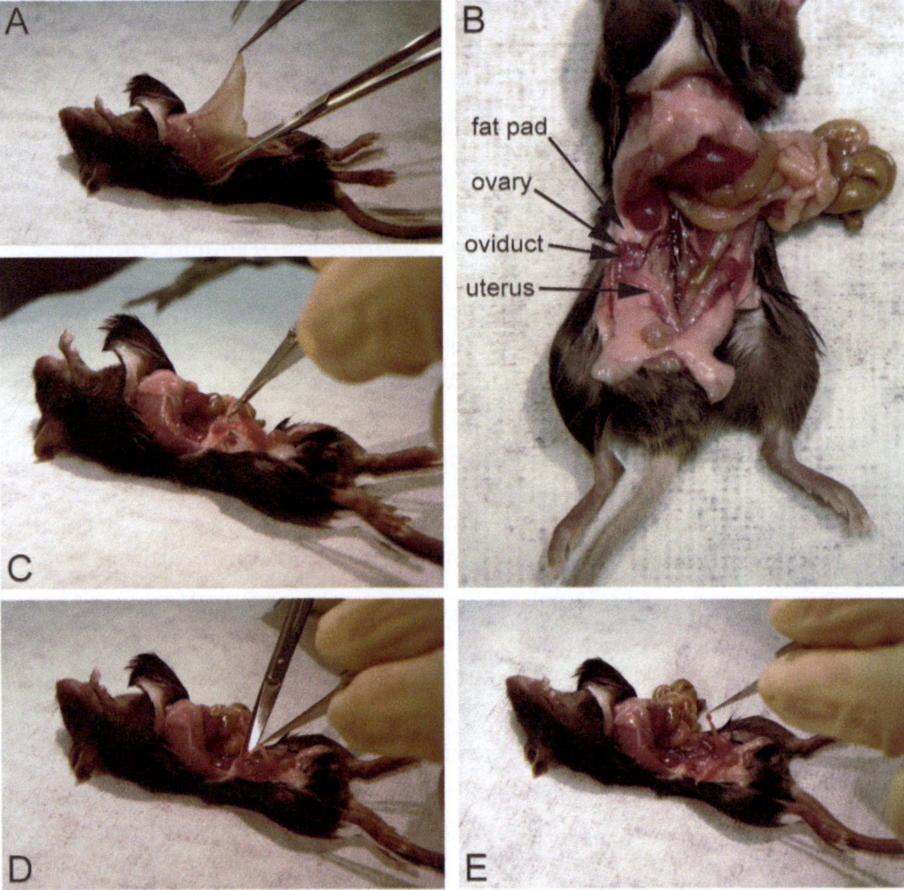

Fig. 1 Harvesting oviducts to isolate fertilized embryos. (**a**) After making an incision through the skin and pulling the skin anteriorly, an incision is made in the peritoneum to expose the body cavity. (**b**) Here the viscera are moved to the side and the organs of interest indicated. (**c**) The top part of the uterus is being held with fine forceps while scissors are used to remove the mesentery. (**d**) A cut is made between the ovary and oviduct using fine scissors. (**e**) Grasping the most anterior part of the oviduct with fine forceps, a second cut is made at the top of the uterus and this tissue moved to a 35 mm culture dish containing M2 medium for the isolation of embryos

With a pair of fine forceps in each hand, tear open the ampulla to release the embryos. It may help to gently squeeze the oviduct with the forceps to help release the embryos.

14. Repeat with each oviduct. The embryos will be surrounded by a mass of cumulus cells. Allowing the mass to incubate with the hyaluronidase in the M2 medium at room temperature for about 2 min will cause the cumulus cells to disaggregate.
15. Using a mouth pipette, collect the embryos in as little medium as possible with each transfer/movement of embryos.
16. Move the embryos through the M2 drop of medium covered in mineral oil (Culture dish 2).

17. Move the embryos from this M2 drop dish and wash the embryos in the KSOM wash dish (Culture dish 4).
18. Carefully observe the embryos in the KSOM wash dish and remove any fragmented, dead, or unfertilized embryos (Fig. 2). Embryos that appear uniform in size and shape and appear to have pronuclei (Fig. 2c) are identified and moved to the KSOM culture dish. Embryos can then be further selected for injection suitability and are placed in the KSOM drop culture dish (Culture dish 5) (Fig. 2). Move about 50 (or the number of embryos you are comfortable injecting within 30 min) to one dot of the KSOM drops covered in mineral oil.

    Continue moving the other fertile injectable embryos to the remaining dots of KSOM. Place the KSOM culture dishes in a humidified 5 % CO_2 incubator at 37 °C.

3.5 Preparation of DNA for Microinjection

1. Prepare the 1× TE Microinjection Buffer.
2. Purify DNA using a Qiagen Column (QIAquick PCR Purification Kit).
3. Determine the size of the DNA fragment. If it is over 10 kb, it is too big to run over a Qiagen column and should be diluted to injection concentration. If the fragment is under 10 kb, proceed with running it over a column to further clean up the DNA for injection.
4. Using a fluorometer, measure the initial concentration of DNA. Multiply this number by the volume to calculate the total amount of DNA.
5. The amount needed to run over a column is 1–5 μg of DNA.
6. Make a 1:5 dilution of DNA to PBI buffer (all buffers are provided in the Qiagen kit), and follow the manufacturer's protocols for the column.
7. Transfer the eluent to a clean, labeled microfuge tube and re-quantify the DNA using a fluorometer.
8. Calculate and make a 3 ng/μl dilution of DNA in 1× TE microinjection buffer.
9. Centrifuge the 3 ng/μl dilution at 10,000 RPM for 15 min.
10. Remove the top 50 μl and transfer to a clean, labeled 1.5 ml microfuge tube.
11. Label 4–5 0.5 ml microfuge tubes for injection. Add 5 μl aliquots to each tube.
12. Store all DNA and aliquots at −20°C until ready for use.

3.6 Microinjection of DNA

1. Using World Precision glass and a Sutter pipette puller (Model P1000), pull glass injection needles. (This should be done just prior to injection; approximately 6–10 needles should be available for an average injection day.)

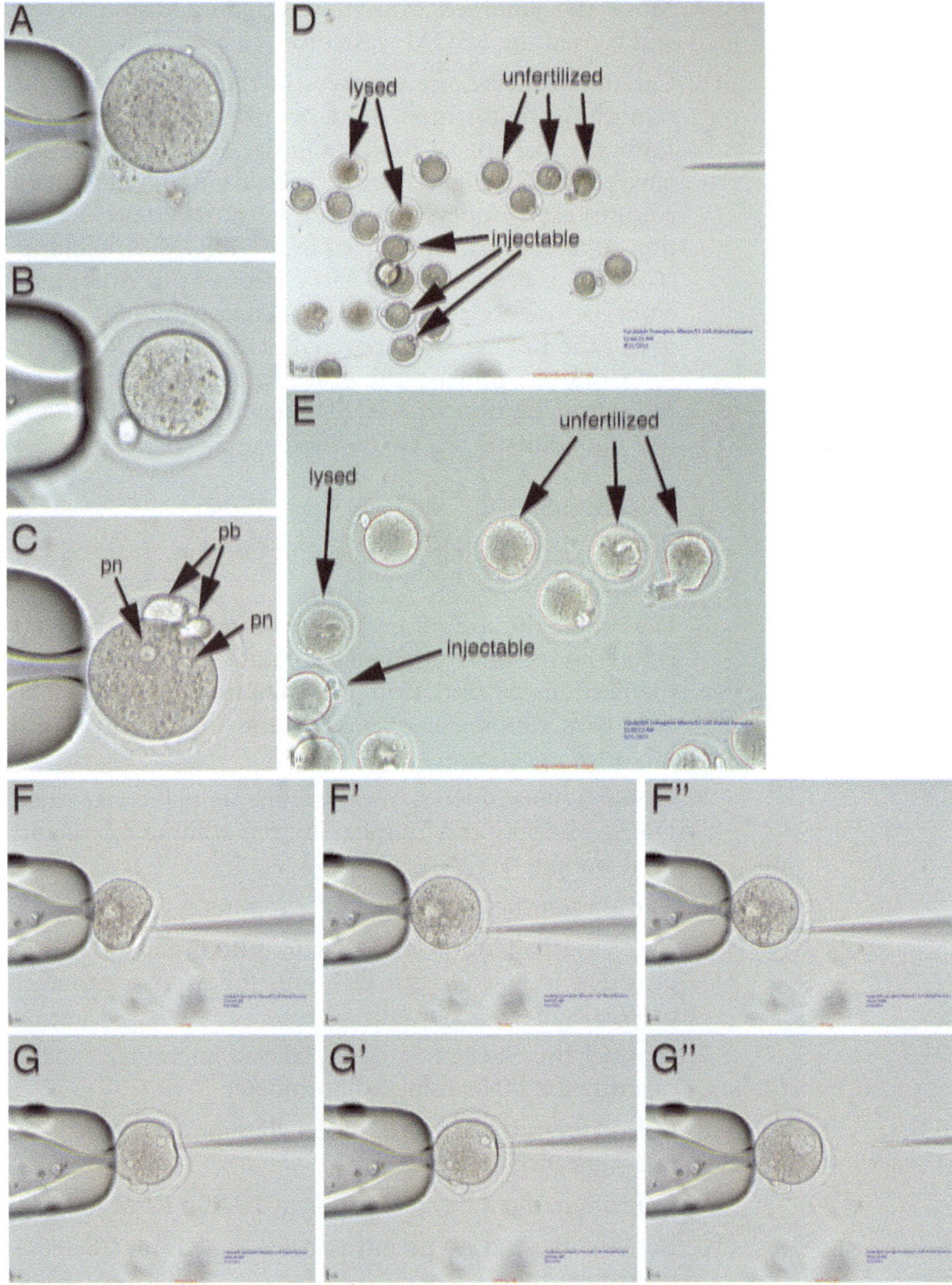

Fig. 2 Morphology of mouse embryos and microinjection. (**a** and **b**) Examples of poor quality embryos lacking clear pronuclei. (**c**) Example of an ideal fertilized one-cell embryo. Note the presence of two polar bodies (pb) and obvious pronuclei (pn). (**d** and **e**) Embryos are sorted and the unfertilized or lysed embryos discarded; these panels show examples of good and bad embryos. Panel **d** is 20× and panel **e** is 40×. (**f**–**g**″) Two series of successful pronuclear injection are shown here. Note how the pronucleus is swollen in the final frame of the injection series. In series **f**–**f**″ and **g**–**g**″ the injected pronucleus is located at approximately 5 o'clock and 2 o'clock, respectively

2. Set up the microinjection microscope by placing a holding pipette on the left manipulator and an injection pipette on the right micromanipulator.
3. Injection needles are loaded with prepared DNA using capillary action by inserting the open end (back end) of the injection needle into the DNA sample for a few seconds. Remove and secure the injection pipette with the sharp end pointed down, to allow the DNA solution to flow into the point of the needle. We use UHU tack, which is a sticky adhesive tack, to hold the pulled needles.
4. Place a 20 μl (or enough to form a drop approximately ¼″ in diameter) dot of M2 medium on a depression slide. Using a sterile transfer pipette, cover the M2 dot with just enough mineral oil to cover the drop of medium. Place and center the depression slide on the microscope.
5. Lower a holding pipette into the M2 medium and center it in the field of view. Allow the M2 medium to fill the holding pipette (1/4 or just past the bend in the holding pipette).
6. Place an injection needle on the right manipulator, lower it into the M2 medium and center the tip of the injection needle in the field of view.
7. Injection needles have closed tips when pulled on the pipette puller. The tip must be manually broken off. Carefully tap the injection needle against the holding pipette to create a small opening in the end of the needle.
8. Transfer the embryos from the culture dish in the incubator and place the desired number of embryos to be injected in one period (usually 30–50) into the medium on the depression slide.
9. Pick up an embryo using the holding pipette and rotate the embryo so that the pronuclear body is clearly visualized. The embryo should be in such an orientation that the larger of the two pronuclei (the male pronucleus) is located at the edge closest to the injection needle.
10. Slowly insert the injection needle into the pronucleus, avoiding nucleoli, inject the DNA until the pronucleus swells, then remove the injection needle. This is illustrated in the two series of injections shown in Fig. 2f, g. Note how the pronucleus is swollen in the last frame.
11. Move the embryo to a designated injected embryo area on the depression slide.
12. Repeat this process until all embryos are successfully injected within a 30-min time frame.
13. Remove the injected embryos from the depression slide and wash through the KSOM culture dish (Culture dish 4).

14. Remove the injected embryos from the KSOM wash dish and place in an appropriate dot of KSOM culture medium (Culture dish 5). Place the dishes containing embryos in a 37 °C incubator until the embryos are ready for transfer.

3.7 Surgical Transfer of Embryos to Foster Dams

1. Determine how many embryos survived the injection process. Viable embryos will maintain a good shape and appearance. Usually, twenty to twenty-five 0.5-day injected embryos are transferred into a pseudopregnant female.
2. Set up a clean cage on a warming pad so that it is prewarmed.
3. Set up a surgical field.
4. Weigh the mouse and administer the appropriate anesthetic/analgesic injection (*see* **Note 1**).
5. Place the mouse in a clean cage until it is fully anesthetized. This can be checked by monitoring for a pedal reflex (i.e., gently pinching the tail or hind foot).
6. To load the pipette with embryos, the pipette should be loaded with oil up to the larger shaft. An air bubble is then added and followed by a small amount of medium. Then a second air bubble, followed by another small amount of medium is added. Next, as carefully and precisely as possible, load the viable embryos in the transfer pipette. Load the embryos so that the embryos are as close to each other as possible with minimal extra medium between them. Finish loading the pipette by adding another air bubble and a small amount of medium.
7. Once the mouse is anesthetized, shave the hair on the back of the mouse. Make sure to shave beyond the surgical borders to enable good surgical preparation and apply eye ointment to the mouse's eyes (Fig. 3a).
8. Wet the shaved area with 95 % alcohol, taking care not to wet the entire mouse as this will unnecessarily lower body temperature.
9. Using a Chlorascrub stick, start in the center of the surgical field and draw concentric circles out from the incision site toward the outer edges of the shaved area (Fig. 3b).
10. Rewet the area with 95 % alcohol, again being careful not to wet the entire mouse.
11. Repeat the Chlorascrub step three times.
12. Repeat the scrub with an iodine swab one time in the same manner.
13. Place Tegaderm drape over the incision area (Fig. 3c, d).
14. The site is now sterile and the surgery pack may now be opened. Don the sterile gloves and begin the surgery.

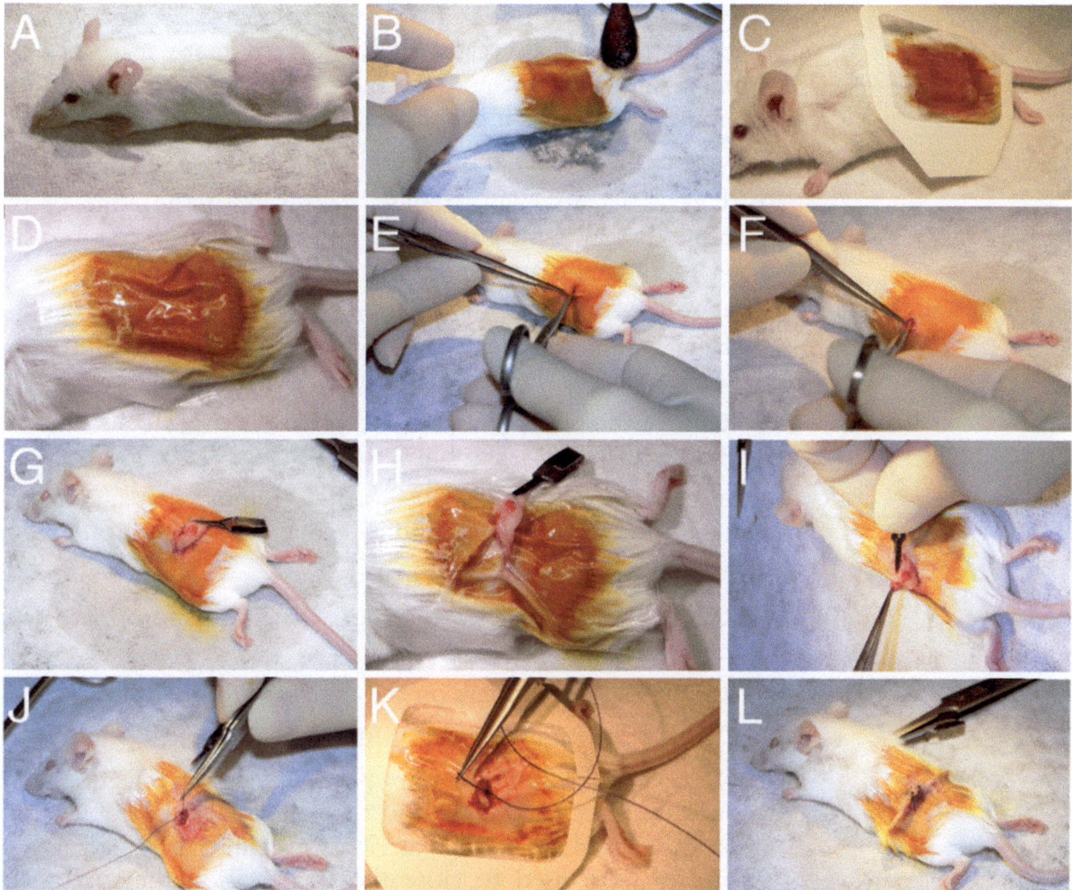

Fig. 3 Surgical transfer of injected embryos into recipient mouse. (**a**) View of mouse shaved for surgery. (**b**) Chlorascrub swabs and iodine swab are used to sterilize the incision site. (**c** and **d**) Tegaderm drape may be used to isolate the surgical field, this will likely be dictated by the local IACUC. (**e**) Initiate the surgery by making a small transverse (~1 cm) incision through the skin, on the side of the body, halfway between the most posterior rib and the hip. (**f**) Incise the peritoneum and locate the fat pad attached to the ovary. It will appear *orange*. Gently pull it out of the body along with the oviduct and ovary. (**g** and **h**) A serraphine clip is attached to the fat pad and stabilizes the reproductive organs for the transfer. (**i**) After the embryo transfer, gently place the organs back into the abdominal cavity. (**j** and **k**) Suture the abdominal wall, and (**l**) close the skin using either a wound clip (as shown) or surgical glue (not shown). *Note*: Some of these pictures feature a Tegaderm drape and some do not

15. Make a small transverse incision in the skin on the side just below the spine and halfway between the last rib and the hip using dissecting scissors and forceps (Fig. 3e).
16. Using fine scissors and forceps, make an incision into the peritoneum and locate the ovarian fat pad (Fig. 3f).
17. Place a serraphine clip on the fat pad and exteriorize the ovary, oviduct, and attached fat pad on a drape to keep the ovary in the visual field (Fig. 3g, h).

18. Place the mouse under a stereomicroscope. Focusing on the ovary and oviduct area, with fine forceps gently tear open the bursa surrounding the ovary and oviduct just above the infundibulum avoiding, if possible, any blood vessels.
19. Locate the oviduct and infundibulum.
20. If necessary to help stabilize, gently grasp the edge of the infundibulum with #5 forceps, and insert the tip of a transfer pipette into the opening of the swollen ampulla.
21. Blow gently and deposit the embryos into the oviduct. Observing the air bubbles inside the oviduct assures the successful transfer of the embryos. Pull the bursa back over the opening.
22. Remove the serraphine clip and place the ovary back into the abdominal cavity using blunt forceps (Fig. 3i).
23. Suture the abdominal wall (Fig. 3j, k) remove drape, and close the skin with either a wound clip (Fig. 3l) or a surgical glue.
24. Place the mouse in a prewarmed cage.
25. Record the anesthesia and analgesics used in appropriate drug logs.
26. Record all relevant data on the cage card for identification.
27. Observe the mouse until it is fully ambulatory.
28. Observe daily for 7–10 days post-surgery for infection, redness, swelling, pain, etc. Report any postsurgical complications to the Veterinarian or Veterinary Technician. If staples or sutures were used to close the skin incision they are to be removed at the end of the 7–10-day observation period.

4 Notes

1. The Department of Animal Care in your institution will likely dictate what anesthetic and analgesic agents you use, but here we list the following options that we have used with success:

   Anesthetic Option 1: Rompun/Ketaset (Xylazine/Ketamine) (Table 1). Administer 100 mg/kg Ketamine and 10 mg/kg Xylazine intraperitoneally (IP) to prepare the mice for survival surgery procedures. Dosage: 0.1 ml/10 g body weight per mouse IP.

Table 1
Rompun/Ketaset (Xylazine/Ketamine)

Dilution directions	50 mg/ml Ketamine	2.0 ml	4.0 ml
	100 mg/ml Xylazine	0.1 ml	0.2 ml
	0.9 % Saline	7.9 ml	15.8 ml
	Total	10 ml	20 ml

Table 2
Avertin (2,2,2-Tribromoethanol and *tert*-amyl alcohol)

Dilution directions for 20 mg/ml working solution	1.6 g/ml Avertin stock solution	0.5 ml
	0.9 % Saline	39.5 ml
	Total	40 ml

Table 3
Buprenex

Dilution directions	0.3 mg Buprenex	1 ml	0.5 ml
	0.9 % Saline	19 ml	9.5 ml
	Total	20 ml	10 ml

Table 4
Metacam

Dilution directions	5 mg/ml Metacam	1 ml
	0.9 % Saline	9 ml
	Total	10 ml

Anesthetic Option 2: Avertin (2,2,2-Tribromoethanol and *tert-amyl* alcohol (2-methyl-2-butanol)) (Table 2). Generate a stock solution of avertin (1.6 g/ml) by dissolving 25 g of 2,2,2-Tribromoethanol in 15.5 ml of *tert*-amyl alcohol. Mix at room temperature for ~12 h in a dark bottle on a rocker. The stock solution can be stored at room temperature for up to 1 year. Filter the solution though a 0.2 μm filter into a dark or foil-covered container and store at 4 °C. The working solution should be replaced monthly. Dosage: 250–500 mg/kg (0.25–0.5 mg/g) should be given IP to the mice. Avertin is lipid soluble so obese mice may require a larger dose.

Analgesia Option 1: Buprenex (controlled substance available through Webster Veterinary) (Table 3). Administer 0.05–0.1 mg/kg per mouse IP or SC every 8–12 h as needed.

Analgesia Option 2: Metacam (5 mg/ml). (Webster Veterinary) (Table 4). Generate a 1:10 dilution to yield a concentration of 0.5 mg/ml. Dosage: Administer 1 mg/kg per mouse IP, IM, or SC every 24 h as needed.

Analgesia Option 3: Rimadyl/Carprofen (50 mg/ml) (Table 5). (Webster Veterinary). Generate a 1:10 dilution to yield a concentration of 5 mg/ml. Dosage: Administer 5–10 mg/kg per mouse SC every 12–24 h as needed.

Table 5
Rimadyl/Carprofen

Dilution directions	50 mg/ml Rimadyl/Carprofen	0.2 ml
	0.9 % Saline	9.8 ml
	Total	10 ml

2. Caution: Avertin is hygroscopic and subject to photo degradation. The degradation products are lethal to mice. Always store in the dark at 4 °C or prepare fresh before use. Never use a solution that is yellow or contains a precipitate. This indicates that oxidation has occurred.
3. Fertilized embryos from superovulated female mice are typically used to maximize the number of embryos recovered per donor. Superovulated females are mated with fertile males so that 0.5-day post-coitum embryos can be acquired for pronuclear DNA microinjection. The desired result is for mating to occur at a time so that fertilization has occurred and that pronuclei will be visible during the injection period.
4. The goal of timed superovulated matings is to produce a large number of fertilized embryos at a specific time. This is achieved by the injection of pregnant mare's serum gonadotropin (PMSG) and human chorionic gonadotropin (hCG). PMSG and hCG mimic follicle-stimulating hormone (FSH) and luteinzing hormone (LH) and increase the number of oocytes ovulated per female.
5. The superovulated females should be mated with fertile males the night before the scheduled microinjection. Mice can be set up to mate after the administration of hCG. The fertile males (studs) used for matings are singly housed. One superovulated female is added to each male's cage and the following morning the female is checked for the presence of a copulatory plug. The stud males' ability to plug female mice is tracked to monitor the reproductive efficiency of each male.
6. Populations of vasectomized CD-1 males are used to mate with CD-1 females in estrous to produce pseudopregnant females. The morning after mating with the vasectomized males, the females are checked for a copulatory plug. Those that have plugged are used for the transfer of injected 0.5-day embryos from the pronuclear DNA microinjection.
7. A typical schedule is to inject PMSG on Monday, inject HCG and mate both superovulated females and females for pseudopregnant foster dams on Wednesday, and harvest embryos and perform the microinject on Thursday.

8. The light cycle is 12 h on/12 h off. The lights come on at 6 a.m. during daylight savings time and 7 a.m. during the summer. Mice to be superovulated are fed a high-fat diet to help stimulate egg production.

References

1. Jaenisch R, Mintz B (1974) Simian virus 40 DNA sequences in DNA of healthy adult mice derived from preimplantation blastocysts injected with viral DNA. Proc Natl Acad Sci USA 71(4):1250–1254
2. Gordon JW, Scangos GA, Plotkin DJ, Barbosa JA, Ruddle FH (1980) Genetic transformation of mouse embryos by microinjection of purified DNA. Proc Natl Acad Sci USA 77(12): 7380–7384
3. Brinster RL, Chen HY, Trumbauer M, Senear AW, Warren R, Palmiter RD (1981) Somatic expression of herpes thymidine kinase in mice following injection of a fusion gene into eggs. Cell 27(1 Pt 2):223–231
4. Costantini F, Lacy E (1981) Introduction of a rabbit beta-globin gene into the mouse germ line. Nature 294(5836):92–94
5. Wagner EF, Stewart TA, Mintz B (1981) The human beta-globin gene and a functional viral thymidine kinase gene in developing mice. Proc Natl Acad Sci USA 78(8): 5016–5020
6. Palmiter RD, Brinster RL (1986) Germ-line transformation of mice. Annu Rev Genet 20: 465–499

Chapter 2

Pulmonary Antigen Presenting Cells: Isolation, Purification, and Culture

Hideki Nakano and Donald N. Cook

Abstract

Antigen presenting cells (APCs) such as dendritic cells (DCs) and macrophages comprise a relatively small fraction of leukocytes residing in lymphoid and non-lymphoid tissues. Accordingly, functional analyses of these cells have been hampered by low cell yields. Also, alveolar macrophages share several physical properties with DCs, and this has complicated efforts to prepare pure populations of lung APCs. To overcome these difficulties, we have developed improved flow cytometry-based methods to analyze and purify APCs from the lung and its draining lymph nodes (LNs). In this chapter, we describe these methods in detail, as well as methods for culturing APCs and characterizing their interactions with T cells.

Key words Antigen presenting cells, Dendritic cells, Macrophages, Monocytes, Lung, Lymph nodes, Gradient centrifugation, Flow cytometry, Autofluorescence, Sorting, Culture

1 Introduction

Pulmonary APCs take up inhaled antigens, process them, and present antigen-derived peptides to T and B lymphocytes to initiate adaptive immune responses [1]. In keeping with their ability to acquire antigens from the airspace or parenchymal tissue, DCs and macrophages are located within the airway epithelium, lung parenchyma, and alveolar spaces [2, 3]. To maintain their positions within the lung, many DCs and macrophages adhere tightly to tissue stromal cells. Protocols that yield large numbers of lung APCs must therefore disrupt molecular interactions that hold APCs and stromal cells together. Although collagenase D has been widely used for this purpose, the yield of DCs obtained from procedures that employ this enzyme has been suboptimal. To improve cell yields, we have modified a tissue digestion method that was originally designed for cardiovascular tissue digestion [4], and found that this new protocol dramatically improves the yield of APCs from the lung [5].

Irving C. Allen (ed.), *Mouse Models of Allergic Disease: Methods and Protocols*, Methods in Molecular Biology, vol. 1032,
DOI 10.1007/978-1-62703-496-8_2, © Springer Science+Business Media, LLC 2013

Lung APCs are highly diverse in terms of both size and density. For example, alveolar macrophages are large and light, while monocytes are relatively small and dense, with lymphocytes and non-leukocytes having even higher densities. Therefore, gradient centrifugation provides a convenient and effective method to enrich for APCs [6]. We have developed simple methods that enrich for different APCs, depending on which type is needed for the individual experiment at hand. After this enrichment step, APCs are often analyzed by flow cytometry to determine their frequency and their display of cell surface molecules. Unlike most other macrophages in the body, alveolar macrophages display the pan-DC marker, CD11c, as well as MHC class II [7, 8]. Consequently, if other markers are not used, alveolar macrophages can be easily mistaken for pulmonary DCs. According, many investigators now use the autofluorescent properties of macrophages and their display of high levels of Siglec-F to distinguish them from DCs [7, 9]. In addition, pulmonary DCs are heterogeneous [2] and include plasmacytoid, inflammatory, and conventional DCs. The latter category includes the two major lung DC subsets, which express high levels of CD11b and CD103, respectively. $CD11b^{hi}$ DCs can be further segregated into pre-DC-derived and monocyte-derived DCs (moDCs) [10, 11]. In this chapter, we describe how to distinguish each DC subset from the others by flow cytometry. This technology is useful not only for characterizing APCs but also for purifying individual APC populations. Purified APCs can be subsequently studied ex vivo to identify their biologic functions. Here, we describe methods to culture lung APCs with naïve T cells to study APC-mediated T helper cell differentiation.

2 Materials

2.1 Tissue Digestion

1. Digestion buffer: PBS (Mg^- Ca^-) with 0.5 % BSA (pH 7.2–7.4), filter-sterilized and stored at 4 °C.
2. Preparation buffer: PBS (Mg^- Ca^-) with 0.5 % BSA and 2 mM EDTA (pH 7.2–7.4), filter-sterilized and stored at 4 °C.
3. 5 mg/ml Liberase TM (Roche) in PBS, stored at −20 °C.
4. 25 mg/ml Collagenase XI (approx. 12,500 U/ml) in PBS, stored at −20 °C.
5. 100 mg/ml Hyaluronidase type I-S (approx. 6,000 U/ml) in PBS, stored at −20 °C.
6. 20 mg/ml DNase I in water, stored at −20 °C (*see* **Note 1**).
7. 120 mM EDTA in PBS (pH 7.2), stored at 4 °C.
8. Nycodenz (Accurate Chemical).
9. Incubator, 37 °C.
10. Cell strainer 70 μm.

2.2 Staining of Leukocytes

1. Preparation buffer: PBS (Mg- and Ca-free) with 0.5 % BSA and 2 mM EDTA (pH 7.2–7.4).
2. FACS buffer: 0.5 % BSA, 0.1 % NaN_3, and 2 mM EDTA in PBS.
3. Normal mouse serum.
4. Normal rat serum.
5. Antibody dilution buffer (5 % normal mouse serum, 5 % normal rat serum, and 5 μg/ml anti-CD16/32 in FACS buffer).
6. Antibodies [12–14]

   Fc block: anti-mouse CD16/CD32 (2.4G2).

   Pan DC markers: CD11c (N418 or HL3), MHC class II I-A^b (AF6-120.1), or I-A^d (AMS-32.1) (*see* **Note 2**).

   DC subset markers: CD11b (M1/70), CD14 (Sa2-8), CD103 (M290 or 2E7), CD317 (JF05-1C2.4.1, 120G8, or eBio927), Ly-6C (AL-21), Siglec-H (eBio440c).

   Macrophage markers: CD11b (M1/70), CD11c (N418 or HL3), F4/80 (BM8), Siglec-F (E50-2440).

   Monocyte markers: CD115 (AFS98), Ly-6C (AL-21), CD11b (M1/70).

   Activation/maturation markers: CD40 (1C10), CD80 (16-10A1), CD86 (GL1), CD197/CCR7 (4B12).

   Lymphocyte markers: CD3e (145-2C11), CD19 (6D5 or eBio1D3), CD49b (DX5).
7. Round- (U) bottom 96-well plate.
8. Plate rotor.
9. 15 ml conical tubes.
10. FACS tubes.
11. Flow cytometer (e.g., FACS LSR-II (Becton Dickenson))

2.3 Cell Sorting and Culture

1. Cell sorter (e.g., FACS-ARIA-II (Becton Dickenson)).
2. RPMI 1640.
3. Fetal bovine serum, certified (low endotoxin).
4. β-Mercaptoethanol.
5. Penicillin/Streptomycin.
6. Round- (U) bottom 96-well plate.
7. Flat-bottom 96-well plate.
8. CO_2 incubator, 5 % CO_2, 37 °C.

3 Methods

3.1 Tissue Digestion

1. Collect lungs from mice and place in tissue culture dish (60 mm) or 6-well plate containing 1 ml of digestion buffer (Reagent #1) in Section 2.1. Up to four lungs per dish can be included.
2. Mince tissue using scissors, razor blade, and/or forceps (Fig. 1). Scissors are recommended.
3. Add 1 ml of digestion buffer (*see* **Note 3**). Add: 40 μl of Liberase, 20 μl of DNase I, 20 μl of collagenase XI, and 20 μl of hyaluronidase.
4. Swirl the dish gently, then incubate dish at 37 °C for 60 min.
5. During the incubation, prepare Nycodenz solution. Weigh Nycodenz according to your target cell types (Fig. 2): 1.45 g for Dendritic cells (excluding pDCs) and macrophages; 1.6 g for Dendritic cells (including pDCs), macrophages, large monocytes, and large B cells; 1.8 g for Dendritic cells (including pDCs), macrophages, monocytes, and large T and B cells. Add Nycodenz to 9.5 ml PBS in 15 ml tube. Place the tube on a shaker or a rotator.
6. To stop tissue digestion, add 0.4 ml of cold 120 mM EDTA to dish.
7. Add 5 ml of preparation buffer (Reagent #2 in Section 2.1) to 15 ml empty conical centrifugation tube (or 25 ml in 50 ml tube if you have multiple dishes). Keep the tubes on ice.

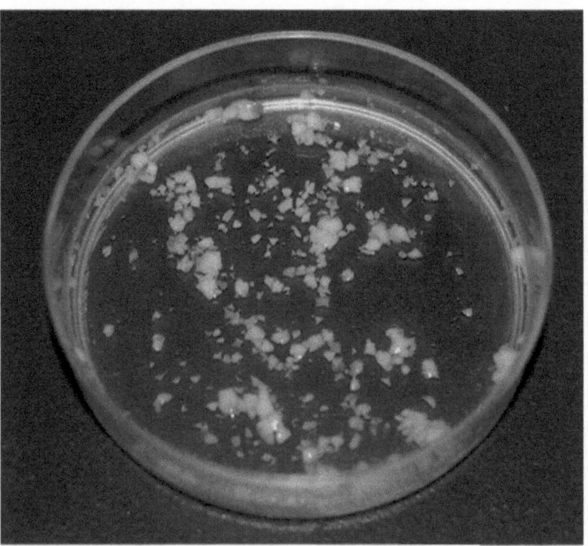

Fig. 1 Minced lung tissue. Lung tissue was minced by scissors in a 60 mm tissue culture dish. Smaller pieces (<1 mm) will result in higher cell yield

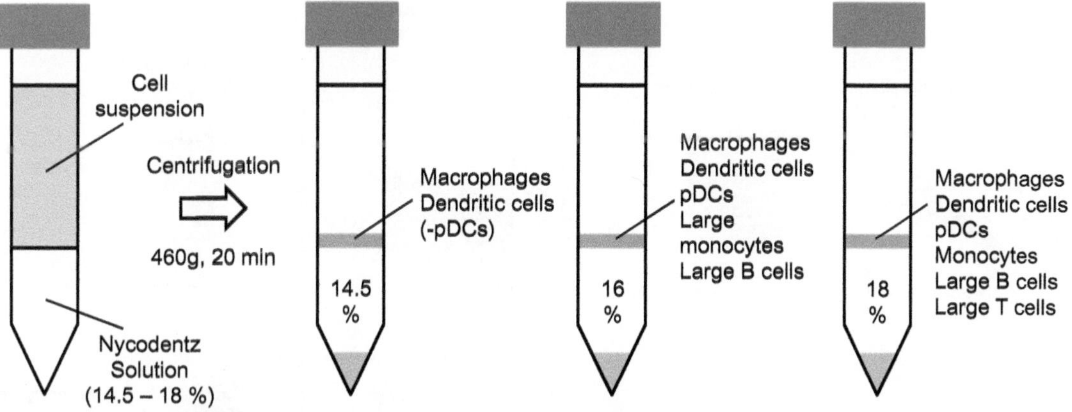

Fig. 2 Gradient centrifugation for enrichment of dendritic cells and macrophages from lung. Different concentration of Nycodenz enriches different cell types. Higher concentrations increases contamination of lymphocytes

8. Meanwhile, add 5 ml cold preparation buffer (Reagent #2 in Section 2.1) to dish. Transfer minced tissue onto a cell strainer in dish and using rubber-tipped plunger of a 3 ml syringe, push tissues through the cell strainer onto the dish.
9. Pipette the liquid in the dish back through the strainer several times to ensure a single cell suspension. Then pipette the cells several times to detach cells from dish, transfer cells (in 7 ml now) to 15 ml tube containing 5 ml of preparation buffer on ice (or 50 ml tube with 25 ml preparation buffer).
10. Centrifuge at $500\times g$ for 5 min at 4 °C. This is equivalent to 1,600 rpm in a table top Sorvall centrifuge.
11. Resuspend cells in 10 ml preparation buffer. Carefully layer 3 ml of gradient solution (e.g., 14.5–18 % Nycodenz solution in PBS) *under* the cell suspension, and spin at $450\times g$ for 20 min at room temperature with the brake OFF.
12. The enriched dendritic cells form a fuzzy white layer at the interface of the gradient solution and buffer. Remove the media until 1.5 ml of liquid is left above the interface. Collect the cell layer carefully (avoid the pellet in sample).
13. Wash cells with 5 ml preparation buffer. Spin cell suspension at $450\times g$ for 5 min at 4 °C with brake ON.
14. Resuspend cell pellets in 500–1,000 μl of preparation buffer. Count cells.

3.2 Staining of Leukocytes

1. Place 1×10^5–2×10^6 cells in each well of round-bottom 96-well plate. Afterwards, use a multichannel pipette. Spin the plate at $800\times g$ for 3 min, and then discard supernatant.
2. Add 50 μl of Ab dilution buffer, and then incubate the cells on ice for 5–10 min.

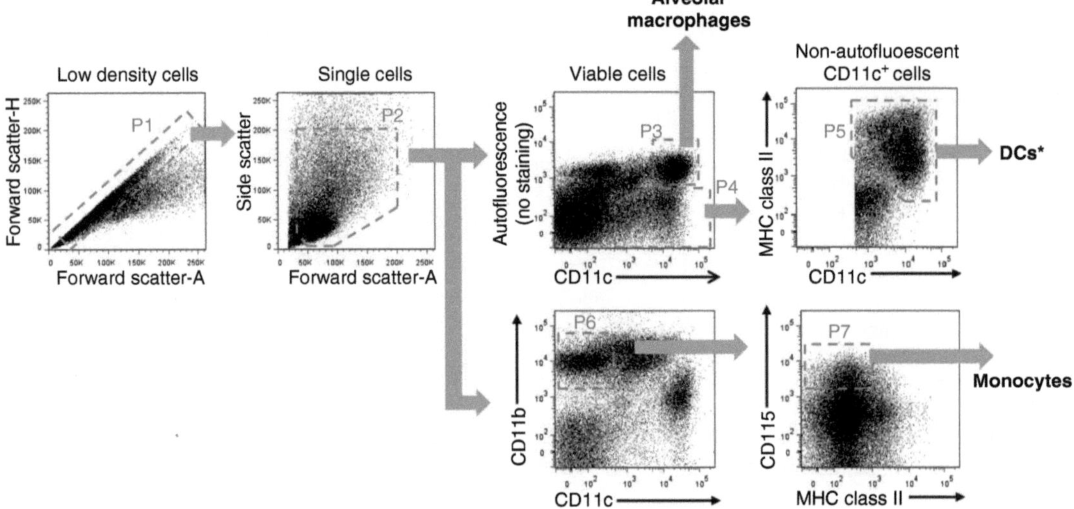

Fig. 3 An example gating strategy for lung APC analysis using flow cytometry. Gatings shown are for segregation of conventional DCs (P5) (*pDCs are not included in this gating), alveolar macrophages (P3), and monocytes (P7). Single cell gating (P1) excludes cell aggregates. P2 is the gate for viable cells. Conventional DCs are CD11c^{+} MHC-II^{+} autofluorescence^{lo} (pDCs are CD11c^{int} MHC-II^{lo}). Alveolar macrophages are CD11c^{hi} autofluorescence^{hi}. Monocytes are CD11b^{+} CD115^{+} MHC-II^{lo} (P7). For lymph node APC analysis, CD3 and CD19 are used instead of autofluorescence to exclude lymphocytes. More details and additional cell markers are described in **Note 6**

3. Prepare Ab cocktail with Ab dilution buffer (2× of final concentration). The optimal final concentration is usually 0.5–2 μg/ml. Add 50 μl of 2× Ab solution to cells then mix well.

   The Ab composition of the cocktail depends on the goal of the experiment, but an example is as follows: I-A^{b}—eFluor 450; CD11b—eFluor 605NC; CD103—Phycoerythrin; CD11c—PerCP-Cy5.5; CD115—APC; and Ly-6C—APC-Cy7. FITC-labeled Ab is not used because this channel will be used for detection of autofluorescence signals (*see* **Note 4**). Protect cells from light and incubate on ice for 30 min.

4. Wash cells with FACS buffer twice. The first time, add 100 μl FACS buffer, and the second time, resuspend the pellet with 200 μl of FACS buffer. Pipette cells every time to resuspend cells.

5. Suspend cells in 200 μl FACS buffer, and transfer cells to FACS tube.

3.3 Flow Cytometric Analysis

1. Gate on single cells (P1 in FSC-A vs. FSC-H) and viable cells (P2 in FSC-A vs. SSC) (Fig. 3).

2. Set voltage of each channel (*see* **Note 5**).

3. Run compensation samples (unstained cells and cells stained with single dye).

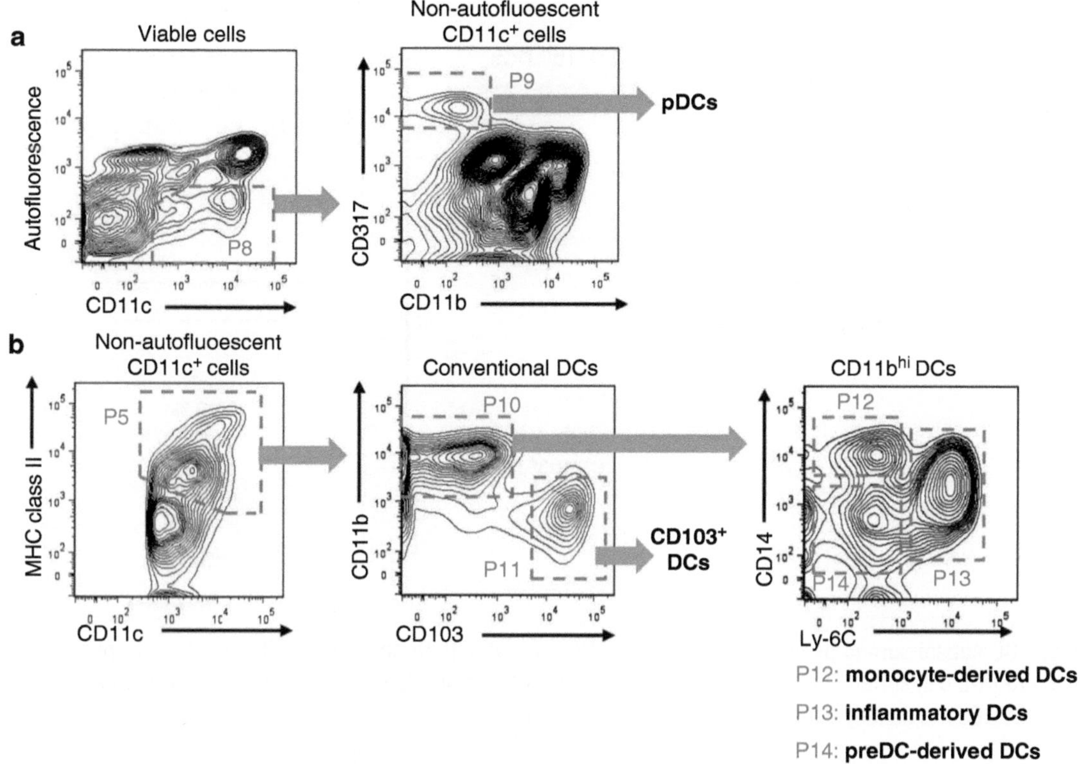

Fig. 4 Analysis of lung DC subsets. (**a**) Gating for pDC analysis; $CD11b^{lo}CD11c^{int}CD317^{+}$ (P9). (**b**) Gating for conventional DC subset analysis. Total $CD11b^{hi}$ DCs: $CD11b^{hi}CD11c^{+}MHC\text{-}Ii^{+}$ (P10); $CD103^{+}$ DCs: $CD11b^{lo}CD11c^{hi}CD103^{+}MHC\text{-}II^{hi}$ (P11); Monocyte-derived DCs: $CD11b^{hi}CD11c^{int}CD14^{hi}Ly\text{-}6C^{lo}MHC\text{-}II^{hi}$ (P12); Inflammatory DCs: $CD11b^{hi}CD11c^{int}Ly\text{-}6C^{hi}MHC\text{-}II^{+}$ (P13); PreDC-derived $CD11b^{hi}$ DCs: $CD11b^{hi}CD11c^{int}CD14^{int/lo}Ly\text{-}6C^{lo}MHC\text{-}II^{hi}$ (P14). More details and additional markers can be found in **Note 6**

4. Adjust compensation manually (*see* **Note 5**). We do not recommend using "Auto Comp," which cannot adjust compensation for DCs or macrophages. Set gates for positive cells (not autofluorescent cells) and negative cells, and then adjust the compensation value in each channel. Repeat same procedures for all channels.
5. Gate on DCs (P4 and P5; e.g., $CD11c^{+}MHC\text{-}II^{+}autofluorescence^{-}$ cells for LN DCs and/or alveolar macrophages (P3; $CD11c^{hi}$ autofluorescent)) (Fig. 2) (*see* **Notes 4** and **6**).
6. Gate on DC subsets (e.g., P10: $CD11b^{+}$, P11: $CD103^{+}$) (Fig. 4) (*see* **Note 6**).
7. Collect 10,000 cells (or as many as possible) in P5.

3.4 Sorting of Dendritic Cells

1. Place up to 1×10^8 cells in 15 ml conical tube. Fill the tube with preparation buffer (Reagent #2) in section 2.1.

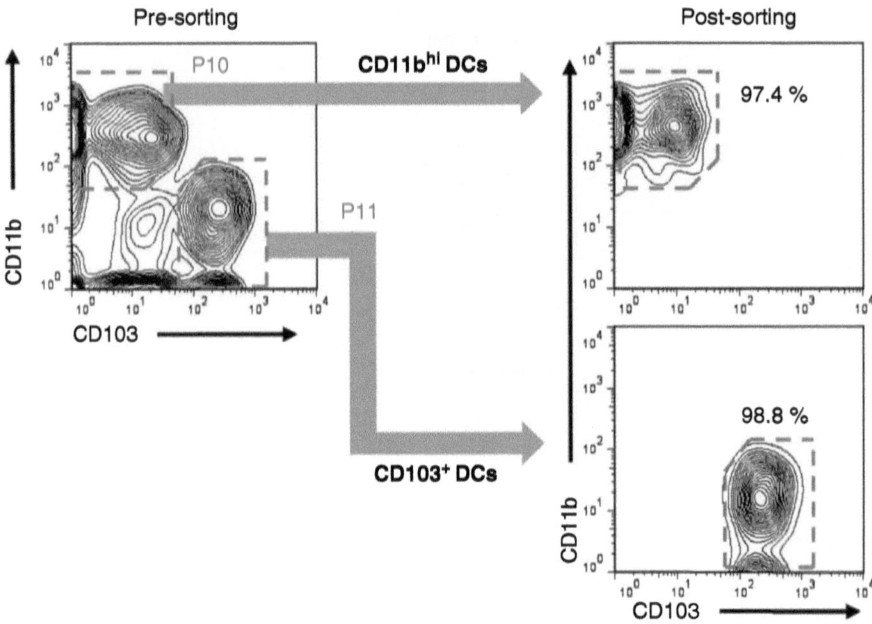

Fig. 5 DC subset sorting by flow cytometry. Total CD11b^{hi} DCs (P10) and CD103^{+} DCs (P11) were purified in a FACS ARIA-II cell sorter. Purified sorted cells are shown. Approximately 1–2 × 10^4 CD11b^{hi} DCs and 2–4 × 10^4 CD103^{+} DCs are usually obtained per mouse lung after sorting

Spin the tube at 500 × *g* for 5 min, and then remove supernatant.

2. Resuspend cells with 1 ml of Ab dilution buffer containing antibodies. Protect cells from light and incubate on ice for 30 min.
3. Meanwhile, add 4 ml of complete culture medium to each FACS collection tube.
4. Wash cells with preparation buffer (Reagent #2 in section 2.2) twice. The first time, add 14 ml of buffer, and the second time, resuspend pellet with 15 ml of buffer. Thoroughly resuspend cells every time.
5. Suspend cells in 1 ml of preparation buffer (Reagent #2 in section 2.2), and transfer cells to FACS filter cap tube.
6. Place 1 ml of preparation buffer (Reagent #2 in section 2.2) on the top of the tube three times to rinse the filter.
7. Remove 3 ml of complete culture medium from each collection tube.
8. Sort cells on FACS ARIA-II (Fig. 5) (*see* **Note 7**).

3.5 Culture of Dendritic Cells with T Cells

1. Transfer sorted dendritic cells or macrophages from the FACS tube to a 15 ml conical tube containing 10 ml of culture medium. Spin the tube at 500 × *g* for 5 min.

2. Wash cells twice with culture medium and then count the cells.
3. Resuspend dendritic cells with culture medium at 5×10^5/ml (*see* **Note 8**). Plate 5×10^4 dendritic cells (100 μl) in each well of a round-bottom, 96-well plate.
4. Add 50 μl of culture medium containing antigens, cytokines, or antibodies.
5. Adjust concentration of purified T cells to 2×10^6 cells/ml. Add 50 μl of T cell suspension to each well (final number: 1×10^5 cell/well)(*see* **Note 9**).
6. Culture cells in a CO_2 incubator (5 % CO_2, 37 °C) (*see* **Note 10**).
7. On day 3, split cells from one well into two wells. Add 100 μl of fresh culture medium to each well.
8. T cell proliferation can be assessed on day 3–5 by counting cell number, CFSE-dilution assay, or [^{3}H]-thymidine incorporation assay.
9. On day 5–6, collect cells with supernatant and centrifuge at $500 \times g$ for 5 min. Save supernatant for cytokine assay.
10. If T cell restimulation is desired, continue with **steps 11–15** (*see* **Note 11**).
11. Wash the cells with culture medium twice then count.
12. Resuspend the cells with culture medium and adjust the cell concentration to 5×10^5/ml.
13. Put 200 μl of T cell suspension (1×10^5) into a flat-bottom 96-well culture plate coated with anti-CD3e (1 μg/ml) and anti-CD28 (1 μg/ml) mAbs.
14. Culture cells in a CO_2 incubator (5 % CO_2, 37 °C).
15. 24 h later, collect supernatants for cytokine assay.

4 Notes

1. Use distilled water to dissolve DNase I. Do not use PBS.
2. Because binding of anti-I-A/I-E mAb (M5/114) alters the phenotype and function of APCs, we recommend using anti-I-Ab (AF6-120.1), anti-I-A^d (AMS-32.1), or anti-I-E (14-4-S) mAb to detect MHC class II.
3. 1.1 ml of premixed enzymes in digestion buffer can be added.
4. Because alveolar macrophages are autofluorescent, they display positive signals in channels in which cells were not stained. Autofluorescence signal is detected in channels with violet and blue lasers (e.g., Pacific blue, AmCyan, FITC, and PE channels).

5. We recommend eliciting advice from an expert in flow cytometry to set voltage and compensation. Because different cell populations have different signal backgrounds (including autofluorescence), Auto-comp cannot adjust the compensation appropriately.
6. Surface makers of pulmonary APC populations are shown below [12–14].
   - Alveolar macrophages: CD11b^{lo}, CD11c^{hi}, F4/80^{+}, Siglec-F^{hi}, autofluorescence^{hi}.
   - Interstitial macrophages: CD11b^{hi}, CD11c^{lo}, F4/80^{+}.
   - Monocytes: CD11b^{hi}, CD115^{hi}, Ly-6C^{hi}, MHC-II^{lo}, autofluorescence.
   - Inflammatory DCs: CD11b^{hi}, CD11c^{int}, Ly-6C^{hi}, MHC-II^{+}.
   - Monocyte-derived DCs: CD11b^{hi}, CD11c^{int}, CD14^{hi}, Ly-6C^{lo}, MHC-II^{hi}.
   - PreDC-derived CD11b^{hi} DCs: CD11b^{hi}, CD11c^{int}, CD14^{hi}, Ly-6C^{lo}, MHC-II^{hi}.
   - CD103^{+} DCs: CD11b^{lo}, CD11c^{hi}, CD24^{+}, CD103^{+}, CD117^{+}, CD207^{+}, MHC-II^{hi}.
   - Plasmacytoid DCs: CD11b^{lo}, CD11c$^{int/lo}$, CD45R/B220^{+}, CD317^{+}, Ly-6C^{+}, MHC-II^{lo}, Siglec-H^{+}.
   - CD8^{+} DCs (LNs): CD8a^{+}, CD11b^{lo}, CD11c^{hi}, MHC-II^{hi}.
   - B cells: CD19^{+}, CD45R/B220^{+}, sIgM^{+}.
7. After sorting lung DCs by flow cytometry, approximately $1–2 \times 10^4$ CD11b^{hi} DCs and $2–4 \times 10^4$ CD103^{+} DCs are usually obtained per mouse, although cell yields vary among different experiments depending on the treatments the mice received. Multiply mouse number based on DC number needed for experiment.
8. Complete RPMI 1640 with 10 % FBS (low endotoxin) is recommended.
9. A 1:2 ratio of DCs to T cells induces robust T cell proliferation and differentiation, although T cell responses can be detected with wide range of ratios (1:1–1:100) of DCs to T cells.
10. T cell response is affected by medium pH. Check the concentration of CO_2 in the incubator and the pH of culture medium prior to culture.
11. Restimulation allows assessment of T cell responses following their differentiation without transfer of cytokines produced by naïve or differentiating T cells during the primary culture. In addition, because an equal number of T cells are typically restimulated, this method allows measurements of T cell responses on a per-cell basis.

Acknowledgments

We thank Rhonda Wilson, Keiko Nakano, Seddon Thomas, Maria Sifre, and Carl Bortner for help with flow cytometric analysis. This work was supported by the Intramural Research Program of the National Institutes of Health and the National Institute of Environmental Health Sciences.

References

1. Sertl K, Takemura T, Tschachler E, Ferrans VJ, Kaliner MA, Shevach EM (1986) Dendritic cells with antigen-presenting capability reside in airway epithelium, lung parenchyma, and visceral pleura. J Exp Med 163:436–451
2. Lambrecht BN, Hammad H (2009) Biology of lung dendritic cells at the origin of asthma. Immunity 31:412–424
3. Sung SS, Fu SM, Rose CE Jr, Gaskin F, Ju ST, Beaty SR (2006) A major lung CD103 (alphaE)-beta7 integrin-positive epithelial dendritic cell population expressing langerin and tight junction proteins. J Immunol 176:2161–2172
4. Galkina E, Kadl A, Sanders J, Varughese D, Sarembock IJ, Ley K (2006) Lymphocyte recruitment into the aortic wall before and during development of atherosclerosis is partially L-selectin dependent. J Exp Med 203: 1273–1282
5. Nakano H, Free ME, Whitehead GS, Maruoka S, Wilson RH, Nakano K, Cook DN (2012) Pulmonary CD103(+) dendritic cells prime Th2 responses to inhaled allergens. Mucosal Immunol 5:53–65
6. Inaba K, Witmer-Pack MD, Inaba M, Muramatsu S, Steinman RM (1988) The function of Ia+dendritic cells and Ia- dendritic cell precursors in thymocyte mitogenesis to lectin and lectin plus interleukin 1. J Exp Med 167: 149–162
7. Stevens WW, Kim TS, Pujanauski LM, Hao X, Braciale TJ (2007) Detection and quantitation of eosinophils in the murine respiratory tract by flow cytometry. J Immunol Methods 327: 63–74
8. Jakubzick C, Randolph GJ (2010) Methods to study pulmonary dendritic cell migration. Methods Mol Biol 595:371–382
9. Vermaelen K, Pauwels R (2004) Accurate and simple discrimination of mouse pulmonary dendritic cell and macrophage populations by flow cytometry: methodology and new insights. Cytometry A 61:170–177
10. Naik SH, Sathe P, Park HY, Metcalf D, Proietto AI, Dakic A, Carotta S, O'Keeffe M, Bahlo M, Papenfuss A, Kwak JY, Wu L, Shortman K (2007) Development of plasmacytoid and conventional dendritic cell subtypes from single precursor cells derived in vitro and in vivo. Nat Immunol 8:1217–1226
11. Onai N, Obata-Onai A, Schmid MA, Ohteki T, Jarrossay D, Manz MG (2007) Identification of clonogenic common Flt3+M-CSFR+plasmacytoid and conventional dendritic cell progenitors in mouse bone marrow. Nat Immunol 8:1207–1216
12. Cheong C, Matos I, Choi JH, Dandamudi DB, Shrestha E, Longhi MP, Jeffrey KL, Anthony RM, Kluger C, Nchinda G, Koh H, Rodriguez A, Idoyaga J, Pack M, Velinzon K, Park CG, Steinman RM (2010) Microbial stimulation fully differentiates monocytes to DC-SIGN/CD209(+) dendritic cells for immune T cell areas. Cell 143:416–429
13. Nakano H, Lin KL, Yanagita M, Charbonneau C, Cook DN, Kakiuchi T, Gunn MD (2009) Blood-derived inflammatory dendritic cells in lymph nodes stimulate acute T helper type 1 immune responses. Nat Immunol 10:394–402
14. Nakano H, Burgents JE, Nakano K, Whitehead GS, Cheong C, Bortner CD, Cook DN (2013). Migratory properties of pulmonary dendritic cells are determined by their developmental lineage. Mucosal Immunol. 2012 Nov 21. doi: 10.1038/mi.2012.106. [Epub ahead of print]

Chapter 3

Evaluation of T Cell Function in Allergic Disease

Brianne R. Barker

Abstract

T lymphocytes play positive and negative roles in the pathogenesis of allergic disease. Isolation and functional characterization of T lymphocyte subpopulations is an important aspect of understanding allergy models and allergy therapies. Measurement of the T cell surface proteins and T cell proliferation can provide insight into T cell activation. T cell function and the identities of T cell subsets can be determined by measuring cytokine production, either via intracellular cytokine staining or ELISPOT. This chapter outlines protocols for T cell isolation as well as the evaluation of surface protein expression, proliferation, intracellular cytokine staining, and ELISPOT.

Key words T cells, Allergy, Flow cytometry, Intracellular cytokine staining, ELISPOT, CFSE

1 Introduction

Allergy is classically defined as a misdirected Th2-type response directed against noninfectious environmental stimuli, suggesting that the understanding of Th2 responses in any model of allergic disease is critical [1, 2]. Measurement of the production of Th2 cytokines including IL-4, IL-5, IL-9, IL-13, and GM-CSF is particularly important in assessing allergic disease [2]. These cytokines function to modulate many of the other effector cell populations acting during an allergic response. However, T cell subpopulations other than Th2 cells can also contribute to the development of or protection from allergic disease. IL-9, originally described as a Th2 cytokine, has more recently been shown to be a product of Th9 cells, which may also produce IL-10 [3]. The production of IL-17 by Th17 cells has been shown to contribute to some forms of allergy [4]. The balance between Th1 and Th2 cells is thought to be dysregulated in allergy, thus resulting in a decrease in Th1 cytokines in allergic disease [5]. Based on these data, therapies to induce immune deviation towards the Th1 phenotype are being attempted to ameliorate allergic disease [6]. In addition, regulatory T cells

Irving C. Allen (ed.), *Mouse Models of Allergic Disease: Methods and Protocols*, Methods in Molecular Biology, vol. 1032,
DOI 10.1007/978-1-62703-496-8_3, © Springer Science+Business Media, LLC 2013

may play a role in protection from allergic disease, likely via their production of TGF-β or IL-10 [7, 8]. NK T cells may also play a role in allergy [2]. Thus, the evaluation of T cells and their function are particularly important in models of allergic disease.

Before measuring T cell function, these cells must be isolated from the mouse. Protocols to isolate leukocytes from peripheral blood, spleen, and lymph nodes are presented below. These organs allow the assessment of systemic immune responses and responses in the draining lymph node. As T cell trafficking to effector sites also plays a key role in the progression of allergic disease, many investigators will also want to isolate T cells from unique organs of interest, such as the skin or the lungs [9]. T cells isolated from these organs may be used in a diverse range of assays; however, the number of isolated cells may be limited. Secondary lymphoid organs, particularly the spleen, allow for the isolation of large numbers of cells that can be used for all of the assays described below. The large numbers of cells recovered from these organs reduce the numbers of mice needed for each assay. All of these protocols result in the isolation of total leukocytes from the organs, which should be kept in mind during subsequent assays. The use of T cell-specific stimuli or flow cytometric analysis of T cell-specific surface proteins is often necessary to ensure specificity of the responses measured. Likewise, magnetic bead-based selection protocols may be used to isolate T cells from these bulk cell populations, but these protocols should be based on negative selection to avoid background activation of T cells before analysis. These selection procedures should be tested to ensure that they result in high yields of unactivated T cells.

The simplest way to evaluate T cells in an allergic model is via surface staining and flow cytometric analysis. This technique allows for the simple measurement of the proportion of T cells or specific T cell subsets among the isolated leukocytes possibly from an effector site or measurement of absolute cell numbers when combined with cell counts. The expression of specific trafficking molecules or activation molecules associated with individual disease phenotypes is often of interest as well [2, 5, 9]. This simple method also underlies some of the more complex protocols that follow. T cell activation can also be measured by examining T cell proliferation, here presented as the measurement of carboxyfluorescein diacetate succinimidyl ester (CFSE) dilution using a flow cytometer. Not only is the measurement of T cell proliferation important for understanding T cell activation, but this technique also allows for an understanding of regulatory T cell activity. Regulatory T cells can control the proliferation and responsiveness of conventional T cells as well as regulate high-dose tolerance in allergy treatment models [6, 7]. In this technique, isolated cells are labeled with the cell-permeant dye CFSE, which labels all cellular proteins. These cells are then stimulated with peptide antigen or other T cell-specific stimuli in in vitro culture. At varying time points following stimulation, cells are removed from culture and analyzed by flow cytometry and

CFSE fluorescence is measured. Lower levels of CFSE fluorescence indicate more rounds of cell division. This method has an advantage over other proliferation assays, including ^{3}H-thymidine incorporation or MTT (3-(4,5-dimethylthiazol-2-yl)-2,5-diphenyl-tetrazolium bromide) metabolism assays in that surface staining for other T cell-specific markers can be used to ensure that the proliferation of T cells is being measured.

The diverse T cell subpopulations described above are most commonly distinguished based on cytokine production. Two common methods to measure cytokine production are presented here: intracellular cytokine staining (using flow cytometry) and ELISPOT. These methods allow for measurement of cytokines from specific cell populations or following specific stimulation, unlike cytokine ELISAs of serum, which only provide information about systemic cytokine levels. Both intracellular cytokine staining and ELISPOT can be performed on cells taken directly ex vivo or on cells that are stimulated with a specific antigen to measure in vitro cytokine production. Intracellular cytokine staining involves the utilization of cell permeabilization techniques and flow cytometry. This technique can be combined with cell surface staining to allow for the determination of cytokine production from specific T cell subsets or for the conservation of experimental animals. These permeabilization techniques can also be modified for the detection of signal transduction molecules and transcription factors like FoxP3 [10]. Intracellular cytokine production evaluation techniques have the advantage of providing cell subpopulation-specific data regarding cytokine production. ELISPOT involves culturing cells in multiscreen plates onto which cytokines may be secreted. Secreted cytokines are then measured via an ELISA-like protocol. ELISPOT has the advantage of providing data on how many cells in a population are producing a cytokine of interest. The user should decide which of these two techniques are more appropriate for measuring the levels of different cytokines in their studies based on each assay's sensitivities and unique advantages.

2 Materials

2.1 Harvesting Leukocytes from Peripheral Blood

1. Mice to be assessed.
2. Blood collection media: RPMI 1640 with 40 units/ml of heparan sulfate (*see* **Note 2**).
3. Lympholyte M or other types of Ficoll (*see* **Note 3**).
4. 15 ml polystyrene conical tubes.
5. Equipment for the collection of mouse blood (*see* **Note 4**).
6. Centrifuge capable of spinning 15 ml conical tubes.
7. Sterile and pyrogen-free PBS with 2 % fetal bovine serum (sterile filtered) (*see* **Notes 1** and **5**).

2.2 Harvesting Leukocytes from Spleen and Lymph Nodes

1. Mice to be assessed.
2. Equipment to euthanize mice (*see* **Note 6**).
3. Sterile surgical instruments: Forceps; scissors; dissection tray; and dissection pins. Jeweler's forceps may be particularly useful to isolate lymph nodes.
4. 70 % ethanol.
5. Spleen/lymph node collection media: Hanks' Balanced Salt Solution with 4 % fetal bovine serum and 10 mM of HEPES (sterile filtered).
6. Lympholyte M or other types of Ficoll (*see* **Note 3**).
7. 15 ml polystyrene conical tubes.
8. Centrifuge capable of spinning 15 ml conical tubes.
9. Sterile and pyrogen-free PBS with 2 % fetal bovine serum (sterile filtered) (*see* **Note 5**).
10. Hemocytometer and trypan blue (optional).
11. Light microscope.
12. 100 μm cell strainer per mouse (*see* **Note** 7).
13. Plunger from a 1 cc syringe per mouse (*see* **Note** 7).
14. Petri dishes or 6-well tissue culture plates (*see* **Note** 7).
15. R10 media: RPMI 1640 plus 10 % fetal bovine serum, 1 % MEM nonessential amino acids, 0.1 % β-mercaptoethanol, 1 % sodium pyruvate, and 1 % penicillin/streptomycin.

2.3 Surface Staining

1. 12×75 mm 5 ml test tubes (*see* **Note 8**).
2. Centrifuge capable of spinning 5 ml conical tubes.
3. Sterile and pyrogen-free PBS with 2 % fetal bovine serum (sterile filtered) (*see* **Note 5**).
4. Ca- and Mg-free PBS or Ca- and Mg-free PBS with 2 % formaldehyde (*see* **Note 9**).
5. Flow cytometer and flow cytometry analysis software.
6. Fluorescence-conjugated antibodies against surface molecules of interest.
7. Vortex.

2.4 Proliferation

1. All materials listed in Subheading 2.3 for surface staining.
2. Hanks' Balanced Salt Solution.
3. 15 ml conical tubes.
4. CFSE. Stock solutions should be generated at 1 mM CFSE in DMSO. This solution is frozen at −20 °C (*see* **Note 10**).
5. R10 media: RPMI 1640 plus 10 % fetal bovine serum, 1 % MEM nonessential amino acids, 0.1% β-mercaptoethanol, 1 % sodium pyruvate, and 1 % penicillin/streptomycin.

6. Rat IL-2.
7. 37 °C incubator.
8. Specific antigenic peptide or overlapping peptide pools.
9. Anti-CD3ε (BD Biosciences).
10. Round-bottom 96-well tissue culture plates.

2.5 Intracellular Cytokine Staining

1. All materials listed under Subheading 2.3 for surface staining.
2. Stimulation media (*see* **Note 11**): RPMI 1640 plus 10 % fetal bovine serum, 1 % MEM nonessential amino acids, 0.1 % β-mercaptoethanol, 1 % sodium pyruvate, 1 % penicillin/streptomycin, 2 μg/ml of anti-CD28 (azide free; BD Biosciences), and 2 μg/ml of anti-CD49d (azide free; BD Biosciences).
3. Fluorescence-conjugated antibodies against cytokines or other intracellular molecules of interest (*see* **Note 12**).
4. Phorbol 12-myristate 13-acetate (PMA).
5. Ionomycin.
6. Specific antigenic peptide or overlapping peptide pools.
7. Cytofix/Cytoperm solution (BD Biosciences). This is a fixation/permeabilization buffer containing formaldehyde and saponin for cell permeabilization.
8. Brefeldin A or Monensin (BD Biosciences).
9. 37 °C incubator.
10. Perm/Wash Buffer (BD Biosciences). This is saponin-containing wash buffer to aid in saponin-based permeabilization.

2.6 ELISPOT

1. PMA.
2. Ionomycin.
3. Specific antigenic peptide or overlapping peptide pools.
4. 96 well multiscreen plates (i.e., Millipore Immobilon-P PVDF plates).
5. Ca- and Mg-free PBS (sterile and pyrogen-free).
6. Anti-cytokine antibodies for coating plates (i.e., anti-IL-4).
7. PBS containing 0.25 % Tween 20 (PBS/Tween).
8. PBS containing 10 % fetal bovine serum.
9. Multichannel pipette.
10. 96-well plate washer (optional).
11. 37 °C incubator.
12. Distilled water.
13. Biotinylated anti-cytokine antibody (i.e., biotinylated anti-IL-4).
14. Streptavidin alkaline phosphatase.

15. Nitroblue tetrazolium (NBT)/5-bromo-4-chloro-3-indolyl-phosphate (BCIP) chromogen solution (Pierce).
16. Automated ELISPOT reader and image processing software. Commonly used readers are from Hitech Instruments or CTL Analyzers LLC. Commonly used software packages are Image-Pro Plus image processing software (Media Cybernetics) or CTL software.

3 Methods

3.1 Harvesting Leukocytes from Peripheral Blood

1. Fill one 15 ml conical tube with 3 ml blood collection media per mouse (*see* **Notes 2** and **4**).
2. Collect peripheral blood and immediately place in a 15 ml tube with blood collection media.
3. Underlay 1 ml Lympholyte M with a 2 ml pipette (*see* **Notes 3** and **13**).
4. Centrifuge at 1,875 × *g* for 20 min without brake.
5. Remove the cell layer from the Lympholyte M and add this layer to 10 ml of PBS/2 % FCS to a new 15 ml conical tube.
6. Centrifuge at 500 × *g* for 10 min.
7. Aspirate and resuspend the resulting cell pellet for downstream applications (*see* **Note 14**).

3.2 Harvesting Leukocytes from Spleen and Lymph Nodes

1. Fill one 15 ml conical with 5 ml of spleen/lymph node collection media per mouse per organ to be isolated.
2. Euthanize mice one at a time and isolate the spleen or the lymph nodes from each mouse immediately after sacrifice (*see* **Note 6**). Immediately place the organ in a 15 ml tube with spleen/lymph node collection media. Collect all organs from all mice and place them on ice before proceeding to the next step.
3. Gently homogenize the spleen or the lymph nodes through the 100 μm cell strainer into a small Petri dish using the plunger from the 1 cc syringe until a single-cell suspension is produced. Pipette the single-cell suspension into a 15 ml conical tube. Wash the strainer, plunger, and dish with 5 ml of mouse R10 and add to the same conical tube (*see* **Note** 7).
4. Centrifuge at 500 × *g* for 5 min.
5. Underlay 1 ml of Lympholyte M with a 2 ml pipette (*see* **Notes 3** and **13**).
6. Centrifuge at 1,875 × *g* for 20 min without brake.
7. Remove the cell layer from the Lympholyte M and add this layer to 10 ml of PBS/2 % FCS tubes in a new 15 ml conical tube.

8. Centrifuge at 500 × *g* for 10 min.
9. Aspirate and resuspend the resulting cell pellet in 10 ml of 2 % PBS/2%FCS and count cells for downstream applications (*see* **Note 14**).

3.3 Surface Staining

1. Transfer at least 1×10^6 cells per sample to 12 × 75 mm 5 ml test tubes. Adjust the volume to 100 μl of PBS/2 % FCS. Also transfer at least 1×10^6 cells to a 12 × 75 mm 5 ml test tube to use for unstained controls, single-color controls, and possibly FMO controls. Adjust the volume to 100 μl with PBS/2 % FCS (*see* **Note 15**).
2. Prepare a cocktail containing the appropriate amounts of all of the surface staining antibodies before staining and add this cocktail to the cells (*see* **Notes 16** and **17**). Add individual diluted antibodies to the single-color control tubes. Vortex all samples and incubate them for 30 min on ice in the dark.
3. To wash, add 3 ml of PBS/2 % FCS to each tube and centrifuge at 500 × *g* for 5 min.
4. Aspirate and resuspend in 500 μl of PBS or PBS/2 % formaldehyde while vortexing to reduce clumping (*see* **Note 9**). Store the cells at 4 °C until analyzing on the flow cytometer.

3.4 Proliferation

1. Add 10×10^6 cells to a 15 ml conical tube. Wash cells twice with 10 ml of HBSS (*see* **Notes 18** and **19**). Resuspend 10×10^6 cells/900 μl in HBSS with no serum. Be sure to set up additional cells for unstained and single-color controls for later flow cytometry analysis.
2. Incubate in HBSS with 1 μM of CFSE for 30 min at 37 °C. Mix by flicking with finger vigorously, but not vortexing.
3. After the 30-min incubation, wash cells twice with R10 media (*see* **Note 18**).
4. Resuspend cells at 1.5×10^6 cells/ml in R10 media. Plate the cells in a round-bottom 96-well plate at 200 μl/well. Add 100 ng/ml of peptide antigen or anti-CD3 as a control (*see* **Note 20**). Be sure to set up additional wells without peptide as a control.
5. Add 25 U/ml rat IL-2 on day 2 of culture (*see* **Note 21**).
6. Take cells for staining as desired (anytime between day 0 and day 8) and utilize the surface staining protocol described under Subheading 3.3.

3.5 Intracellular Cytokine Staining

1. Transfer at least 4×10^6 cells per sample to 12 × 75 mm 5 ml test tubes (*see* **Note 8**). Adjust the volume to 500 μl of stimulation media. Also transfer at least 4×10^6 cells to a 12 × 75 mm 5 ml test tube to utilize as controls for staining per experiment

(unstained controls, single-color controls, and possibly FMO controls) and controls for stimulation per sample (unstimulated, antigen stimulated, and PMA/ionomycin stimulated). Adjust the volume to 500 μl of stimulation media (*see* **Notes 11, 15**, and **20**).

2. Add 1 μl of Golgi-stop to each sample. Add 1 μg of antigenic peptide or peptide pool to each sample to be stimulated with antigen. Add 0.5 μg of PMA and 2.5 μg of ionomycin to each positive control (PMA/ionomycin sample).
3. Vortex cells, place caps on loosely, and incubate for 6 h at 37 °C (*see* **Note 22**).
4. Add 3 ml of PBS/2 % FCS to each tube and centrifuge at 500 × *g* for 5 min to wash. Adjust the volume to 100 μl of PBS/2 % FCS.
5. Prepare a cocktail containing the appropriate amounts of all of the surface staining antibodies before staining and add this cocktail to the cells (*see* **Note 17**). Add individual diluted antibodies to the single-color control tubes. Vortex all samples and incubate them for 30 min on ice in the dark.
6. Add 3 ml of PBS/2 % FCS to each tube and centrifuge at 500 × *g* for 5 min to wash. **Steps 4–6** are optional and are only necessary if you are interested in staining for surface antigens in addition to intracellular antigens.
7. Vortex each sample. Add 500 μl of Cytofix/Cytoperm to each sample while vortexing. Incubate at room temperature for 45 min (*see* **Note 22**).
8. Vortex each sample. Add 2 ml of perm/wash buffer. To wash, centrifuge the samples at 800 × *g* for 7 min. Aspirate and wash with another 2 ml of perm/wash buffer.
9. Vortex each sample. Prepare a cocktail containing the appropriate amounts of all of the intracellular staining antibodies before staining and add this cocktail to the cells (*see* **Notes 12** and **17**). Vortex all of the samples and incubate them for 30 min on ice in the dark.
10. Add 2 ml of perm/wash buffer. Centrifuge at 800 × *g* for 7 min to wash.
11. Aspirate and resuspend the cells in 500 μl of PBS or PBS/2 % formaldehyde while vortexing to reduce clumping (*see* **Note 9**). Store the cells at 4 °C until ready to analyze using a flow cytometer.

3.6 ELISPOT

1. Coat 96-well multiscreen plates with 100 μl per well of 5 μg/ml anti-cytokine antibody diluted in PBS. Incubate plates overnight.
2. Wash plates three times with PBS containing 0.25 % Tween 20 (PBS/Tween) (*see* **Note 23**).

3. Add 200 μl per well of PBS containing 10 % fetal bovine serum to block. Incubate the plate for 2 h.
4. Add 2×10^5 cells and the appropriate antigenic peptides (1 μg/ml) or other stimuli to each well. It is advisable to set up triplicate wells for each condition. Unstimulated cells should also be included in the assay to allow for an assessment of background cytokine production. Incubate the plate for 18 h at 37 °C (*see* **Note 20**).
5. Wash the plates nine times with PBS/Tween and once with distilled water.
6. Add 2 μg of biotinylated anti-cytokine antibody diluted in PBS to a total volume of 100 μl per well. Incubate the plate for 2 h at room temperature.
7. Wash the plate six times with PBS/Tween.
8. Incubate the plate with a 1:500 dilution (100 μl total volume per well, dilute in PBS) of streptavidin alkaline phosphatase for 2.5 h.
9. Wash the plate five times with PBS/Tween and once with PBS only.
10. Develop the plate by adding NBT/BCIP chromogen solution. Stop the reaction once color has developed with tap water and air-dry the plate.
11. Read the pate with an automated ELISPOT reader and quantitate the number of spots apparent using appropriate software. Data from an ELISPOT assay are usually expressed as spot-forming cells (SFC) per 10^6 cells added to the well and compared to background levels seen in unstimulated cells.

4 Notes

1. Prepare all solutions using ultrapure water and pyrogen-free, tissue culture-grade reagents. Store all reagents at 4 °C unless indicated otherwise. Pay careful attention to waste disposal recommendations of your institution; some prepackaged kits or reagents contain preservatives that may require special collection and disposal. We perform all assays using sterile technique in a laminar flow hood, although terminal assays in which cells will not be cultured may be performed on a bench top. Be sure to wear appropriate personal protective equipment throughout the procedure.
2. Blood should be collected in the presence of anticoagulant; however, we have used anticoagulants other than heparin in our blood collection media with generally good results. Calcium chelators such as EDTA can adversely affect some

functional assays including intracellular cytokine staining and should be tested carefully.

3. We use Lympholyte M as a standard way of separating peripheral blood mononuclear cells from other cell types found in peripheral blood or secondary lymphoid organs. We find that this technique provides the cleanest cell population without debris that can cause problems in cytometry. Instead of using Lympholyte M or another type of Ficoll, it is possible to lyse the red blood cells in a single-cell suspension with NH_4Cl lysis buffer (ACK). Further, some tissues, particularly spleen, contain large numbers of red blood cells and cell preparations from these tissues may be improved by adding an ACK lysis step following Lympholyte treatment. ACK buffer is made as follows: Add nine parts 0.16 M NH_4Cl to 1 part of 0.17 M Tris base pH 7.65 and then adjust the pH of the resulting solution to 7.2 and sterile filter. The ACK lysis protocol is as follows:
   (a) Centrifuge heparinized blood or single-cell suspension generated from spleen or lymph node.
   (b) Add approximately 5 ml of ACK solution to the cell pellet. The specific amount will vary based on the number of cells.
   (c) Invert tubes to mix well and incubate for approximately 3 min. The amount of time will also vary based on the number of cells and tissue. Do not overlyse.
   (d) Centrifuge tubes immediately to remove ACK buffer. Overlysis of cells can cause problems with surface staining and functional assays, or can result in poor cell yield.
4. Appropriate techniques for the collection of mouse blood vary among institutions and IACUC committees. We have successfully used blood obtained via retroorbital (generally disfavored among IACUC committees), submandibular, and cardiac puncture routes. Submandibular blood collection utilizing Goldenrod Animal Lancets can be performed on live mice and allows the investigator to follow the same mice throughout the course of disease but results in smaller volumes of blood for experimentation. Blood volume may be replaced with Ringer's lactate solution. Blood collection via cardiac puncture results in larger volumes of blood for experimentation but does not allow mice to be followed.
5. Throughout this protocol, PBS with 2 % fetal bovine serum can be substituted with PBS with BSA.
6. Appropriate techniques for mouse euthanasia vary among institutions and IACUC committees.
7. There are multiple methods of dissociating spleens and lymph nodes to generate single-cell suspensions. We tend to use syringe plungers and disposable cell strainers in either Petri

dishes or wells of 6-well tissue culture plates. We have also used syringe plungers or autoclavable glass rods with autoclavable mesh screens in a similar fashion to the method described here or homogenized spleens between two frosted glass slides.

8. Flow cytometry staining and analysis are traditionally performed in 5 ml test tubes. However, the use of these tubes may be cumbersome when staining large numbers of samples. Alternatively, we have stained cells in round-bottom 96-well plates or strips of PCR tubes. Either of these methods allows for the use of a multichannel pipette. Both alternatives require additional wash steps as cells cannot be washed with large volumes of liquid. A centrifuge capable of spinning 96-well plates is also necessary. Cells can then be transferred into 5 ml test tubes for analysis or may be analyzed directly in a 96-well plate if appropriate flow cytometer hardware is available.
9. We fix our flow cytometry samples with formaldehyde as a standard procedure. Cells do not need to be fixed and can be resuspended in PBS alone provided there are no biosafety concerns and the samples will be analyzed on a flow cytometer immediately. Formaldehyde fixation can alter some fluorophores, so fixed and unfixed samples should not be compared.
10. When attached to proteins, the emission and excitation peaks of CFSE are 492 and 517 nm and it is typically read in the FITC channel. CFSE should be carefully titrated to ensure that spillover into other channels does not occur. Similar compounds with different emission and excitation peaks (i.e., Molecular Probes, Cat. No. 34557) have been developed and allow good results.
11. Stimulation media is the R10 media listed above with the addition of purified, azide-free anti-CD28 and anti-CD49d antibodies. These antibodies allow for co-stimulation of T cells during antigenic stimulation to result in optimal cytokine production. The specific antibodies used in this stimulation media, particularly with regard to the use of CD49d, vary among investigators. If direct ex vivo cytokine analysis is desired, this media is not necessary.
12. The protocol presented here is specific for staining for intracellular cytokines. Other intracellular molecules, particularly transcription factors like the regulatory T cell transcription factor FoxP3 or other signal transduction molecules, can also be assessed by flow cytometry. The protocols for these techniques are generally similar to those presented here with two changes: in vitro cell stimulation is not used and alcohol-based permeabilization methods are sometimes necessary. Specific protocols vary for individual signaling molecule and often require optimization.

13. Lympholyte M and other Ficolls are sucrose solutions that allow for cell separation based on density. Lympholyte M should be stored at 4 °C to prevent contamination once it has been opened. Lympholyte M should then be at room temperature when used to separate cells to ensure that it is at the correct density.
14. Cells at this stage can be stored for short periods of time at 4 °C or may be cryopreserved for later use. Cryopreservation may influence cell performance in functional assays.
15. Flow cytometry experiments require unstained cell controls and controls stained with each of the antibodies individually for setting voltages and compensation. We often stain compensation control beads instead of cells for our single-color controls (BD Biosciences 552843 or 552845 depending on the antibody isotype). This allows conservation of cells and measurable staining with even those antibodies that stain rare populations. Unstained cells are still required to properly set up the flow cytometer. For complex experiments, we also use fluorescence minus one (FMO) gating controls. In an FMO control, all antibodies in a panel except for one are used to stain cells. This aids in setting negative gates [11].
16. We sometimes include MHC–peptide tetramers to allow for staining of antigen-specific T lymphocytes. If staining with tetramers, the protocol should be modified as follows:
    (a) Add appropriate amount of tetramer to cells to stain. Vortex all samples and incubate them for 30 min on ice in the dark.
    (b) Prepare a cocktail containing appropriate amounts of all of the surface staining antibodies before staining and add this cocktail to cells to stain. Add individual diluted antibodies to single-color control tubes. Vortex all samples and incubate them for 30 min on ice in the dark.

    Tetramers should always be added before antibodies, particularly anti-CD3, to allow tetramer access to TCR without hindrance from other antibodies.
17. The concentrations listed on the data sheets included with antibodies are often a useful place to start with staining. Antibodies can usually be further diluted and careful titration can save on reagents and allow for cleaner staining.
18. CFSE is a cell-permeant dye that labels proteins. Staining must be performed in serum-free media to ensure that cellular proteins and not serum proteins are labeled. Once staining is complete, the cells should be washed with a large volume of media containing serum to quench the staining reaction. We have used different types of media (HBSS, PBS, RPMI) for the staining reaction with no adverse effects as long as the staining

was in a serum-free media and the wash was in a serum-containing media.

19. The CFSE staining protocol listed utilizes large numbers of cells. It is also possible to stain smaller numbers of cells with protocol modifications including adding serum to the staining reaction. This helps the cells survive the toxicity associated with CFSE staining.
20. Stimulation of all T cells in a mixed population can be achieved with azide-free anti-CD3 antibody or a mixture of PMA/ionomycin. PMA/ionomycin is preferred for short-term cytokine production but does result in substantial cell death. Anti-CD3 is preferred for proliferation of cells in culture but must be azide-free to allow cells to proliferate. These reagents are useful positive controls to determine the maximum capacity of your cells to produce cytokine or proliferate as compared to cells stimulated with specific antigen. Unstimulated cells are also important negative controls. Stimulation is not necessary when measuring cytokine production directly ex vivo and stimulation steps may be excluded in that case.
21. Rat IL-2 allows for optimal T cell survival in culture.
22. Intracellular cytokine staining is a lengthy procedure. We have had good luck with the following modifications in order to spread the procedure over two days:

    *Protocol 3.5, **step** 3*: Utilize a heat block on a timer to incubate at 37 °C for 6 h, followed by cooling to 4 °C until the next day or manually moving cells to 4 °C following the 6-h incubation.

    *Protocol 3.5, **step** 7*: Incubate at 4 °C overnight.
23. While using multichannel plates and plate washers makes the ELISPOT protocol less laborious, they are also the cause of many problems with the protocol. Be sure not to touch the membrane with your pipette tips or the plate washer. Multiscreen plates are generally quite sensitive and should be treated with care.

References

1. Palm NW, Rosenstein RK, Medzhitov R (2012) Allergic host defenses. Nature 484: 465–472
2. Holgate ST (2012) Innate and adaptive immune responses in asthma. Nat Med 18: 673–683
3. Jabeen R, Kaplan MH (2012) The symphony of the ninth: the development and function of Th9 cells. Curr Opin Immunol 24:303–307
4. Wang Y, Wills-Karp M (2011) The potential role of interleukin-17 in severe asthma. Curr Allergy Asthma Rep 11:388–394
5. Galli SJ, Tsai M, Piliponsky AM (2008) The development of allergic inflammation. Nature 454:445–454
6. Maggi E (2010) T cell responses induced by allergen-specific immunotherapy. Clin Exp Immunol 161:10–18

7. Hawrylowicz CM, O'Garra A (2005) Potential role of interleukin-10-secreting regulatory T cells in allergy and asthma. Nat Rev Immunol 5:271–283
8. Lloyd CM, Hawrylowicz CM (2009) Regulatory T cells in asthma. Immunity 31:438–449
9. Islam SA, Luster AD (2012) T cell homing to epithelial barriers in allergic disease. Nat Med 18:705–715
10. Krutzik PO, Irish JM, Nolan GP, Perez OD (2004) Analysis of protein phosphorylation and cellular signaling events by flow cytometry: techniques and clinical applications. Clin Immunol 110:206–221
11. Roederer M (2002) Compensation in flow cytometry. Curr Protoc Cytom Chapter 1 Unit 1.4

Chapter 4

Evaluating B-Cells: From Bone Marrow Precursors to Antibody-Producing Cells

M. Manuela Rosado, Marco Scarsella, Simona Cascioli, Ezio Giorda, and Rita Carsetti

Abstract

Lymphocyte characterization is primarily based on the differential expression of surface markers. In this context, flow-cytometry analysis (FACS) is an exceptional technique that not only allows the identification of B-cell subsets, but can also be used to evaluate cell function, activation, and division. Here, we will combine the use of FACS analysis and ELISA techniques to identify murine bone marrow and peripheral B-cell subsets. The main function of B cells, derived through a multistage differentiation process from precursor cells, is to produce antibodies. This task is performed by terminally differentiated B cells called antibody-secreting cells (ASC) present at mucosal sites, in the bone marrow and in the spleen. The number and specificity of ASC can be measured by Enzyme-linked immunosorbent spot (ELISPOT) assay, a variation of the enzyme-linked immunosorbent assay (ELISA) used to quantify serum immunoglobulins.

Key words Flow-cytometry, Mouse B cell subsets, Antibodies

1 Introduction

B-lymphocytes can be classified in different subsets according to their origin, function, and localization. Each B-cell subset expresses a combination of cell surface markers that allows for their identification/purification using FACS analysis and cell sorting. The B-cell identity is given by the B-cell receptor (BCR). In the mouse, the first BCR expressing cells appear as early as at the embryonic day 16 (ED16) of gestation and are generated from fetal liver haematopoietic stem cells (HSCs) [1]. Although HSCs start to colonize the embryonic spleen at ED12 and bone marrow at ED15-16, the fetal liver retains haematopoietic functions until birth [2, 3]. At birth, the main districts responsible for B cell production is the bone marrow and, to a lesser extent, the spleen. In the bone marrow, commitment to the B cell lineage starts at the pro-B cell stage, when cells start to rearrange BCR genes. If the

Irving C. Allen (ed.), *Mouse Models of Allergic Disease: Methods and Protocols*, Methods in Molecular Biology, vol. 1032,
DOI 10.1007/978-1-62703-496-8_4,

gene rearrangement is productive, pro-B cells differentiate into pre-B-cells. Surface expression of the BCR identifies immature B cells (Fig. 1). Immature/transitional B cells exit the bone marrow and migrate to the peripheral organs [4] where they differentiate into mature, memory, and antibody-secreting cells (ASC). Bone marrow-derived B cells preferentially replenish B cell pools in charge of the acquired immune responses, mainly follicular B cells and B2 cells (Fig. 2a, b) [5]. Although B cell turnover at the periphery is low, the daily B-cell out-put from the bone marrow allows a continuous "refreshment" of antigenic specificities. Moreover, B cell precursors present in the spleen can generate B cells "on demand." These precursors sustain the production of the so-called innate B cells, specifically B-1a B cells, in the body cavities (Fig. 3) and marginal zone B cells in the spleen. B-1a B cells produce antibodies through a T cell-independent mechanism and are responsible for generating the majority of the IgM natural antibody compartment. B-1a B cells are generated at a very low rate from fetal-derived precursor cells residing in the adult spleen. The B-1a B cells also supply the gut with IgA plasma cell precursors and are responsible for maintaining the secretory IgA compartment at mucosal sites [3].

In spite of the lack of consensus on the origin of certain B cell subsets, such as the dichotomy of B-1 versus B2 B cells, characterization of the mouse B cell compartments are well established. Indeed, through multiparametric FACS analyses it is now possible to identify almost all of the B cell subsets. Table 1 shows a combination of useful markers for each subset with some suggested bibliography.

2 Materials

2.1 Solutions for Cell Preparation

1. PBS (10×): PBS (10×) washing buffer pH = 7.2, indicated amounts for 10 L: dissolve 43 g of $NaH_2PO_4 \cdot 2H_2O$; 258 g of $Na_2HPO_4 \cdot 12H_2O$ and 850 g of NaCl in 500 ml of distilled H_2O. Adjust the volume by adding distilled H_2O, check the pH, and store at 4 °C.
2. Incomplete medium: RPMI 1640 supplemented with heat inactivated 2 % FCS (*see* **Note 1**).
3. Culture medium B cell stimulation: RPMI 1640 supplemented with heat inactivated 10 % FCS, 2 % L-glutamine, 5×10^{-5} M 2-β mercaptoethanol and antibiotics (either gentamicin or penicillin/streptomycin).
4. Culture medium for antibody secretion: RPMI 1640 supplemented with heat inactivated 2 % FCS, 2 % L-glutamine, 5×10^{-5} M 2-β mercaptoethanol and antibiotics (either gentamicin or penicillin/streptomycin).

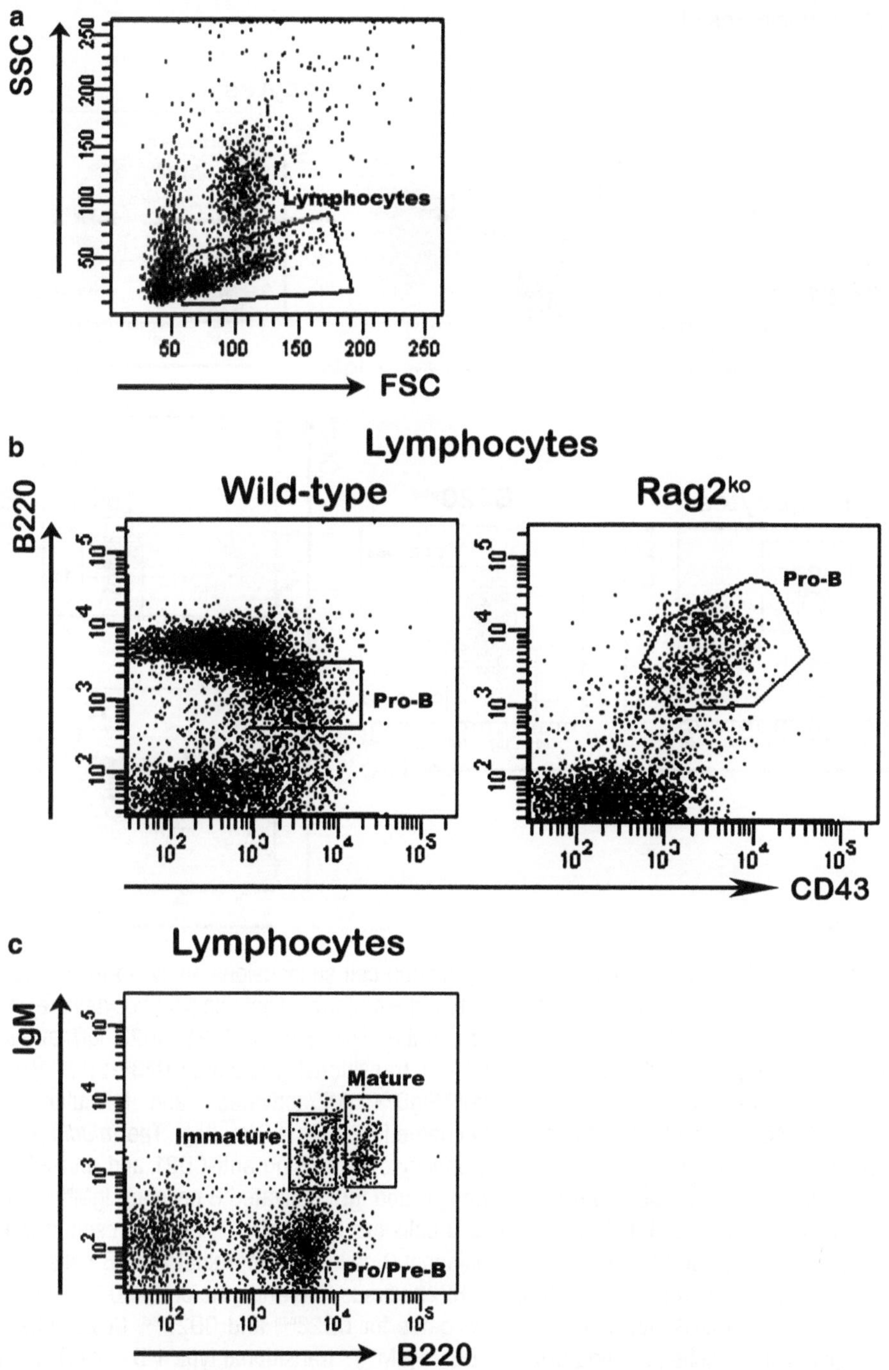

Fig. 1 Representative flow-cytometry dot plots showing the expression of B220 (formally CD45), CD43, and IgM in the bone marrow. (**a**) Shows a forward (FSC)/side scatter (SSC) plot. FSC correlates to cell volume and SSC to cell complexity, i.e., shape of nucleus, amount and type of cytoplasmic granules, or membrane roughness. FSC/SSC plotting allows the exclusion of dead cells and debris from the analysis. It is also helpful to define and select the lymphocyte gate used later for analysis of the different fluorescent cell markers. (**b**) Plot shows the expression of B220 and CD43 in the bone marrow of wild-type (*left*) and Rag2-deficient mice (*right*) inside the lymphocyte gate. Pro-B cells on the way to rearrange Ig genes are identified as B220^{low}CD43^{low}. This is the only B cell population present in Rag2-deficient mice, because lack of *Rag* genes impairs BCR and TCR gene rearrangement, blocking the development before the pre-B or pre-T cell stage. (**c**) Plots show the expression of B220 and IgM: B220^{pos}IgM^{neg} correspond to pro/pre-B cells, B220^{pos}IgM^{pos} are immature B cells and B220^{bright}IgM^{pos} represent mature B cells that recirculate with the blood

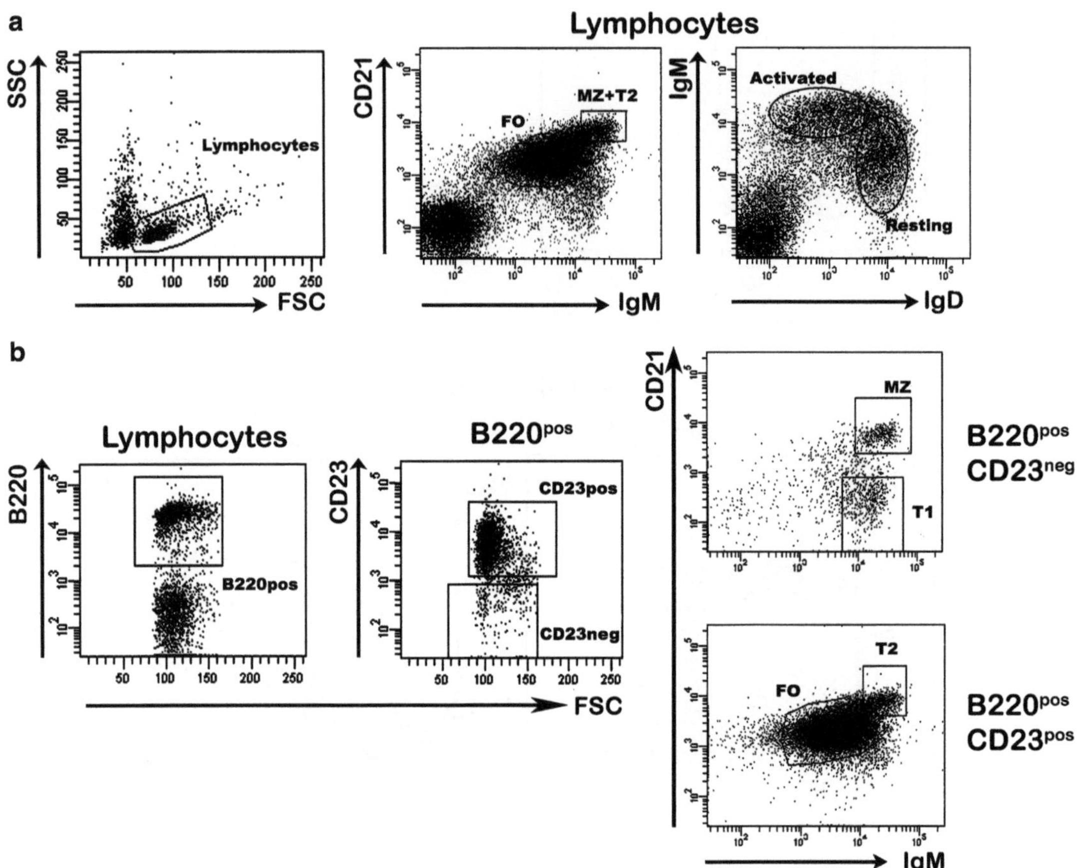

Fig. 2 Representative flow-cytometry plots showing spleen cell suspensions analyzed for the expression of CD21, CD23, B220, IgM, and IgD. (**a**) *First plot* shows that the majority of splenic lymphocytes are small. Spleen B cells can be classified in various subsets according to the expression of CD21, CD23, IgD, and IgM. Briefly, transitional type 1 B cells are $CD23^{neg}CD21^{neg}IgM^{bright}$ (T1), transitional type 2 are $CD23^{pos}CD21^{bright}IgM^{bright}$ (T2), marginal zone B cells are $CD23^{neg}CD21^{bright}IgM^{bright}IgD^{low}$ (MZ/activated), and follicular B cells are $CD23^{pos}CD21^{pos}IgM^{pos}IgD^{pos}$ (in other districts are also named B2 cells, FO/resting). The *middle plot* shows FO, MZ, and transitional B cells analyzed inside the lymphocyte gate using anti-CD21 and anti-IgM antibodies. *Right plot* exemplifies another type of analysis using IgM and IgD: activated B cells are $IgM^{bright}IgD^{dull}$, contain MZ and transitional B cells and B-1 B cells; resting B cells are $IgM^{dull}IgD^{bright}$, that correspond to FO or B2 B cells. (**b**) Analysis strategy used to distinguish transitional 2 cells from marginal zone B cells that share the CD21 markers and are both bright for IgM: first plot B220 versus FSC and gate on $B220^{pos}$, inside the $B220^{pos}$ check the expression of CD23 and define two new gates for $CD23^{neg}$ and $CD23^{pos}$. $CD23^{neg}CD21^{high}IgM^{bright}$ identifies marginal zone B cells (MZ) and $CD23^{neg}CD21^{neg}IgM^{bright}$ transitional type 1 B cells (T1). The majority of the $CD23^{pos}$ cells are $CD21^{pos}IgM^{pos}$ follicular B cells (FO) and a small population of transitional type 2 cells (T2) that are $CD21^{high}IgM^{bright}$

5. Gey's solution: It is useful to deplete erythrocytes from the peripheral blood and spleen. Gey's solution destroys erythrocytes while maintaining membrane integrity of mononuclear cells. Solutions should be prepared fresh each time by mixing 14 ml of sterile H_2O + 4 ml of solution A + 1 ml of solution B + 1 ml of solution C.

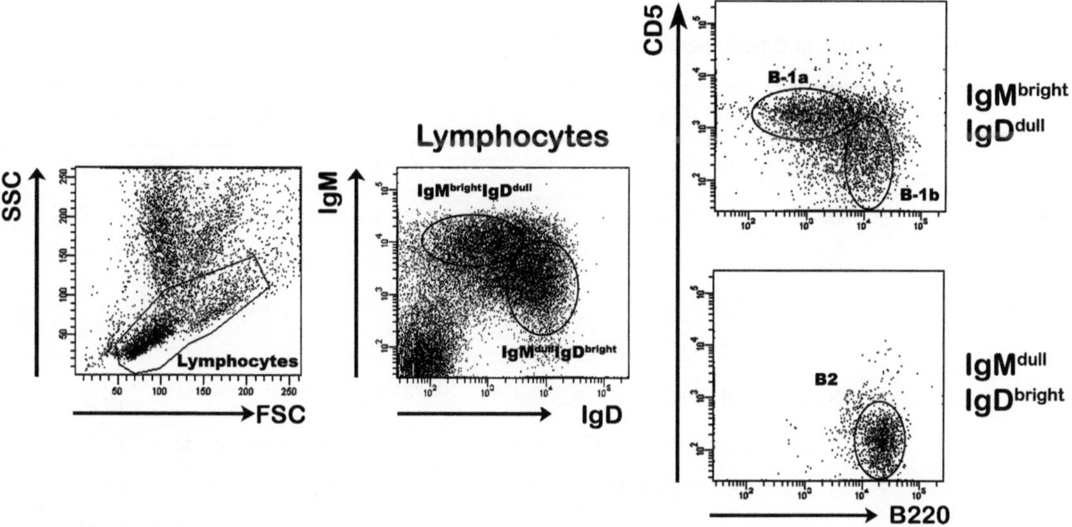

Fig. 3 Representative example of flow-cytometry analysis showing B cell subsets present in the peritoneal cavity. Cell suspensions were stained for CD5, B220, IgM, and IgD. SSS/FSC plot, mouse peritoneal cavity is composed of a large fraction of macrophages and large lymphocytes corresponding to activated cells. *Middle plot* shows the expression of IgM and IgD in total lymphocytes, activated B cells are indicated as $IgM^{bright}IgD^{dull}$ and resting B cells as $IgM^{dull}IgD^{bright}$. Expression of CD5 surface markers and the amount of B220 allows the separation of the B-1a and B1b B cells contained in the activated pool. B-1a cells are $CD5^{pos}B220^{dull}$ whereas B-1b cells are $CD5^{neg}B220^{pos}$. $IgM^{dull}IgD^{bright}$ B cells correspond to B2 cells that are $B220^{bright}$ and do not express CD5 molecule

Solution A (for 1 L of water): Dissolve 35 g of NH_4Cl + 1.85 g of KCl + 1.5 g of $Na_2HPO_4{\cdot}12H_2O$ + 0.119 g of KH_2PO_4 + 5.0 g of glucose + 25 g of gelatine in distilled H_2O. Add 0.05 g of phenol red to the solution. Adjust the volume to 1 L, autoclave at 120 °C and store at 4 °C.

Solution B (for 100 ml water): Dissolve 0.14 g of $MgSO_4{\cdot}7H_2O$ + 0.42 g of $MgCl_2{\cdot}6H_2O$ + 0.34 g of $CaCl_2{\cdot}2H_2O$ in distilled H_2O. Adjust the volume to 100 ml with distilled H_2O, autoclave at 120 °C and store in dark at 4 °C.

Solution C (for 100 ml of water): Dissolve 2.25 g of $NaHCO_3$ in distilled H_2O. Adjust the volume to 100 ml with distilled H_2O, autoclave at 120 °C and store in dark at 4 °C.

2.2 Flow Cytometry Analysis

1. FACS buffer: PBS 1×, 2 % FCS, and 0.01 % Sodium azide (*see* **Note 2**).

2.3 Solutions for ELISA and ELISA Spot Assay

1. K_2HPO_4 (0.5 M solution): Dissolve 87.05 g of K_2HPO_4 in 500 ml distilled H_2O and adjust the volume to 1 L with dH_2O.
2. KH_2PO_4 (0.5 M solution): Dissolve 68.045 g of KH_2PO_4 in 500 ml of distilled H_2O and adjust the volume to 1 L with dH_2O.

Table 1
B cell subsets in central and peripheral lymphoid organs

	Main surface markers	Main localization	References
Pro-B[a]	$B220^{pos}CD43^{pos}IgM^{neg}$	Bone marrow	[7, 8]
Pre-B[a]	$B220^{pos}CD43^{neg}IgM^{neg}$	Bone marrow	[9, 10]
Immature B	$B220^{pos}IgM^{pos}$	Bone marrow	
Re-circulating B	$B220^{bright}IgM^{pos}IgD^{pos}$	Bone marrow/blood	
Transitional 1	$B220^{pos}IgM^{bright}CD21^{neg}CD23^{neg}$	Spleen	[4]
Transitional 2	$B220^{pos}IgM^{bright}CD21^{bright}CD23^{pos}$	Spleen	[4]
Follicular	$B220^{pos}IgD^{pos}IgM^{pos}CD21^{pos}CD23^{pos}$	Spleen/lymph node	[11]
Marginal zone	$B220^{pos}IgM^{bright}CD21^{bright}CD23^{neg}$	Spleen	[12]
B-1a	$B220^{low}IgM^{bright}IgD^{dull}CD5^{pos}CD11b^{pos}$	Peritoneal cavity	[13]
B-1b	$B220^{low}IgM^{bright}IgD^{dull}CD5^{neg}CD11b^{pos}$	Peritoneal cavity	[14]
B2	$B220^{pos}IgM^{dull}IgD^{bright}CD5^{pos}$	Peritoneal cavity	
ASC	$B220^{low}CD138^{pos}PNA^{low}Ig^{low}$	Spleen, bone marrow mucosal sites	

[a]pro-B/pre-B cells can be subdivided in fractions according to the expression of BP-1, CD24, CD25 surface markers, the state of Ig gene rearrangement and expression of the recombination enzymes. For further details *see* refs. 15, 16
Because we still lack a unique phenotypic marker able to distinguish memory B cells from naïve B cells in the mouse, memory B cell subset was not included in the table

3. Coating buffer: 0.5 M K_2HPO_4 pH = 8.0 (stock solution, 10×). Add the KH_2PO_4 solution to the K_2HPO_4 solution until pH 8.0. Autoclave and filter the solution or store at 4 °C. Always visually inspect each solution to ensure that no contamination is present. The working concentration of the coating buffer should be 0.05 M.
4. ELISA blocking solution: PBS (1×) + 1 % gelatin (100 ml). In a microwave oven, dissolve 1 g of gelatin in an Erlenmeyer flask with 50 ml of dH_2O. Place the flask on ice until the solution reaches room temperature. Add 10 ml of PBS (10×) and adjust to the final volume (100 ml) with dH_2O. This buffer cannot be stored for more than overnight at 4 °C.
5. ELISpot blocking solution: PBS (1×) + 1 % gelatin + 0.05–0.1 % Tween-20 (100 ml) (*see* **Note 3**).
6. ELISA substrate buffer:

   Solution A: Dissolve 38.82 g of $Na_2HPO_4 \cdot 12H_2O$ in dH_2O and adjust the volume to 500 ml.

   Solution B: Dissolve 10.53 g of citric acid in dH_2O and adjust the volume to 500 ml.

   Substrate buffer: Add buffer solution B to solution A until pH = 5.6. Autoclave the solution and store at 4 °C. Prepare

0.5 mg/ml of OPD (*ortho*-phenylenediamine) in substrate and add 1 μl/ml of H_2O_2 (30 %) (*see* **Note 4**).

7. ELISpot substrate buffer: *AMP 10× buffer* (2-amino-2-methyl-L-propanol, pH 10.25). Add to 100 ml AMP (1.5 M, pH 10.3)+752 μl of $MgCl_2$ (1 M)+152 μl of Triton X-405+1.5 ml of NaN_3 (10 %)+47.6 ml of dH_2O and adjust the pH to 10.25 with HCl. Store the solution at 4 °C. Dissolve 500 mg of BCIP in 50 ml of AMP 10× buffer+450 ml of dH_2O. Stir the solution at room temperature for 1 h, protected from the light, and filter through a 0.45 μm filter. The solution should be stored in the dark at 4 °C.
8. SDS (10 %) stop solution: Add 50 g of Dodecylsulfate–Na salt in 350 ml of dH_2O. Stir the solution overnight and adjust the volume to 500 ml with dH_2O.

3 Methods

3.1 Cell Preparation

1. Collect peripheral blood from the retro-orbital sinus using a Pasteur pipette (*see* **Note 5**) and transfer into 1.5 ml eppendorf tubes containing 50 μl of heparin. Deplete erythrocytes by incubating the blood sample with 1 ml of Gey's solution for 1 min. Add 1 ml of incomplete RPMI and spin at 250×*g* for 5 min at 4 °C. Discard the liquid by inverting the tube or by aspiration and resuspend the pellet in 300 μl of FACS medium. Leave the tubes on ice.
2. To obtain serum, collect the blood into 1.5 ml eppendorf tubes, leave overnight at 4 °C. The following day, remove and discard the clot with the help of a needle or a toothpick. Spin the tubes at 700×*g* for 2 min and transfer the serum to new 1.5 ml eppendorf tubes. Store the serum at −20 °C until analysis.
3. Sacrifice the animals after blood withdrawal by cervical dislocation (*see* **Note 5**).
4. Collect peritoneal cavity cells by injecting 5 ml cold PBS (1×) into the peritoneum (10 ml syringe with a 21 G×1.5″ needle). Allow the PBS to move in the cavity by gentle shaking and recover it in 15 ml tubes prefilled with 5 ml of cold PBS (1×) 2 % FCS. Spin tubes at 250×*g* for 10 min at 4 °C. Discard the liquid by inverting the tube or by aspiration and resuspend the pellet in 1 ml of FACS medium. Leave the tubes on ice.
5. Collect femurs and place into Petri dishes containing 5 ml of RPMI supplemented with 2 % FCS. Prepare single cell suspensions by flushing the bones with incomplete culture medium into 15 ml tubes using a 1 ml syringe with 26 G×0.5″ needle.

6. Prepare spleen and lymph node cell suspensions by smashing the organ between two frosted slides in 5 ml of incomplete culture medium. Leave the spleen cells on ice for 5 min to allow debris to sediment and transfer cells into new tubes. Wash the cells by centrifuging the tubes at 250×*g* for 10 min at 4 °C. Resuspend the pellets in 5 ml incomplete culture medium and keep the tubes on ice (*see* **Note 6**).
7. Count the nucleated cells. For each tissue take 10 µl of the cell suspension and mix it with 90 µl of Trypan blue (stock solution should be diluted 1:1 in PBS (1×)). Count living cells using the Burker counting chamber.

3.2 Cell Cultures

1. Prepare duplicates for each culture condition in order to evaluate cell proliferation at day 3 and Ig secretion at day 7.
2. Take 4×10^6 spleen cells spin and centrifuge at 250×*g* for 7 min at 4 °C.
3. Resuspend the cell pellet in 4 ml of 5-chloromethylfluorescein diacetate (CellTracker CMFDA) [6] at a final concentration of 2.5 µg/ml in PBS (1×). Incubate the sample for 30 min at 37°C in the water bath. Protect the sample from the light.
4. Add 10 ml of PBS (1×) and centrifuge the sample at 250×*g* for 5 min at 4 °C.
5. Discard the supernatant, resuspend the pellets in 800 µl of complete culture medium and distribute 200 µl (1×10^6 cells)/well into 96-well flat-bottom plates. Add 10 µl of LPS (10 µg/ml) in two wells.
6. Incubate the plates at 37 °C and 5 % CO_2 for 3 or 7 days.
7. After 3 days of stimulation, collect the LPS-stimulated and nonstimulated cells from the two wells by gently pipetting up and down. Transfer the cells into 15 ml tubes and add 10 ml of FACS medium. Centrifuge the tubes at 250×*g* for 7 min at 4 °C. Resuspend the cells in 1 ml of FACS medium and follow the staining procedures indicated below.
8. After 7 days of stimulation, centrifuge the plate at 250×*g* for 5 min at 4 °C. Collect supernatants into 1.5 ml eppendorf tubes and store at −20 °C until analysis by ELISA.

3.3 Staining Procedures for Flow-Cytometry Analysis

1. Carry out all procedures on ice and protect the samples from light.
2. Collect 1×10^6 cells/staining in a round-bottom 96-well plate (*see* **Note 7**).
3. Centrifuge plate at 250×*g* for 5 min at 4 °C and remove the supernatant by inverting the plate (*see* **Note 8**).
4. Add 10 µl of each antibody diluted in FACS medium to the cell pellet (Table 2) and shake gently. Make sure that the cell pellet is resuspended.

Table 2
Monoclonal antibodies used to characterize B cell subsets

	Clone
CD5	53-7.3
CD16 (FcγIII/IIR)	2.4G2
CD21	7G6
CD23	B3B4
CD43	S7
CD45R (B220)	RA3-6B2
IgD	11.26c
IgM	2911

5. Incubate the cells on ice for 20 min and protect from light. At the end of the incubation, add 200 μl of FACS medium and spin as described under Protocol 3.3.
6. Remove supernatant and resuspend the pellet in 200 μl of FACS medium. Transfer the cells into FACS tubes. Wash the wells with an additional 200 μl of FACS medium to recover all the cells and add to the tubes. Analyze using a flow-cytometer (*see* **Note 9**).
7. Dead cells can be excluded from the analysis by side/forward scatter gating.

3.4 ELISpot

1. Coating: Distribute 50 μl per well of antibody or antigen diluted in coating buffer in a flat-bottom 96-well plate. Vortex the plate and seal it to avoid evaporation. Incubate at 4 °C overnight (or 37 °C for 1 h). The typical protein concentration for coating is 1–10 μg/ml
2. Washing: Submerge the plate in a container with PBS (1×). Empty the plate by inversion over a sink. Tap the inverted plate against some layers of soft paper tissue to remove residual liquid. There is no need to change PBS between washes, just add more to the container. Repeat the washing procedure three times.
3. Blocking agent: Add 200 μl of PBS (1×) + 1 % gelatin/well and incubate the plates at 37 °C for 1 h.
4. Washing: Remove the plates from the incubator and wash three times as described above in **step 2**.
5. Incubation with cells: Prefill the plate with 100 μl/well of RPMI containing 2 % FCS. Adjust the cell concentration to 2×10^6 cells/ml in incomplete medium. Add 100 μl of cells to

the first row and mix gently by pipetting up and down. Collect 100 µl from the first row of the plate and mix in the second row. Repeat the 1:2 dilution series until the end of the rows. Discard the last 100 µl. Incubate plates at 37 ° C, 5 % CO_2 for 4–6 h. The plate should not move during the incubation.

6. Washing: Remove plates from the incubator and submerge them in a container filled with water + 0.05 % Tween20. Empty the plate by inversion over a sink. Submerge the plate in a container with PBS-0.05 % Tween20 and leave the plate with washing solution on the bench for 10 min. Repeat the washes three times with PBS + 0.05 % Tween20 (total washing time 30 min). Tap the inverted plate against some layers of soft paper tissue to remove residual liquid.
7. Incubate with biotin or alkaline phosphatase-labeled antibody: Prepare the antibody dilution in PBS + 1 % gelatin + 0.05 %Tween20 and distribute 50 µl/well. Seal the plates and incubate overnight at 4 °C.
8. Remove the plates from 4 °C and leave them at room temperature for 10 min. Wash the plates three times with PBS + 0.05 %Tween20. Allow the plates to sit on the bench for 10 min between each wash with PBS-Tween20 in each well (the total washing time is 30 min).
9. Add 8 ml of ESA substrate solution to 3 ml of dH_2O. Distribute 50 µl/well of the diluted substrate solution and incubate overnight at 4 °C or 2 h at 37 °C (*see* **Note 10**).
10. Wash the plates three times with dH_2O as described above in **step 2**.
11. Air-dry the plates and count spots using a dissection microscope (Fig. 4a).

3.5 Quantification of Serum Igs by ELISA

1. Coating: Distribute 50 µl of antibody or antigen diluted in coating buffer into each well of a flat-bottom 96-well plate. Vortex and seal the plate to avoid evaporation. Incubate the plate at 4 °C overnight (or 37 °C for 1 h). The typical protein concentration for coating is 1–10 µg/ml.
2. Washing: Wash the plate three times with PBS (1×) as described for ELISpot under Protocol 3.4, **step 2**.
3. Blocking agent: Add 200 µl of PBS + 1 % gelatin/well and incubate the plates at 37 °C for 1 h.
4. Washing: Remove the plates from the 37 °C incubator and wash three times as described above under **step 2**.
5. Incubation with serum or culture supernatant: Generate a "masterplate" for dilutions using a round-bottomed 96-well plate. Fill all of the wells with 100 µl of PBS + 1 % gelatin + 0.05 % Tween20 and add 10 µl of serum to the

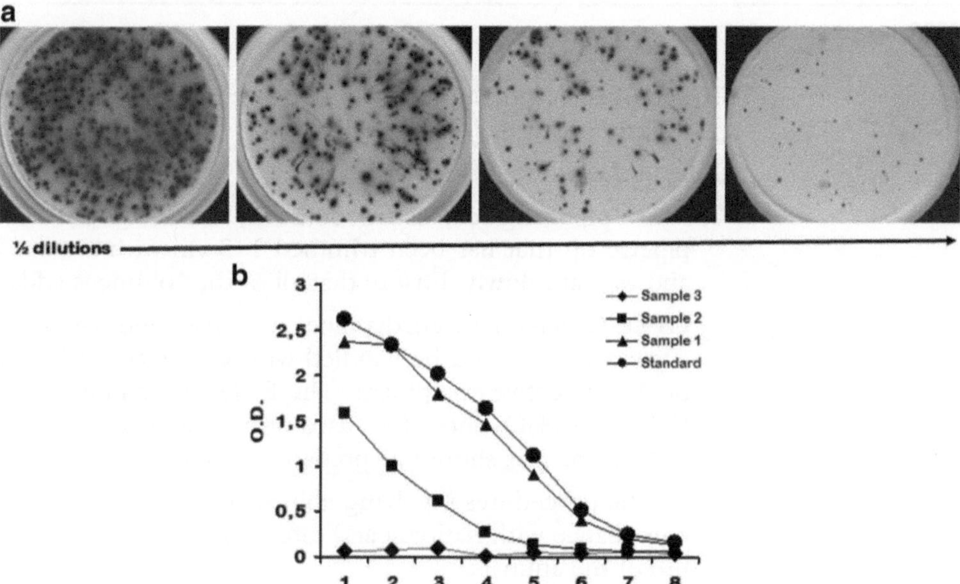

Fig. 4 Antibody-secreting cells (ASC) and serum/supernatant antibodies. (**a**) Images represent 1:2 serial dilutions of IgM-producing cells present in the spleen of an adult mouse. Each *dark spot* corresponds to a single cell that secreted IgM. The number of spots can be reported to the number of cells seeded in order to have the number of ASC/10^6. (**b**) Graph represents the optical density (OD) measured at 450 nm at the end of the ELISA. To calculate serum or culture supernatant Ig concentration is sufficient to extrapolate OD values of the exponential phase curve from the standard curve

first row (for the supernatant, *see* **Note 11**). Mix by pipetting up and down. Collect 50 μl from the first row and mix in the second row. Repeat the 1:3 dilution series for each row on the plate. Discard the last 50 μl. Transfer 50 μl of the dilutions to the coated, blocked, and washed ELISA plate. Incubate the plates at 37 °C for 1 h.

6. Washing: Remove the plates from the 37 °C incubator and wash three times as described above in **step 2**.
7. Incubate with biotin- or peroxidase-conjugated antibody: Prepare the antibody dilution in PBS + 1 % gelatin + 0.05 % Tween20 and distribute 50 μl/well. Incubate the plates at 37 °C for 1 h.
8. Washing: Remove the plates from the 37 °C incubator and wash three times as described above under **step 2**.
9. Substrate reaction: Add 100 μl/well of substrate solution (*see* **Note 11**). Incubate at room temperature for 10–45 min and protect the plates from light using aluminum foil or a box.
10. Stop the enzymatic reaction: Add 50 μl/well of 10 % SDS.
11. Read plates using a spectrophotometer at 450 nm (Fig. 4b).

4 Notes

1. Fetal calf serum should be heat inactivated by incubating for 30 min in a water bath at 56 °C.
2. Handle sodium azide with care.
3. When pipetting very dense solutions, such as Tween-20, use a pipette tip that has been trimmed 1–3 cm with a razor blade and aspirate slowly. Ensure that all of the volume is added.
4. OPD (*ortho*-phenylenediamine) is toxic and carcinogenic. Therefore it should be handled with gloves and other appropriate protective equipment. The ELISA substrate buffer with OPD and H_2O_2 should be used immediately after mixing the H_2O_2. The mix should be prepared fresh each time.
5. All the procedures involving animals have to be performed in compliance with national and international laws on the ethical use of the animals.
6. Quality of the FACS staining may be improved with the depletion of erythrocytes, in particular for peripheral blood and spleen samples. The use of Gey's solution is also recommended when there is a need to analyze or quantify minute cell subsets.
7. Before the use of labeled or unlabeled antibodies, make sure they specifically bind to the receptor of interest and that the antibodies are appropriately diluted. Antibodies to be used in the FACS analysis should be diluted in FACS medium each time. To remove fluorescent precipitates we recommend centrifuging the antibody dilution for 10 min at 9,600 × *g* before use.
8. Quality of the FACS staining can be improved by preincubating the cells with CD16-FcγIII/IIR (Fc-block reagent).
9. If cell acquisition is not possible shortly after the staining procedure, consider fixing the cells. After the surface staining and the last wash, add 200 μl of 1 % paraformaldehyde in PBS (1×) to the cell pellet and incubate at 4 °C for 20 min in the dark. Transfer cells from the plate into FACS tubes and add 200 μl of FACS medium.
10. Check the quality of ESA substrate solution before use. The solution should be transparent and without precipitates. Precipitates can be removed by filtering the stock solution with a 0.45 μm filter before diluting in dH_2O.
11. As Ig concentration in culture supernatants is expected to be lower than Ig concentration in sera from healthy subjects, the starting dilution in the ELISA plate should be lower. Fill all wells with 100 μl of PBS + 1 % gelatine + 0.05 %Tween20, except the first row of wells that should get only 50 μl of PBS + 1 % gelatine + 0.05 % Tween20. Take 50 μl of culture

supernatant and add to the first row. Proceed in the following steps as discussed for the serum.

12. Make sure the substrate buffer is at room temperature before adding the OPD and H_2O_2. ELISA substrate is unstable and should be used immediately.

Acknowledgments

We thank Dr. Claudio Pioli for his critical review of the manuscript. R.C. is supported by EUROPAD NET (EC Grant Nr. 201549).

References

1. Godin I, Cumano A (2002) The hare and the tortoise: an embryonic haematopoietic race. Nat Rev 2(8):593–604
2. Ghosn EE, Sadate-Ngatchou P, Yang Y, Herzenberg LA, Herzenberg LA (2011) Distinct progenitors for B-1 and B-2 cells are present in adult mouse spleen. Proc Natl Acad Sci USA 108(7):2879–2884
3. Rosado MM, Aranburu A, Capolunghi F, Giorda E, Cascioli S, Cenci F, Petrini S, Miller E, Leanderson T, Bottazzo GF, Natali PG, Carsetti R (2009) From the fetal liver to spleen and gut: the highway to natural antibody. Mucosal Immunol 2(4):351–361
4. Carsetti R, Kohler G, Lamers MC (1995) Transitional B cells are the target of negative selection in the B cell compartment. J Exp Med 181(6):2129–2140
5. Carsetti R, Rosado MM, Wardmann H (2004) Peripheral development of B cells in mouse and man. Immunol Rev 197:179–191
6. Quah BJ, Warren HS, Parish CR (2007) Monitoring lymphocyte proliferation in vitro and in vivo with the intracellular fluorescent dye carboxyfluorescein diacetate succinimidyl ester. Nat Protoc 2(9):2049–2056
7. Hardy RR, Carmack CE, Shinton SA, Kemp JD, Hayakawa K (1991) Resolution and characterisation of pro-B and Pre-Pro-B cell stages in normal mouse bone marrow. J Exp Med 173:1213–1225
8. Hardy RR, Li YS, Allman D, Asano M, Gui M, Hayakawa K (2000) B-cell commitment, development and selection. Immunol Rev 173:23–32
9. Rolink A, Grawunder U, Winkler TH, Karasuyama H, Melchers F (1994) IL-2 receptor alpha chain (CD25, TAC) expression defines a crucial stage in pre-B cell development. Int Immunol 6(8):1257–1264
10. Kitamura D, Roes J, Kuhn R, Rajewsky KA (1991) B cell-deficient mouse by targeted disruption of the membrane exon of the immunoglobulin mu chain gene. Nature 350(6317): 423–426
11. Casola S, Otipoby KL, Alimzhanov M, Humme S, Uyttersprot N, Kutok JL, Carroll MC, Rajewsky K (2004) B cell receptor signal strength determines B cell fate. Nat Immunol 5(3):317–327
12. Chen X, Martin F, Forbush KA, Perlmutter RM, Kearney JF (1997) Evidence for selection of a population of multi-reactive B cells into the splenic marginal zone. Int Immunol 9(1): 27–41
13. Hayakawa K, Hardy RR, Honda M, Herzenberg LA, Steinberg AD, Herzenberg LA (1984) Ly-1 B cells: functionally distinct lymphocytes that secrete IgM autoantibodies. Proc Natl Acad Sci USA 81(8):2494–2498
14. Baumgarth N (2011) The double life of a B-1 cell: self-reactivity selects for protective effector functions. Nat Rev Immunol 11(1): 34–46
15. Hardy RR, Kincade PW, Dorshkind K (2007) The protean nature of cells in the B lymphocyte lineage. Immunity 26(6):703–714
16. Rolink AG, Andersson J, Melchers F (2004) Molecular mechanisms guiding late stages of B-cell development. Immunol Rev 197:41–50

Chapter 5

Protocols for Identifying, Enumerating, and Assessing Mouse Eosinophils

Kimberly D. Dyer, Katia E. Garcia-Crespo, Caroline M. Percopo, Eva M. Sturm, and Helene F. Rosenberg

Abstract

Eosinophils are prominent in allergic diseases, and their effector functions are studied in numerous gene-deleted and transgenic mouse models. However, mouse eosinophils and human eosinophils are not structurally or functionally equivalent, and assays designed to evaluate the properties of human eosinophils may or may not be reliable or effective in experiments targeting their murine counterparts. In this chapter, we emphasize methods focused on detection, isolation, and functional assessment of eosinophils from mouse tissue and present a protocol that promotes the growth and differentiation of eosinophils from unselected mouse bone marrow progenitors. Overall, these protocols provide a scaffold on which the relative contributions of mouse eosinophils can be evaluated.

Key words Piece-meal degranulation (PMD), Eosinophil peroxidase (EPO), Major basic protein (MBP), Eotaxin, Ribonuclease, IL5-Rα, CCR3

1 Introduction

Although eosinophil-related biomedical research relies substantially on the use of mouse models of human disease, mouse eosinophils and human eosinophils are actually quite different from one another. One must not assume that protocols designed to evaluate human eosinophils will be appropriate or even adequate for the study of mouse eosinophils. Some of the most prominent differences between these cells are listed in Table 1. For instance, human eosinophils from peripheral blood have characteristic bilobed nuclei and prominent refractile granules that stain vividly with acidic dyes. However, mouse eosinophil morphology is somewhat more subtle; the nucleus can take on different shapes (Fig. 1), and the granules are smaller and less refractile than those found in human eosinophils [1]. Many methods are available to stain eosinophils that distinguish them from the other granulocytes, primarily neutrophils

Irving C. Allen (ed.), *Mouse Models of Allergic Disease: Methods and Protocols*, Methods in Molecular Biology, vol. 1032, DOI 10.1007/978-1-62703-496-8_5, © Springer Science+Business Media, LLC 2013

Table 1
Mouse and human eosinophils are not identical

Characteristic	Human	Mouse
Nuclear morphology	Bilobed	Bilobed and donut shaped
Granule morphology	Large, refractile	Smaller, less refractile
Secretory ribonucleases	Cationic ECP; more neutral EDN	Highly divergent mEAR cluster
Galectin-10/Charcot-Leyden crystal protein	Present in high concentration	Absent; no identifiable ortholog
High affinity IgE receptor	Present; surface expression	Absent
Cell surface Siglec expression	Siglec 8	Siglec F
Degranulation	Highly responsive; multiple secretagogues	Minimally responsive; few identified secretagogues

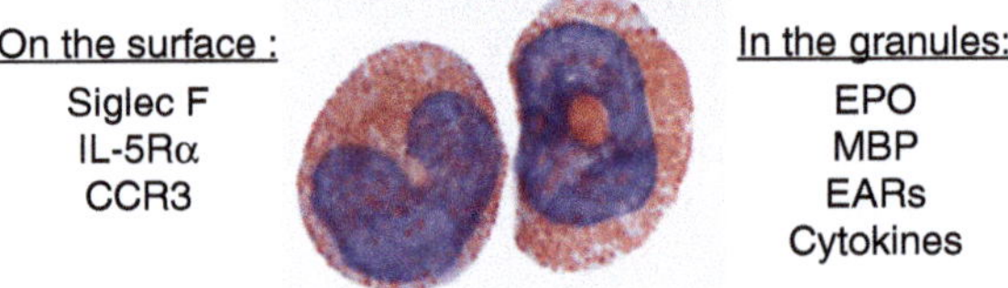

Fig. 1 Freshly isolated naïve mouse bone marrow eosinophils stained with Diff Quik (*see* Protocol 3.6). Note the two nuclear phenotypes. Also indicated are select surface markers and some contents of the granules that are stained here in *red*

and basophils [2]. The protocol provided here has been optimized so that mouse eosinophil granules stain prominently.

Eosinophils possess a few relatively specific proteins that can be used as markers for confocal microscopy or flow-cytometric-based identification. The granule major basic protein (MBP) and eosinophil peroxidase (EPO) and cell surface proteins Siglec F, CCR3, and IL-5Rα have all been used to identify mouse eosinophils. We present a protocol for intracellular staining of MBP [3] and a protocol that utilizes antibodies directed against Siglec F for the identification of eosinophils by flow cytometry. Human eosinophils degranulate readily in response to many stimuli but mouse eosinophils differ in that they do not release their granule contents under similar conditions or in response to similar secretagogues. Mouse eosinophils, similar to human eosinophils, exhibit piecemeal degranulation; therefore any one secretagogue may not stimulate the release of all granule components equally. We have provided several protocols that assess the release of eosinophil contents. The first is an assay that detects the activity of EPO using a cell-impermeable substrate as first reported by Adamko et al. [4]. The second assay utilizes multibead cytokine assays or ELISAs to measure cytokine release. And the third method is an assay that detects the activity of the eosinophil-associated ribonucleases against a tRNA substrate as reported by Rosenberg and Domachowske [5]. Finally, we provide the protocol for a chemotaxis assay that utilizes eotaxin-2 as a stimulant.

The protocols included in this chapter are organized into three sections. The first set of protocols (3.1–3.5) focuses on isolation of source material; specifically, single cell suspensions from mouse bone marrow, spleen, lung, and bronchoalveolar lavage fluid, typically from interleukin-5 (IL-5) transgenic or antigen sensitized and challenged mice, from which eosinophils can be enumerated, isolated, and evaluated. This group also includes a protocol that describes methods to grow and differentiate eosinophils from the bone marrow of wild-type and gene-deleted mice (bmEos). The second set of protocols (3.6–3.9) is directed at evaluating the physical attributes of the eosinophils found in this source material. We provide protocols for staining eosinophils in single cell suspensions, for isolation of RNA and analysis of eosinophil gene expression by quantitative RT-PCR, protocols for analysis of immunoreactive proteins by confocal microscopy and immunohistochemical analyses and methods to detect eosinophils by flow cytometry. We also provide protocols for functional assays such as eosinophil degranulation (3.10–3.12) and chemotaxis (3.13).

2 Materials

2.1 Buffers and Reagents

1. BSA/PBS: 0.1 % or 1 % BSA (as specified) in PBS.
2. RPMI-1640 without phenol red.
3. RPMI-1640 (with phenol red).
4. Hanks' Buffered saline solution (HBSS).
5. Fetal bovine serum (FBS): heat inactivated for 1 h at 56 °C.
6. FBS/HEPES/HBSS: 1 % fetal bovine serum in HBSS with 10 mM HEPES.
7. EDTA/PBS: 10 mM EDTA in PBS.
8. Lung isolation media: RPMI-1640, 0.05 % DNase, 20 mM HEPES, 2 mMl-glutamine 100 IU penicillin and 10 μg/ml streptomycin, 60 μl of 50 mg/ml Liberase.
9. FBS/RPMI: 3 % FBS in RPMI-1640.
10. Percoll: 40 % Percoll and 70 % Percoll.

11. ACK: ammonium chloride lysis buffer.
12. OPD (*o*-phenylene-diamine): 800 μl 5 mM OPD in 4 ml 1 M Tris–HCl (pH 8.0), 5.2 ml H_2O and 1.25 μl 30 % H_2O_2.
13. SDS: 0.2 % sodium dodecyl sulfate.
14. H_2SO_4, 4 M.
15. Pertussis toxin, 100 ng/ml.
16. Platelet-activating factor (PAF): 1 mM in DMSO, store at −20 °C. Use at final concentration 1–5 μM.
17. IL-6: 20 ng/ml in 0.1 % BSA/PBS, store in single-use aliquots at −80 °C.
18. Cycloheximide, 5 μg/ml.
19. Multibead cytokine assay (Millipore, BioRad).
20. Deoxyribonuclease (DNase) I.
21. Diethyl-pyrocarbonate (DEPC)-treated water.
22. First Strand cDNA Synthesis Kit for RT-PCR.
23. Real time PCR primer probe sets (Applied Biosystems, ABI): EPO, MBP, IL-5Rα/CD125, CCR3, and GAPDH.
24. Cell permeabilization and fixation reagent (i.e. Fix and Perm (Caltag Laboratories)).
25. 4 % paraformaldehyde.
26. Methanol—ice cold.
27. DAPI—4′,6-diamidino-2-phenylindole dihydrochloride.
28. Cell differential staining reagents (i.e. Diff-Quik).
29. Cell viability stain (i.e. Live-Dead Stain (Invitrogen)).
30. Antibodies: anti-CD16/CD32, Rabbit anti-MBP (#509, provided on request from Dr. Nancy A. Lee and Dr. James J. Lee, Mayo Clinic, Scottsdale, Arizona), goat anti-rabbit IgG-Alexa Fluor 647, anti-Siglec-F, anti-CD11c, anti-CD45.
31. Base media: RPMI-1640 with 20 % FBS, 25 mM HEPES, 1 mM sodium pyruvate, 2 mM glutamine, 1× NEAA, 50 μM β-mercaptoethanol, 100 IU/ml penicillin, 10 μg/ml streptomycin.
32. Chemotaxis assay media: RPMI-1640 media supplemented with 1 % Fetal Calf Serum (FCS) and 10 mM HEPES Buffer.
33. Chemoattractants such as eotaxin: suspended in chemotaxis assay media.
34. RNA stabilization buffer (i.e. RNAlater).
35. Qiagen RNeasy kit.
36. Real-time quantitative PCR buffer, such as ABI 2× Taqman reagent.

37. Phosphate buffer: 100 mM sodium phosphate in DEPC water, pH 7.4.
38. 40 mM Lanthanum nitrate in DEPC water.
39. 6 % perchloric acid in DEPC water.
40. 20 mg/ml yeast tRNA in DEPC, aliquot immediately and store in single-use aliquots at −80 °C.
41. T and B bead buffer: 0.5 % BSA and 2 mM EDTA, pH 7.2 in PBS.
42. T and B cell microbeads: CD90.2 (Thy1.2, Miltenyi) and CD45R (B220, Miltenyi).
43. RNase Assay STOP solution: 1:1 v/v mixture of 40 mM lanthanum nitrate and 6 % perchloric acid, prepare immediately prior to use.
44. Bovine ribonuclease A: 100, 1,000, and 10,000 ng/ml in PBS.
45. bmEos base media: 20 % FBS (heat inactivated), 25 mM HEPES, 100 IU/ml penicillin and 10 μg/ml streptomycin, 2 mM glutamine, 1× NEAA, 1 mM sodium pyruvate, 50 μM β-ME all in RPMI-1640.
46. Mouse Interleukin-5: (mIL-5, R&D): resuspend in 0.1 % BSA/PBS at 5 μg/ml and use at 10 ng/ml. Store in single-use aliquots at −80 °C.
47. Mouse Stem Cell Factor (mSCF, Peprotech): resuspend in 0.1 % BSA/PBS at 10 μg/ml and use at 100 ng/ml. Store in single-use aliquots at −80 °C.
48. Mouse Flt3L (PeproTech): resuspend in 0.1 % BSA/PBS at 10 μg/ml and use at 100 ng/ml. Store in single-use aliquots at −80 °C.

2.2 Supplies

1. Cytofunnels.
2. 96-well flat bottom plates.
3. Cell strainers, 40 and 70 μm.
4. HTS Transwell®-96 Permeable Support System with 5.0 μm pore polycarbonate membrane.
5. 5 ml Polystyrene Round-Bottom Tubes.
6. CS column (Miltenyi).
7. Small feeding needle (22 × 1″ Cadence, Inc.).

2.3 Equipment

1. Centrifuge.
2. Cytospin centrifuge.
3. Light microscope with 64× oil immersion objective.
4. ELISA Plate reader with 492 nm filter.
5. 37 °C, 5 % CO_2 humidified incubator.
6. BioRad BioPlex multibead plate reader.

7. Confocal microscope.
8. Flow cytometer.
9. Tissue homogenizer.
10. Real-time quantitative PCR instrument.
11. Spectrophotometer capable of reading absorbance at 260 nm.
12. Vario MACS Magnet (Miltenyi).
13. Hemacytometer.

3 Methods

3.1 Isolation of Total Bone Marrow Cells

1. This protocol is generally applicable to all strains of mice. Recovery from a wild-type naïve mouse is typically $10–20 \times 10^6$ cells with about 5 % eosinophils; this percentage will increase to 40–60 % eosinophils when using bone marrow from IL-5 transgenic mice [6].
2. Euthanize mice according to approved animal care procedures. Remove the femurs and tibias, remove the flesh from the bones, with a scalpel cut off the ends of the bones as distally as possible. Insert a 25 gauge needle into the end of the bone and flush the marrow into a 15 ml tube with a total of 12 ml of RPMI-1640 per four mouse bones.
3. Centrifuge the cells and lyse the red blood cells by suspending the pellet in 9 ml of dH_2O for 30 s and then add 1 ml of 10× PBS to adjust tonicity to normal, centrifuge and repeat two more times.
4. Suspend the cells in 10 ml of HBSS and then count the cells to determine the total cell number. Eosinophils and eosinophil progenitors from bone marrow can be enumerated by direct staining (*see* Protocol 3.6), by immunohistochemical staining (*see* Protocol 3.7), and/or by flow cytometric methods (*see* Protocol 3.8).

3.2 Isolation of Cells from the Spleen

1. The spleen of the IL-5 transgenic (tg) mouse is an excellent source of mature eosinophils. This protocol, modified from that of Aizawa et al. [7] and Shen et al. [8] provides a method for the isolation of 10^7 cells with >90 % eosinophils from spleens of IL-5tg mice.
2. Euthanize mice according to approved animal care procedures. Place the spleen in cold 1 % FBS/10 mM HEPES/HBSS until ready to process.
3. Once the isolation of single cells begins, keep cells at room temperature and use reagents brought to room temperature. Move the spleen into a petri dish or six-well plate and cut into small pieces. Place the spleen fragments in a 70 μm strainer

inserted into a 50 ml tube. Force the tissue through the mesh using the plunger of a 3 ml syringe. Rinse the strainer with 10 ml of 1 % FBS/10 mM HEPES/HBSS and repeat process using a 40 μm strainer.

4. Centrifuge the cells, resuspend the pellet in 1 ml of cold FBS/HEPES/HBSS and lyse the red blood cells with ACK lysis buffer or with 45 ml of dH_2O for 30 s followed by 5 ml of 10× PBS, centrifuge and repeat two more times.
5. After the last centrifugation, suspend the cells in 50 ml of HBSS prior to the determination of total cell number. Approximately $2–10 \times 10^7$ cells will be recovered from the spleen of a wild-type naïve mouse [9].
6. From this point, eosinophils are isolated by negative selection. B and T cells are removed via interactions with anti-CD45R and anti-CD90.2 microbeads, respectively. Centrifuge 10^7 cells at $300 \times g$ for 10 min and completely remove the supernatant. Suspend cells in 90 μl of ice-cold T and B bead buffer and add 10 μl anti-CD45R/B220 and 10 μl anti-CD90.2 microbeads (*see* **Note 1**).
7. Incubate exactly 15 min at 4 °C tumbling end over end.
8. Wash the cells in 2 ml of ice-cold T and B bead buffer and pass through a 70 μm sieve and centrifuge.
9. While centrifuging, set up the CS column per manufacturer's directions. Flush the CS column with T and B bead buffer through the syringe and then elute 10–30 ml of T and B bead buffer through the column from the top. Attach a 20–25-gauge needle to act as a flow regulator (a smaller needle will yield greater purity, but will diminish the number of cells recovered).
10. After centrifuging the cells, suspend the pellet at 10^8 cells in 500 μl of buffer and apply the cells to the column.
11. Collect the unlabeled cells, which will pass through the column and wash column twice in 1 ml buffer. Then add an additional 10 ml of buffer to the column. The column will retain T and B cells and eosinophils will be unlabeled and pass through the column. Determine the number of collected, unlabeled eosinophils.
12. Eosinophils from the spleen can be assessed by direct staining (*see* Protocol 3.6), by immunohistochemical staining (*see* Protocol 3.7), and/or by flow cytometric methods (*see* Protocol 3.8). These cells can also be used for degranulation studies (*see* Protocols 3.9–3.11) and for chemotaxis assays (*see* Protocol 3.12).

3.3 Isolation of Cells from the Lung

1. This protocol is modified from that of Carlens et al. [10] and generates single cell suspensions from lung tissue for evaluation of eosinophils elicited in response to antigen sensitization

and airway challenge, or in response to systemic and/or local expression of cytokine transgenes. Approximately 2–5 × 10^6 cells are recovered from a pool of two wild-type naïve mouse lungs, and 10 × 10^6 cells from a pool of two lungs from wild-type mice sensitized and challenged with ovalbumin, as described in reference [11].

2. Euthanize mice according to approved animal care procedures. Open the chest cavity and perfuse the lungs by injecting 8 ml of 10 mM EDTA/PBS into the right ventricle of the heart to remove peripheral blood cells and then remove the lungs from the mouse. The lung will turn noticeably whiter in color as the RBCs are flushed out; good perfusion of the lungs is critical for cell recovery (i.e. poor perfusion means reduced yield).
3. Pool the lungs from two mice and mince in a petri dish using a straight razor blade.
4. Transfer lung tissue to a 50 ml beaker containing freshly prepared 15 ml of lung isolation media and add 60 μl of 50 mg/ml Liberase and stir for 30 min at 37 °C.
5. After incubation, put the contents of the beaker through a 70 μm cell strainer. Rinse the strainer two to three times with 5 ml of media with 3 % FBS and then pass the cell/media mixture through a 40 μm strainer.
6. Centrifuge the cells. Pipette off the liquid and lyse the red blood cells by suspending the pellet in 3 ml of ACK lysing buffer and incubate for 5 min at room temperature, add 10 ml of media with 3 % FBS and centrifuge cells again.
7. Suspend the pellet in 8 ml of 40 % Percoll then overlay on 3 ml of 70 % Percoll and centrifuge at 580 × *g* for 30 min at room temperature with the rotor brake off.
8. Collect the cells at the interface and wash with 10 ml HBSS. Centrifuge cells, suspend pellet in 1 ml HBSS and count. Cell populations from the lung can be enumerated by direct staining (*see* Protocol 3.6), by immunohistochemical staining (*see* Protocol 3.7), and/or by flow cytometric methods (*see* Protocol 3.8).

3.4 Isolation of Cells from Bronchial Alveolar Lavage Fluid

1. Naïve wild-type mice have few to no eosinophils in the bronchial alveolar lavage fluid (BALF). BALF collected from wild-type BALB/c mice sensitized and challenged with ovalbumin will have up to 60 % eosinophils [11].
2. Euthanize mice according to approved animal care procedures, but keep in mind that cervical dislocation, if performed, will need to be done gently so as not to damage the trachea and surrounding tissues.
3. Place the mouse on its back with limbs fixed and soak the chest and abdomen with 70 % ethanol. Dissect to open the mouse

from the diaphragm up to the top of the neck and pin down neck skin to immobilize the head in a prone position. When dissected appropriately the trachea should be visible.

4. Put 0.8 ml of 1 % BSA/PBS in a 1 ml syringe and attach a small feeding needle. Insert feeding needle through the mouth into the trachea. Some resistance should be felt and the feeding needle should be visible in the trachea. Fill lungs with 0.7 ml of 1 % BSA/PBS. Lungs should visibly inflate; if not remove needle and try again as the solution is going into the stomach or coming back out of the mouth.
5. When the lungs inflate, carefully pull back on the syringe to remove fluid. Usually you can recover roughly 0.5 ml of BALF. Repeat this process with another 0.8 ml of 1 % BSA/PBS.
6. The total volume of BALF collected is 0.5–1.0 ml per mouse. Collect the cells by centrifugation. Cell populations from the BALF can be enumerated by direct staining (*see* Protocol 3.6), by immunohistochemical staining (*see* Protocol 3.7), and/or by flow cytometric methods (*see* Protocol 3.8).

3.5 Differentiation of Eosinophils from the Bone Marrow

1. This protocol provides a method for generating large numbers of phenotypically mature eosinophils ex vivo from unselected bone marrow progenitors [12]. We [13, 14] and others [15, 16] have used this method to generate eosinophils from a number of gene-deleted strains.
2. Prepare 500 ml of bmEos base media and add SCF and Flt3L to 50 ml of bmEos base media. Prepare concentrated stocks in 0.1 % BSA/PBS and freeze at −80 °C, thaw immediately before use and add to media at 100 ng/ml each. Use cytokine containing media within 1 week.
3. Euthanize mice and collect marrow (as per Protocol 3.1) under sterile conditions. Once all marrow has been collected, centrifuge to pellet cells.
4. Prepare sterile dH_2O and 10× PBS, lyse red blood cells by pipetting up and down two times in 9 ml of dH_2O and then immediately add 1 ml of 10× PBS to make solution isotonic.
5. Centrifuge again.
6. Lyse again if necessary, if not, suspend in 1× PBS or media for counting and preparing slides for differential count. Do not perform lysis procedure more than three times.
7. Centrifuge, remove PBS, and put into bmEos base media + SCF and Flt3L at 10^6 cells/ml.
8. On day 2 of culture, remove ½ volume of media from each culture (will contain cells), centrifuge and suspend the cells in the fresh media containing SCF and Flt3Lthat is equivalent to the volume removed, or more if it is necessary to

adjust the concentration to 10^6 cells/ml, and return all cells to the original flask. On day 2, count the cells and make slides for differential count. The cell count should remain unchanged from day 0.

9. On day 4, make IL-5 media by adding IL5 to base media at 10 ng/ml. Make 50–100 ml and use as needed within 1 week.
10. Remove media and nonadherent cells from the flask. Count the cells and prepare slides for differential staining. Centrifuge cells and remove all the SCF + Flt3L media. Replace with media containing IL-5 such that the concentration is again 10^6 cells/ml. Put all of the cells back into the original flask.
11. On day 6, remove ½ volume of media containing some nonadherent cells from each culture. Count cells and prepare slides for differential count. Centrifuge, remove media, and suspend cells in amount of volume removed or more if it is necessary to adjust the concentration to 10^6 cells/ml. Return all cells to original flask.
12. On day 8, pipette the media over the bottom of the flask to dislodge loosely adherent cells. Remove media and all nonadherent cells from the flask. Count cells, make slides for differential count
13. Centrifuge, remove ½ media, and suspend cells in amount of volume removed or more if it is necessary to adjust the concentration to 10^6 cells/ml. Move all cells into a new flask.
14. On day 10, the cells in culture should be primarily eosinophils. Count and determine eosinophil purity every other day as desired (*see* **Note 2**). Eosinophils obtained from bone marrow culture can be assessed by direct staining (*see* Protocol 3.6), by immunohistochemical staining (*see* Protocol 3.7), and/or by flow cytometric methods (*see* Protocol 3.8). These cells can also be used for the examination of RNA expression (*see* Protocol 3.9), degranulation studies (*see* Protocols 3.10 and 3.11) and for chemotaxis assays (*see* Protocol 3.12).

3.6 Slide Preparation and Cell Counts

1. After generating cells via any of the aforementioned methods, centrifuge 50,000 cells and suspend in 100 μl of 0.1 % BSA/PBS.
2. Pipette the 50,000 cells in 100 μl of 0.1 % BSA/PBS into a cytofunnel assembled with glass slide and labeled in pencil (ink will come off slide in subsequent staining steps). Centrifuge at $500 \times g$ for 5 min.
3. Remove the cytofunnel from the glass slide. The cells should be visible as a round smudge.
4. Stain the slides with Diff Quik as follows: 5 min in fixative, then at least 2 min air dry; 3 min in solution 1 (xanthene dye)

followed by three quick washes in dH_2O, then 2 min air dry; 10 s in solution 2 (thiazine) followed by three washes in dH_2O.

5. Air or blot dry and cover slip.
6. Eosinophils are detected based on the pink to red staining of their specific granules and are readily visible under a 64× oil immersion objective. Eosinophils can be determined as a fraction of the total cells per high-powered field (HPF, counting 10–20) and reported as eosinophils/HPF, or as a fraction of a fixed number of total cells (such as 500) and can be reported as percent of total cells.

3.7 Immunostaining of Eosinophils with Rabbit Anti-mouse MBP for Confocal Analysis

1. This protocol uses the polyclonal rabbit anti-mouse MBP.
2. Wash 10^6 cells isolated or differentiated as described above with 3 ml of 0.1 % BSA/PBS and transfer to a 15 ml tube.
3. Fix and permeabilize cells with FIX & PERM as per manufacturer's protocol or fix with 500 μl 4 % paraformaldehyde followed by washing with 3 ml of 0.1 % BSA/PBS and then adding 500 μl ice-cold methanol to permeabilize. After fixing and permeabilizing the cells, move them to a 1.5 ml tube for staining.
4. Dilute rabbit anti-mouse MBP at 1:5,000 in 0.1 % BSA/PBS and stain cells in a total volume of 100 μl for 1 h at 4 °C. *See* **Note 3** for other antibody choices. Appropriate controls include an irrelevant primary rabbit primary antibody and a sample incubated with only the conjugated secondary antibody.
5. Wash the cells three times in 1 ml of 0.1 % BSA/PBS.
6. Dilute goat anti-rabbit IgG-Alexa Fluor 647 at 1:100 dilution 0.1 % BSA/PBS and stain cells in a total volume of 100 μl for 1 h in the dark at room temperature (*see* **Note 4**).
7. Wash the cells three times in 1 ml of 0.1 % BSA/PBS and add the nuclear stain, 4′,6-diamidino-2-phenylindole dihydrochloride (DAPI) at 1 μg/ml and for 15 min in the dark.
8. Wash the cells three times in 1 ml of 0.1 % BSA/PBS and fix onto glass slides using cytofunnels (*see* Protocol 3.6) and coverslip (*see* **Note 5**).
9. Collect images on a confocal microscope using a 63× oil immersion objective. Fields are selected "blinded" in that the microscope is focused on the DAPI-stained nuclei and that field was imaged regardless of the presence or absence of MBP-Alexa Fluor 647 positive cells as Alexa Fluor 647 is far red and not visible to the eye. Settings are selected based on the negative controls and then are not changed when imaging the sample stained with anti-MBP and the secondary antibody.

3.8 Flow Cytometric Analysis Utilizing the Eosinophil Surface Marker Siglec F

1. Antibodies directed against the cell surface Ig-type lectin, mouse Siglec F, are generally specific and selective for mouse eosinophils, with some exceptions, as noted below.
2. Suspend cells in HBSS and put 10^6/1 ml in flow tubes, with one tube for each sample and each single color control. For one sample and four colors, there will be a total of nine tubes—unstained, Live-Dead, and a tube for each antibody, a tube for each isotype and the sample tube stained with all colors.
3. Incubate with Live-Dead reagent according to manufacturer's suggestions (*see* **Note 6**).
4. Wash cells with 3 ml of 0.1 % BSA/PBS to remove unincorporated stain.
5. Suspend cells in 0.1 % BSA/PBS at 10^6/100 μl.
6. Incubate cells with anti-Siglec F, anti-CD11c, and anti-CD45 in the presence of 0.5 μg of anti-CD16/CD32 blocking antibody in a total volume of 100 μl for 30–60 min at 4 °C in the dark (*see* **Note 7**).
7. Wash with 3 ml of 0.1 % BSA/PBS and flow samples immediately (go to **step 9**) or fix with 500 μl of 4 % formaldehyde in PBS.
8. When ready to perform flow cytometry, remove formaldehyde by washing with 3 ml of 0.1 % BSA/PBS and resuspend samples in 100 μl 0.1 % BSA/PBS.
9. Collect at least 100,000 events on the flow cytometer. Compensation may be performed on the flow cytometer using single color tubes or compensation beads. Compensation can also be performed post-collection as long as the single color controls were collected.
10. All analyses are performed on the living cells since dead cells can be autofluorescent (*see* **Note 8**) and can bind antibody nonspecifically. The data can be reported as percentage of live cells. After gating on live cells, CD45 positive cells are selected; eosinophils will be Siglec F^+ and $CD11c^-$. This method correlates well with direct counting of cells fixed to slides and stained with Diff Quik [9].

3.9 RNA Isolation and Analysis of Eosinophil Transcript Expression by QPCR

1. Quantitative RT-PCR has largely supplanted Northern blots for analysis of RNA. This is a standard protocol in use in our lab; information on several eosinophil-related primer probe sets is also included.
2. Collect tissue or cells of interest and immediately place in a tube containing cold RNAlater and store at 4 °C overnight. The amount of RNAlater used can vary; follow the manufacturer's instructions. For long-term storage move from 4 °C to −80 °C. If making RNA from purified eosinophils, proceed

directly to **step 3** without any homogenization. *See* **Note 9** for specific issues regarding isolation of RNA from eosinophil-enriched sources.

3. Thaw tissue on ice and rinse in DEPC-treated water to remove salts from the RNAlater.
4. Homogenize 30 mg tissue and isolate RNA following the Qiagen RNeasy minikit instructions. Briefly, homogenize tissue in lysis buffer containing β-mercaptoethanol, centrifuge, pass supernatant over column, wash and perform on-column DNase treatment, wash and elute RNA in RNase-free water.
5. Reverse transcribe 2 μg of RNA using a First Strand cDNA Synthesis Kit
6. One or two microliters cDNA can be used per 25 μl Taqman PCR reaction using Fam-labeled probe and primers to each gene of interest. Eosinophil genes of interest might include primer-probe sets for EPO, MBP, IL-5Rα/CD125, and CCR3.
7. All experiments include the following controls: a no reverse transcriptase, no template controls, and mouse GAPDH-VIC is used as the endogenous control (*see* **Note 10**).
8. Expression of eosinophil gene of interest (GOI) is normalized to GAPDH to account for variations in initial template concentration ($\Delta Ct = Ct_{GOI} - Ct_{GAPDH}$) and then expressed relative to data collected from control (condition or time point, $\Delta\Delta Ct = \Delta Ct_{expreimental} - \Delta Ct_{control}$). Generally data is expressed as relative fold (RQ) expression ($RQ = 2^{-\Delta\Delta Ct}$) where the data is reported relative to control time point or condition (*see* **Note 11**).

3.10 Detection of Eosinophil Peroxidase Release from Mouse Eosinophils

1. This colorimetric assay was adapted from the report of Adamko et al. [4] and measures the peroxidase activity of eosinophil peroxidase (EPO) utilizing a substrate that is not cell membrane permeable therefore only degranulated/released EPO is measured, not EPO that remains within granules, inside the cell.
2. Prepare concentrated secretogoue at 100-fold concentrations such that 1 μl used in a 100 μl assay will achieve desired final concentration. For example, two effective secretagogues for mouse eosinophils, C16 platelet-activating factor (PAF), and C16 lysoPAF can be prepared in DMSO at 1 mM and stored at −20 °C. Prior to using, thaw and dilute further in DMSO if desired.
3. Suspend cells in RPMI-1640 without phenol red at 250,000 cells/ml. Put 100 μl in each well of a 96-well plate. In addition to the wells containing the secretagogue, each plate contains a set of cells that remain untreated and a set of wells in which the cells lysed in 0.2 % sodium dodecyl sulfate in order to determine the total EPO content. Perform assay in duplicate or triplicate.

4. Add 1 μl of secretagogue or vehicle to each well as appropriate and 0.2 % SDS to a set of wells to determine total EPO content and incubate at 37 °C, 5 % CO_2 for 30 min.
5. Add 100 μl OPD reagent to each well. Monitor color change in the SDS lysed wells very closely and terminate when these wells achieve a brownish color. Terminate the reaction by adding 100 μl 4 M H_2SO_4 to each well and read at 492 nm (*see* **Note 12**).
6. Data are reported as percent of total EPO [(absorbance of stimulated sample − no treatment) × 100/total EPO from SDS-lysed cells]. All data are presented as mean ± SEM.

3.11 Detection of Cytokines Released from Eosinophils

1. Eosinophils store a number of cytokines in the granules. We have successfully used recombinant mouse IL-6 as a secretagogue to elicit the release of these cytokines from eosinophils [14]. The relatively short incubation period (1 h) and the inclusion of cycloheximide will assure that the cytokine measured is from intracellular stores and not from *de novo* synthesis.
2. Suspend cells in RPMI-1640 without phenol red at 10^6 cells/ml. Put 100 μl in each well of a 96-well plate. Perform assay in duplicate or triplicate.
3. Add 1 μl recombinant IL-6 to achieve a final concentration of 20 ng/ml. This concentration stimulates the release of IL-1β, IL-9, IL-12(p70), IFNγ, TNFα, and MCP-1/CCL2 from bone marrow-derived eosinophils [14]. Cycloheximide can be used at a final concentration of 5 μg/ml and added prior to the addition of IL-6 to inhibit *de novo* protein synthesis and to insure that you are looking at the release of stored products rather than newly synthesized and secreted productions.
4. After addition of the stimulant, incubate cells at 37 °C, 5 % CO_2 for 60 min.
5. After incubation, centrifuge plate and store the cell free supernatant in the freezer at −80 °C until assayed for cytokine content.
6. Thaw samples on ice and proceed to multibead cytokine assays following the manufacturer's (Millipore, BioRad) directions to prepare standards and run assay (*see* **Note 13**).
7. Collect data on a plate reader such as the BioPlex (BioRad) plate reader per manufacturer's suggestions.

3.12 Detection of Ribonuclease Activity

1. This method measures the ribonucleolytic activity of the eosinophil associated ribonucleases [5]. Mouse eosinophils contain several closely related eosinophil-associated ribonucleases (EARs). This assay will not determine which of these ribonucleases is released, but the combined activity can be assessed.

2. Prepare enough ribonuclease assay STOP solution (1:1 v/v mixture of 40 mM lanthanum nitrate and 6 % perchloric acid) for assay. STOP solutions should be prepared fresh and kept on ice. Perform experiment in triplicate; include a negative control (no sample or RNase) and a positive control (bovine RNase) and blank.
3. Put 300 μl $NaPO_4$ and 500 μl DEPC-dH_2O in all tubes.
4. Put up to 50 μl of solution to be tested (BALF or solution containing degranulation products) in each tube except the blank.
5. Add 500 μl STOP solution to the blank tube only.
6. Defrost tRNA (20 mg/ml yeast tRNA) solution on ice and add 10 μl of tRNA to all tubes for appropriate time (3, 5 or 10 min).
7. Once time has elapsed, add 500 μl ice-cold STOP solution to all tubes, mix, and place on ice for 10 min.
8. Precipitate the acid-insoluble undigested tRNA at 16,200 × *g* for 5 min at room temp.
9. Measure the optical density (OD) of the supernatant to assess the production of acid-soluble ribonucleotides at OD_{260}. The OD_{260} is directly proportional to the ribonuclease activity in the product (BALF, cell culture supernatant, etc.) assayed.

3.13 Chemotaxis Assay

1. This is a standard assay that can be used to evaluate the chemotactic responses of isolated mouse spleen eosinophils and/or bone marrow-derived eosinophils. The assay requires the use of a chemokinesis control in which the chemoattractant is placed in both the upper and the lower wells so that the non-directed movement of the eosinophils can also be assessed (*see* **Note 14**).
2. Remove the plastic lip from the Transwell Support System and add 100 μl of chemotaxis assay media into the feeder port of each well of the receiver plate. Incubate the Transwell Support System for at least 1 h at 37 °C in a humidified CO_2 incubator. This initial equilibrium will improve cell attachment.
3. Wash isolated eosinophils in RPMI-1640 and resuspend 10^6 cells/ml in chemotaxis assay media (*see* **Note 15**).
4. Dilutions of the chemoattractants or their solvents are prepared in assay media and kept on ice until use.
5. Transfer the insert plate to a second 96-well plate.
6. Remove the assay media from the receiver plate and add 100 μl of chemoattractant (recombinant eotaxin) or vehicle control to the wells. Perform the experiment in duplicate or triplicate and use a range of concentrations in the nanomolar range.

7. Place the insert plate back into the receiver plate. Take care not to trap air bubbles underneath the inserts. Add 100 μl of the cell suspension to each insert (10^5 cells/well). Remember to add chemoattractant to the chemokinesis control well(s). Put on the plastic lid and incubate the Transwell Support System for at least 2 h at 37 °C in a humidified CO_2 incubator.
8. Carefully remove the insert plate from the receiver plate. Transfer the cells that have migrated through the insert towards the chemoattractant into a 5 ml FACS tube and add 150 μl of PBS to each sample.
9. Enumerate the cells that migrated by counting on a flow cytometer for 30 s at high flow rate or manually with hemacytometer.
10. Migration in response to a chemoattractant is expressed as the chemotactic index, (CI = # cells migrated in response to chemoattractant/# cells migrated in response to vehicle control). Alternatively, data can be reported as percent of vehicle control.

4 Notes

1. Protocol is written for 10^7 cells. If more cells are used, then scale up proportionally. The limit for the CS column is 2×10^8 magnetically labeled beads.
2. BALB/c bone marrow cultures increase in total cell number from D4 to day 10 and continue to increase thereafter and reach approximately 90 % eosinophils or greater by day 10. C57BL/6 bone marrow cultures do not proliferate to the same extent and lag 1–2 days behind in % eosinophils, achieving 90–100 % eosinophils at day 12.
3. Mouse eosinophils express CCR3, IL-5Rα, and Siglec F which can be detected on the cell surface and also store EPO and MBP in the granules.
4. Secondary antibodies conjugated to other fluorochromes may be used for confocal analysis with the exception of PE as it photo-quenches rendering it unusable for this application.
5. The coverslip can be mounted in confocal mounting media to reduce autofluorescence and prolong detection signal. One such mounting media is ProLong (Invitrogen).
6. It is a very good idea to titrate both antibody and Live-Dead reagent as this will reduce cost and increase signal to noise ratio.
7. Siglec F is a fairly specific marker for mouse eosinophils although it is also expressed on alveolar macrophages [17]. Anti-CD11c will differentiate between eosinophils ($CD11c^-$) and alveolar macrophages ($CD11c^+$).

8. Eosinophils are autofluorescent so great care must be taken to include unstained controls and single color controls for all test antibodies. Autofluorescence seems to be the greatest problem in the FITC/Alexa Fluor 488 channel.
9. In our experience, RNA isolated from eosinophil-enriched tissues can yield poor results in the QPCR assays. This method using the RNAeasy mini kit yields RNA that is efficiently transcribed and provides good results in QPCR assay (i.e. GAPDH Ct in the low 20s). RNA isolated with other methods can be re-isolated with the Qiagen kit. If Ct values for GAPDH are not in the low 20s, the RNA should be re-isolated, re-transcribed, and the QPCR assay repeated.
10. The expression of the endogenous control transcript needs to be assessed in each experiment to make certain that its expression is not fluctuating with the experimental conditions. Endogenous controls can be run separately or multiplexed, but this should be determined empirically for each primer-probe set as multiplexing can lead to interference.
11. It is tempting to say expression of one gene is higher than another but this is not correct, as one cannot know *a priori* the relative efficiencies of a different primer-probe pairs. One can be more precise by making standard curve of GOI and the endogenous control and reporting actual copy numbers per GAPDH.
12. It may be necessary to determine the development time empirically so that the SDS lysis control will not be off scale. A final concentration of 5 μM of either C16-PAF or C16-lysoPAF stimulates the release of 40–50 % of total EPO [14].
13. The multibead assays work well with cell culture supernatants as well as BALF. They also work well with serum samples provided the standards are rehydrated according to manufacturer's directions. We have not had great success with multibead assays using plasma samples. Choose a cytokine assay method based on the amount of sample available and expense. Multibead cytokine assays represent a fast and convenient way to determine concentrations of a significant number of cytokines using a relatively small (50 μl) sample. ELISAs take longer to run and require more sample volume. In general, if more than three cytokines are to be assayed, it is probably cheaper to use a multibead kit than individual ELISAs.
14. To explore the possible contributions of the chemokinesis (in addition to chemotactic) responses of eosinophils, it may be desirable to perform checkerboard analysis. In a checkerboard analysis, the concentration of chemotactic agent is increased stepwise from zero (media alone) to highest concentration in both the top and bottom wells. If the response is due

solely or primarily to chemotaxis (not simply chemokinesis), then maximum cell migration will be observed in response to the sharpest gradient (i.e. when the cells are in media alone and the opposite chamber contains chemoattractant). In contrast, chemokinesis would be observed when the cells were immersed directly in increasing concentrations of mediator.

15. In some experiments it might be useful to cytokine-starve the cells by placing them in bmEos base media for 18 h prior to the assay. When assaying single cell suspensions from eosinophil-enriched tissues, gate on the migrated granulocyte population rather than on total cells. Migrated eosinophils can be detected with anti-Siglec F for a more specific analysis.

Acknowledgment

This work is supported by NIAID DIR funding #AI000941 to H.F.R.

References

1. McGarry MP, Protheroe CA, Lee JJ (2010) Mouse hematology: a laboratory manual. Cold Spring Harbor Laboratory Press, Cold Spring Harbor, NY
2. Meyerholz DK, Griffin MA, Castilow EM, Varga SM (2009) Comparison of histochemical methods for murine eosinophil detection in an RSV vaccine-enhanced inflammation model. Toxicol Pathol 37(2):249–255
3. Lee JJ, McGarry MP, Farmer SC, Denzler KL, Larson KA, Carrigan PE, Brenneise IE, Horton MA, Haczku A, Gelfand EW, Leikauf GD, Lee NA (1997) Interleukin-5 expression in the lung epithelium of transgenic mice leads to pulmonary changes pathognomonic of asthma. J Exp Med 185(12):2143–2156
4. Adamko DJ, Wu Y, Gleich GJ, Lacy P, Moqbel R (2004) The induction of eosinophil peroxidase release: improved methods of measurement and stimulation. J Immunol Methods 291(1–2):101–108
5. Rosenberg HF, Domachowske JB (2001) Eosinophil-derived neurotoxin. In: Methods in enzymology: ribonuclease. Academic, New York
6. Dent LA, Daly C, Geddes A, Cormie J, Finlay DA, Bignold L, Hagan P, Parkhouse RM, Garate T, Parsons J, Mayrhofer G (1997) Immune responses of IL-5 transgenic mice to parasites and aeroallergens. Mem Inst Oswaldo Cruz 92(Suppl 2):45–54
7. Aizawa H, Zimmermann N, Carrigan PE, Lee JJ, Rothenberg ME, Bochner BS (2003) Molecular analysis of human Siglec-8 orthologs relevant to mouse eosinophils: identification of mouse orthologs of Siglec-5 (mSiglec-F) and Siglec-10 (mSiglec-G). Genomics 82(5): 521–530
8. Shen HH, Ochkur SI, McGarry MP, Crosby JR, Hines EM, Borchers MT, Wang H, Biechelle TL, O'Neill KR, Ansay TL, Colbert DC, Cormier SA, Justice JP, Lee NA, Lee JJ (2003) A causative relationship exists between eosinophils and the development of allergic pulmonary pathologies in the mouse. J Immunol 170(6):3296–3305
9. Dyer KD, Garcia-Crespo KE, Killoran KE, Rosenberg HF (2011) Antigen profiles for the quantitative assessment of eosinophils in mouse tissues by flow cytometry. J Immunol Methods 369(1–2):91–97
10. Carlens J, Wahl B, Ballmaier M, Bulfone-Paus S, Forster R, Pabst O (2009) Common gamma-chain-dependent signals confer selective survival of eosinophils in the murine small intestine. J Immunol 183(9):5600–5607
11. Dyer KD, Garcia-Crespo KE, Percopo CM, Bowen AB, Ito T, Peterson KE, Gilfillan AM, Rosenberg HF (2011) Defective eosinophil hematopoiesis ex vivo in inbred Rocky Mountain White (IRW) mice. J Leukoc Biol 90(6):1101–1109

12. Dyer KD, Moser JM, Czapiga M, Siegel SJ, Percopo CM, Rosenberg HF (2008) Functionally competent eosinophils differentiated ex vivo in high purity from normal mouse bone marrow. J Immunol 181(6):4004–4009
13. Dyer KD, Percopo CM, Rosenberg HF (2009) Generation of eosinophils from unselected bone marrow progenitors: wild-type, TLR- and eosinophil-deficient mice. Open Immunol J 2:163–167
14. Dyer KD, Percopo CM, Xie Z, Yang Z, Kim JD, Davoine F, Lacy P, Druey KM, Moqbel R, Rosenberg HF (2010) Mouse and human eosinophils degranulate in response to platelet-activating factor (PAF) and lysoPAF via a PAF-receptor-independent mechanism: evidence for a novel receptor. J Immunol 184(11):6327–6334
15. Mueller T, Robaye B, Vieira RP, Ferrari D, Grimm M, Jakob T, Martin SF, Di Virgilio F, Boeynaems JM, Virchow JC, Idzko M (2010) The purinergic receptor P2Y(2) receptor mediates chemotaxis of dendritic cells and eosinophils in allergic lung inflammation. Allergy 65(12):1545–1553
16. Rankin AL, Mumm JB, Murphy E, Turner S, Yu N, McClanahan TK, Bourne PA, Pierce RH, Kastelein R, Pflanz S (2010) IL-33 induces IL-13-dependent cutaneous fibrosis. J Immunol 184(3):1526–1535
17. Stevens WW, Kim TS, Pujanauski LM, Hao X, Braciale TJ (2007) Detection and quantitation of eosinophils in the murine respiratory tract by flow cytometry. J Immunol Methods 327(1–2): 63–74

Chapter 6

Evaluation of Classical, Alternative, and Regulatory Functions of Bone Marrow-Derived Macrophages

Beckley K. Davis

Abstract

The role of macrophage subsets in allergic diseases in vivo is under current investigation. These cells perform sentinel functions in the lung, the skin, and the gastrointestinal mucosa. Their interface with environmental cues influences the initiation, progression, development, and resolution of allergic diseases. Researchers often culture bone marrow-derived macrophages to study macrophage biology. The in vitro maturation of bone marrow precursor cells into mature macrophages is a powerful technique used to study macrophage biology. The polarization or differential activation of macrophages into functionally distinct subsets can provide insight into allergic disease pathologies. Classically activated, alternatively activated, and regulatory macrophages have different effector functions that can affect allergic responses. Understanding macrophage biology during allergen exposure, host sensitization, and disease progression/resolution may lead to improved therapeutic interventions. The purpose of this chapter is to outline protocols used for the culture and polarization of classically activated, alternatively activated, and regulatory macrophages. In addition, the techniques to measure macrophage-specific effector molecules by ELISA, RT-PCR, and immunoblotting are reviewed.

Key words M1 macrophage, M2 macrophage, Regulatory macrophage, Inflammation, Cytokine, Allergy and asthma

1 Introduction

Macrophages may play different roles in allergic responses depending on their location, predisposing genetic factors, and environmental factors. Macrophages are a predominant immune cell of tissues exposed to the environment such as the lung, intestine, and skin [1] and are likely to be one of the first effector cells to come into contact with allergens. Therefore, the response of the macrophage will have profound primary effects on the microenvironment and secondary effects on downstream cell types. After subsequent allergen exposure following an initial sensitization phase, the macrophage can secrete inflammatory cytokines such as interleukin-1β, interferon-γ, tumor necrosis factor-α, and

Irving C. Allen (ed.), *Mouse Models of Allergic Disease: Methods and Protocols*, Methods in Molecular Biology, vol. 1032,
DOI 10.1007/978-1-62703-496-8_6, © Springer Science+Business Media, LLC 2013

interleukin-6. Elaboration of these cytokines causes an influx of additional inflammatory cells and can alter smooth muscle and epithelial cell function. Alternatively, macrophages can secrete anti-inflammatory mediators such as interleukin-10 and prostaglandin E_2 that can dampen allergic responses [2]. Experimental models of asthma and allergy, typically mouse models, have revealed a role for cytokines associated with T helper 2 (Th2) inflammation: interleukin-4, -5, and -13 [3, 4]. Although ex vivo analysis of patient samples has corroborated some conclusions from animal models, they have also illustrated that there is a more complex and variable disease process than was previously understood [5].

The heterogeneity of macrophage functions has led to the classification of three phenotypically distinct populations, the classically activated macrophage (CAM) or M1 macrophage, the alternatively activated macrophage (AAM) or M2 macrophage, and the regulatory macrophage. These designations are analogous with the T helper subsets Th1, Th2, and Treg, respectively. The M1 macrophage is characterized by secretion of proinflammatory cytokines (IL-1β, IL-12, and TNF-α) and increased amounts of reactive oxygen and nitrogen species [6]. These cells become polarized in the presence of IFN-γ and TNF-α or lipopolysaccharide (LPS) and are maintained by Th1 T lymphocytes. In contrast, M2 macrophages are characterized by increased expression of l-arginase, YM1, and RELMα/FIZZ1, which facilitate wound healing and angiogenesis. These cells are induced in the presence of interleukin-4 or interleukin-13. Regulatory macrophages are less well characterized. These cells are anti-inflammatory and secrete immunosuppressive cytokines such as interleukin-10 and transforming growth factor-β. These cells can be generated in vitro by incubation with immune complexes and Toll-like receptor agonists [8]. Their existence in vitro may be reflected in myeloid-derived suppressor cells and tumor-associated macrophages in vivo.

Recent evidence has provided support for the in vivo differentiation of these macrophage subsets [9, 10]. Nonetheless, the dynamic nature of macrophage plasticity suggests that these phenotypes may not be stable in vivo. Transcriptome analysis of in vitro-polarized macrophages and of ex vivo-purified macrophage populations has revealed striking differences in transcriptional programs of these cells [11]. During allergic diseases, aberrant macrophage activation and/or polarization is sometimes seen. These cells play a key role in vivo in the development and resolution of allergic diseases. Macrophages populate the interface of the host with the environment, specifically, the lung, the skin, and the gastrointestinal mucosa. These cells are one of the first cells to come in contact with environmental allergens and provide biomolecules to modulate an allergic response.

The role of macrophage subsets in allergic diseases in vivo is currently under investigation. Much of the data from experimental models fails to present a clear picture. Depending on the model system, each subset has been shown to either promote or inhibit allergic responses. Ex vivo analysis of macrophages from atopic patients has revealed conflicting results [11–14]. The complexity of macrophage responses in allergic disease reflects the relative contributions and balance of M1, M2, and regulatory macrophages. As this area of research will ultimately improve treatment of allergic diseases, the culture of bone marrow-derived macrophages is an important laboratory technique. This is especially true when combined with ex vivo analyses of tissue-specific or tissue-resident macrophages, which will lead to a more complete understanding of disease pathologies.

2 Materials

2.1 Harvest

1. Personal protective equipment, including but not limited to laboratory coat, gloves, and goggles.
2. Age- and sex-matched mice: We typically use 8–12-week-old male mice.
3. Laminar flow hood.
4. Surgical instruments: Forceps and scissors.
5. 20–27 gauge needles.
6. 4. 3 or 5 cc syringes.
7. 100 μm cell strainer.
8. Hemocytometer.
9. Light microscope.

2.2 Culturing

1. Tissue culture incubator.
2. Tabletop tissue culture centrifuge equipped to spin 15 and 50 ml conical tubes.
3. Sterile and pyrogen-free PBS (without Ca^{2+} and Mg^{2+}).
4. Hank's Balanced Salt Solution.
5. Trypsin:EDTA.
6. Base media: DMEM, 10 % heat-inactivated fetal bovine serum, 1 % l-glutamine, 1 % sodium pyruvate, 1 % nonessential amino acids, 1 % penicillin/streptomycin.
7. Macrophage media: 20 % L929 cell (from American Type Culture Collection; CCL-1) conditioned media as a source of Macrophage-Colony-Stimulating Factor (M-CSF), plus base media. Alternatively M-CSF can be purchased commercially and used to supplement base media at 1×10^4 U/ml. L929 cells are a reliable source of inexpensive M-CSF. L929 cells should be cultured in base media until they are 90 % confluent.

Harvest the media by centrifugation and filter through a 0.45 μm filter to sterilize. Store filtered media at −80 °C until use.

8. 1 % Penicillin/streptomycin.
9. Fetal bovine serum (FBS), certified and low endotoxin tested.
10. Ethylenediaminetetraacetic acid (EDTA).
11. 100 × 20 mm tissue culture-treated plates.
12. 150 × 25 mm tissue culture-treated plates.
13. Multi-well tissue culture-treated plates: 6-, 12-, and 24-well plates.
14. Ultralow-bind non-treated tissue culture plates or petri dishes.
15. Pipettes, pipettors, pipette aids.
16. Tubes: 1.5 ml; 15 ml BD Falcon™ conical tubes; 50 ml BD Falcon™ conical tubes.

2.3 Functional Assays

1. Cell scraper.
2. Diff-Quick staining reagents.
3. Microscope slides.
4. Flow cytometer (optional).
5. Anti-F4/80-FITC antibody.
6. Anti-CD11b (Mac-1)-PE antibody.
7. Flow cytometry wash buffer: 1× PBS plus 2 % FBS.
8. Isotype control antibodies.
9. Recombinant mouse interferon-γ (IFN-γ), interleukin-4 (IL-4), interleukin-13, or Macrophage-Colony Stimulating Factor (M-CSF) (Peprotech).
10. Ultrapure LPS.
11. Superscript III (Invitrogen).
12. Oligo dT_{16-18} primer.
13. Phusion™ DNA polymerase (New England Biolabs).
14. ELISA plate reader.
15. ELISA kits capable of quantifying IL-1β, IL-12, and TNF-α.
16. Cell lysis buffer: 1× PBS plus 1 % Triton-X100 and protease inhibitors.
17. BCA assay kit (Thermoscientific) or Bradford protein assay (Biorad).
18. Standard materials for immunoblotting.
19. Endofit ovalbumin (Invivogen).
20. Dialyzed Rabbit anti-ovalbumin (Fitzgerald Industries International).

3 Methods

3.1 Isolation

1. Mice from specific pathogen-free housing should be used (*see* **Note 1**). Euthanize mice according to current Institutional Animal Care and Use Committee (IACUC) guidelines. Animals should be sex matched for minor histocompatibility antigens. We use 8–12-week-old donor mice for all of our experiments.
2. Prepare one mouse (*see* **Note 2**) at a time on a dissection tray and spray down the carcass with 70 % ethanol to sterilize the field.
3. Pin the carcass down with dissecting pins or large-gauge needles with the ventral side facing up.
4. Apply forceps to the skin anterior to the urethral opening. With scissors, cut skin along the ventral midline from the groin to the chin, carefully avoiding the underlying musculature.
5. Next, with scissors, make an incision from the start of the first incision caudally to the ankle on both sides of the animal. Carefully peel the skin off the appendages to the ankle joint.
6. Remove tissue from the legs with scissors and dissect the leg away from the body.
7. Denude the remaining soft tissue from the pelvic and femoral bones and separate proximal to the knee joint and the pelvic girdle (*see* **Note 3**).
8. Immerse the dissected femurs in 70 % ethanol for 1 min (*see* **Note 4**).
9. Wash twice in DPBS with penicillin (500–1,000 U/ml) and streptomycin (500–1,000 μg/ml).
10. While supporting the femur with forceps, use a 25 gauge (*see* **Note 5**) needle fitted to either a 3 or a 5 cc syringe filled with 2 ml of DPBS (*see* **Note 6**). Carefully insert the needle into the bone marrow cavity and gently expel the bone marrow from the bone with a jet of liquid directed into a 15 ml screw top tube with 5 ml of prewarmed 1× DPBS. Repeat and articulate the needle along the bone shaft to ensure that a majority of the bone marrow has been evacuated from the cavity.
11. Centrifuge cells for 10 min at $500 \times g$ at 10 °C. Discard the supernatant.
12. Count bone marrow cells in a hemocytometer and adjust the cells to a density of 5×10^6/ml in macrophage media.

3.2 Culturing

1. Add between 2 and 5×10^5 cells to a sterile tissue culture (100 × 15 cm) or petri dish (*see* **Note 7**).
2. Incubate for 6–7 days (*see* **Note 8**) in a 5 % CO_2-humidified tissue culture incubator. Check cells daily (*see* **Note 9**) and

wash cells one time every 2–3 days with DPBS. Resuspend the washed cells with macrophage media and replate on the same dish.

3. On day 6 or 7, discard the media in the tissue culture dish and wash the adherent cells with DPBS. Add 5–7 ml of 0.05 % trypsin–EDTA solution and incubate for 15–20 min at 37 °C (*see* **Note 10**).
4. Dislodge cells with gentle washing with a pipette aid.
5. Centrifuge the cells to wash and resuspend the pellet in base media.
6. Two femurs from a single mouse (12 weeks of age) should yield $2–6 \times 10^7$ macrophages.

3.3 Phenotyping

1. Resuspend $1–5 \times 10^5$ cells in 100 μl of 1× DPBS supplemented with 2 % FBS and 2 mm EDTA in a 1.5 ml tube.
2. Add fluorescently labeled anti-F4/80 and Mac-1 antibodies (*see* **Note 11**) and incubate on ice in the dark for 30 min.
3. Wash twice with 1× DPBS supplemented with 2 % FCS.
4. Resuspend cells in 500 μl of wash buffer.
5. Analyze the cells by flow cytometry. Macrophages should be positive for both F4/80 and CD11b. Cell purity ranges from 90 to 99 %, as indicated by double-positive staining.

3.4 Polarization to Classically Activated Macrophages (M1) (See Note 12)

1. Culture macrophages for 6–8 days.
2. Add $0.5–1.0 \times 10^6$ cells in 1 ml of media to each well in a 6-well tissue culture plate. Add 10–200 U/ml of recombinant mouse IFN-γ (*see* **Note 13**) for 6–18 h depending on the functional endpoint.
3. The following day add 1–100 ng of ultrapure LPS to stimulate cells. Stimulation times will vary depending on the endpoint assay.
4. For gene induction studies measuring transcription of proinflammatory cytokines, 2–6 h of stimulation with LPS works well. Briefly, cells are washed in 1X DPBS and cells are removed via physical scraping. Total RNA can be isolated using standard techniques. 1 μg of total RNA is reverse transcribed using Superscript III with oligo $dT_{16–18}$ primer following the manufacturer's suggested protocol. We use 2 μl of cDNA reaction for amplification with Phusion™ DNA polymerase (*see* **Note 14**) to amplify the following genes (with primers listed): *Il-12p40*, *Tnfa*, *iNos*, and *Gapdh* (*see* Table 1).
5. For cytokine elaboration: Harvest cell-free tissue culture supernatants (*see* **Note 15**) 6–18 h after stimulation depending on the cytokine assayed. Perform cytokine ELISA (*see* **Note 16**) on serially diluted supernatants.

Table 1
RT-PCR primers

Gene	Forward primer	Reverse primer
Tnfa	5′-CAGCCTCTTCTCATTCCTGCTTGTC-3′	5′-CTGGAAGACTCCTCCCAGGGTATAT-3′
iNos	5′-CCCTTCCGAAGTTTCTGGCAGCAGC-3′	5′-GGCTGTCAGAGCCTCGTGGCTTTGG-3′
Il12p40	5′-ATGGCCATGTGGGAGCTGGAGAAAG-3′	5′-GTGGAGCAGCAGATGTGAGTGGCT-3′
Arg1	5′-CAGAAGAATGGAAGAGTCAG-3′	5′-CAGATATGCAGGGAGTCACC-3′
Fizz1	5′-GGTCCCAGTGCATATGGATGAGACCATAGA-3′	5′-CACCTCTTCACTGCAGGGACAGTTGGCAGA-3′
Il-10	5′-CCAGTTTTACCTGGTAGAAGTGATG-3′	5′-TGTCTAGGTCCTGGAGTCCAGCAGACTCAA-3′
SK-1	5′-ACAGCAGTGTGCAGTTGATGA-3′	5′-GGCAGTCATGTCCGGTGATG-3′
Gapdh	5′-GCACTTGGCAAAATGGAGAT-3′	5′-CCAGCATCACCCCATTAGAT-3′

6. Alternatively, harvest the cell pellet for western blot analysis. Wash cells twice with 1× DPBS. Add 1 ml of 1× DPBS, scrape cells from their respective wells, and place in a 1.5 ml microcentrifuge tube. Centrifuge at 4 °C for 1 min at maximum speed (>10,000 × *g*). Aspirate the supernatant. Lyse cells in 100 μl of lysis buffer with protease inhibitors for 30 min on ice. Spin lysed cells for 15 min at maximum speed (>10,000 × *g*) at 4 °C. Transfer lysate to a new tube and quantitate protein concentration by BCA assay or Bradford protein assay. Load 20–100 μg of total cell lysate on an SDS-PAGE gel (*see* **Note 17**). Gels can be transferred to nitrocellulose or PVDF membranes for immunoblotting. We used standard immunoblotting techniques for the detection of cytokines, cell surface receptors, and intracellular signaling molecules.
7. Functional assays such as phagocytosis, reactive oxygen or nitrogen species generation, and migration are generally performed 24–72 h after polarization.

3.5 Polarization to Alternatively Activated Macrophages (M2) (See Note 12)

1. Culture macrophages for 6–8 days.
2. Add 0.5–1.0 × 10^6 bone marrow-derived macrophages in 1 ml of media to each well in a 6-well tissue culture plate. Add 10–20 U/ml of recombinant mouse IL-4 or IL-13 for 18 h (*see* **Note 13**).
3. Stimulate cells with 1–100 ng ultrapure LPS and incubate (*see* **Note 18**).
4. For gene induction studies measuring transcription of proinflammatory cytokines, 2–6 h of stimulation with LPS works well. Briefly, cells are washed in 1× DPBS and cells are removed via physical scraping. Total RNA can be isolated using standard techniques.
5. 1 μg of total RNA is reverse transcribed using Superscript III with oligo dT_{16-18} primer following the manufacturer's suggested protocol. We use 2 μl of cDNA reaction for amplification with Phusion™ DNA polymerase (*see* **Note 14**) to amplify the following genes: *Arg1*, *Fizz1*, and *Gapdh* (*see* Table 1).
6. It has been reported in the literature that activity and soluble collagen production can be measured in AAM lysates [15].

3.6 Polarization to Regulatory Macrophages (See Note 12)

Regulatory macrophages might represent a heterogenous population of macrophages that arise from different stimulation/polarization protocols. Indeed, there have been regimens that produce "regulatory" macrophages that include immune complexes, glucocorticoids, IL-10, and others [16, 17]. Here, we focus on regulatory macrophages generated in the presence of immune complexes.

1. Add 0.5–1.0 × 10^6 bone marrow-derived macrophages in 1 ml of media to each well in a 6-well tissue culture plate.

2. Prepare ovalbumin immune complexes by adding 20 μl of 1 mg/ml of endofit ovalbumin (*see* **Note 19**) to 500 μl of DMEM. Add 75 μl of 4 mg/ml rabbit anti-ovalbumin IgG dropwise. Nutate for 30–60 min at room temperature to allow complexes to form.
3. Stimulate macrophages with 1–50 ng of ultrapure LPS and with 100 μl endotoxin-free ovalbumin:IgG complexes as prepared above. Control stimulations (including unstimulated, LPS only, OVA only, and OVA-specific IgG only) should be done in parallel.
4. Incubate the macrophages for 18–24 h in a 37 °C incubator.
5. For gene induction studies measuring transcription of proinflammatory cytokines, 2–6 h of stimulation with LPS works well. Briefly cells are washed in 1× DPBS and removed via physical scraping. Total RNA can be isolated using standard techniques.
6. 1 μg of total RNA is reverse transcribed using Superscript III with oligo dT_{16-18} primer following the manufacturer's suggested protocol.
7. We use 2 μl of cDNA reaction for amplification with Phusion™ DNA polymerase (*see* **Note 14**) to amplify the following genes: *Il10*, *Il12p40 SK-1*, and *Gapdh* (*see* Table 1).
8. Collect cell-free supernatants for ELISA measurement of IL-12 p40, IL-10, and either TNF-α or IL-6 (*see* **Note 16**).

4 Notes

1. We use mice housed exclusively in specific pathogen-free (SPF) containment. Mice with underlying inflammatory conditions or infections may affect macrophage function.
2. It is imperative that all solutions remain sterile and pyrogen-free. Bone marrow-derived macrophages are exceptionally sensitive to bacterial components. If possible, all manipulations should be carried out in a laminar flow hood using aseptic techniques. The generation of bone marrow-derived macrophages from novel, transgenic, or gene ablation mice may require individual optimization.
3. Tissue-specific macrophages can be harvested in parallel. Tissues commonly used for macrophage isolation include, but are not limited to, spleen, liver, lung, and intestine. Other immunologically relevant tissues such as spleen, lymph nodes, and thymus can also be harvested at this time to assay different cellular components, making full use of the experimental animal.

4. Tibia bones can be used as an additional source of bone marrow precursor cells.
5. Smaller or larger gauge needles can be used.
6. Different isotonic solutions such as HBSS or DMEM can be used in place of DPBS.
7. We have used both treated and non-treated tissue culture plasticware to cultivate bone marrow-derived macrophages. Using treated plasticware avoids possible confusion while growing different cell types. As a result of using treated tissue culture plasticware, bone marrow-derived macrophages adhere tightly to these dishes and may require physical dissociation with a cell scraper or prolonged treatment with trypsin:EDTA solution.
8. Slight variability in bone marrow-derived macrophage growth and maturation may be due to variability of growth factors (M-CSF) in L929 conditioned media.
9. Daily inspection of cells allows for visual confirmation of cell growth, adherence, and rapid assessment of contamination.
10. Bone marrow macrophages adhere tightly to tissue culture-treated plasticware and may require additional incubation time with 0.05 % trypsin:EDTA, increased concentration (0.25 % vs. 0.05 %) of trypsin:EDTA solution, or mechanical detachment with a cell scraper.
11. We have used many different fluorophores and antibody sources. The fluorophores must not overlap in emission spectra and must be compatible with the flow cytometer laser(s) and filters.
12. After 6–8 days in culture, macrophages can be polarized into one of the three main populations: classically activated, alternatively activated, or regulatory macrophages.
13. Commercial sources of recombinant growth factors such as interleukins are typically expressed in *E. coli*. These preparations have varying amounts of microbial contaminants (i.e., LPS) that may alter macrophage function. Source and lot variation should be evaluated.
14. Other DNA polymerases can be used (for example, Takara LA Taq). We have had success with Phusion™ using different source material and amounts, primer sets, and amplifying conditions.
15. Different effector molecules have different kinetic secretion profiles. Initial time point experiments will better define the appropriate stimulation periods.
16. A series of four twofold serial dilutions of supernatants will allow for experimental values to fall within the linear range of the assay.

17. The level of sensitivity of analyte will depend on the reagents used. Optimization with different detection antibodies and lysate concentrations might be necessary.
18. We have seen lot, source, and experimenter variability with LPS preparations. Single-use aliquots should be stored at −80 °C and quality assured before experimentation.
19. Commercial preparations of ovalbumin contain varying amounts of LPS. We have used endofit ovalbumin; other sources of ovalbumin should be tested for LPS before experimentation.

References

1. Murray PJ, Wynn TA (2011) Protective and pathogenic functions of macrophage subsets. Nat Rev Immunol 11(11):723–737
2. Moreira AP, Hogaboam CM (2011) Macrophages in allergic asthma: fine-tuning their pro- and anti-inflammatory actions for disease resolution. J Interferon Cytokine Res 31(6):485–491
3. Palm NW, Rosenstein RK, Medzhitov R (2012) Allergic host defenses. Nature 484: 465–472
4. Holgate ST (2012) Innate and adaptive immune responses in asthma. Nat Med 18: 673–683
5. Holgate ST (2011) Pathophysiology of asthma: what has our current understanding taught us about new therapeutic approaches? J Allergy Clin Immunol 128(3):495–505
6. Gordon S (2007) The macrophage: past, present and future. Eur J Immunol 37 Suppl: S9–S17
7. Gordon S, Martinez FO (2010) Alternative activation of macrophages: mechanism and functions. Immunity 32(5):593–604
8. Mantovani A (2006) Macrophage diversity and polarization: in vivo veritas. Blood 108(2): 408–409
9. Sica A, Mantovani A (2012) Macrophage plasticity and polarization: in vivo veritas. J Clin Invest 122(3):787–795
10. Lawrence T, Natoli G (2011) Transcriptional regulation of macrophage polarization: enabling diversity with identity. Nat Rev Immunol 11(11):750–761
11. Moreira AP, Cavassani KA, Hullinger R et al (2010) Serum amyloid P attenuates M2 macrophage activation and protects against fungal spore-induced allergic airway disease. J Allergy Clin Immunol 126(4):712–721.e7
12. Bedoret D, Wallemacq H, Marichal T et al (2009) Lung interstitial macrophages alter dendritic cell functions to prevent airway allergy in mice. J Clin Invest 119(12): 3723–3738
13. Shahid SK, Kharitonov SA, Wilson NM et al (2002) Increased interleukin-4 and decreased interferon-γ in exhaled breath condensate of children with asthma. Am J Respir Crit Care Med 165(9):1290–1293
14. Kim CK, Kim SW, Park CS et al (2003) Bronchoalveolar lavage cytokine profiles in acute asthma and acute bronchiolitis. J Allergy Clin Immunol 112(1):64–71
15. Edwards JP, Zhang X, Frauwirth KA, Mosser DM (2006) Biochemical and functional characterization of three activated macrophage populations. J Leukoc Biol 80(6): 1298–1307
16. Mosser DM, Zhang X (2008) Activation of murine macrophages. Curr Protoc Immunol Chapter 14: Unit 14.2
17. Mosser DM, Edwards JP (2008) Exploring the full spectrum of macrophage activation. Nat Rev Immunol 8(12):958–969

Chapter 7

Applications of Mouse Airway Epithelial Cell Culture for Asthma Research

Amjad Horani, John D. Dickinson, and Steven L. Brody

Abstract

Primary airway epithelial cell culture provides a valuable tool for studying cell differentiation, cell–cell interactions, and the role of immune system factors in asthma pathogenesis. In this chapter, we discuss the application of mouse tracheal epithelial cell cultures for the study of asthma biology. A major advantage of this system is the ability to use airway epithelial cells from mice with defined genetic backgrounds. The in vitro proliferation and differentiation of mouse airway epithelial cells uses the air–liquid interface condition to generate well-differentiated epithelia with characteristics of native airways. Protocols are provided for manipulation of differentiation, induction of mucous cell metaplasia, genetic modification, and cell and pathogen coculture. Assays for the assessment of gene expression, responses of cells, and analysis of specific cell subpopulations within the airway epithelium are included.

Key words Asthma, Trachea, Mouse, Air–liquid interface, Mucous cell, Ciliated cell

1 Introduction

1.1 Mouse Airway Epithelial Cell Models for Asthma Research

Asthma is characterized by remodeling and inflammation of the airway epithelium. Experimental models of asthma in mice allow control of genetic and environmental factors. In this chapter, the power of mouse genetics is extended to culture of mouse tracheal epithelial cells (mTEC). The use of airway epithelial cells from defined genetic strains of mice facilitates testing phenotypes relevant to asthma in a highly controlled environment and offers analysis of epithelial–immune interactions using syngeneic cells. Since its introduction, our mTEC protocol has been widely adapted for experimental purposes relevant to the study of asthma [1–12].

Protocols and assays provided in this chapter are diagrammed in Fig. 1. The basic mTEC culture protocol can be used to generate cell preparations with epithelial cell type constituents as found in vivo, including basal, ciliated, and secretory cells. The mTEC culture protocol results in a surface that is similar to that of the native mouse trachea [13]. While the method for the basic culture

Irving C. Allen (ed.), *Mouse Models of Allergic Disease: Methods and Protocols*, Methods in Molecular Biology, vol. 1032,
DOI 10.1007/978-1-62703-496-8_7, © Springer Science+Business Media, LLC 2013

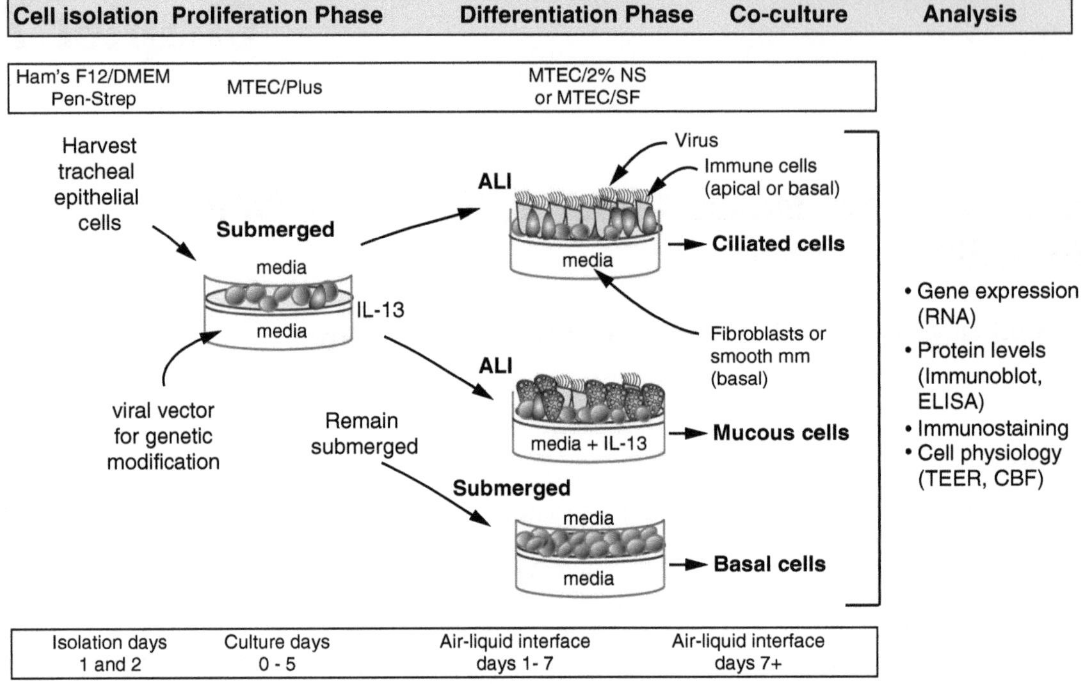

Fig. 1 Overview of culture and manipulation of mTEC. Each phase of the procedure is indicated, the culture media required is listed, and the timeline is noted. Tracheal epithelial cells are seeded onto supported membranes. During proliferation, cells are submerged in mTEC/Plus medium with retinoic acid (RA) for approximately 5 days until confluent. Differentiation uses the air–liquid interface (ALI) condition and either mTEC/NS or mTEC/SF medium (each with RA). Examples of manipulation of differentiation are shown. Mucous cells can be generated by treatment with IL-13 or cells held undifferentiated by submersion. Coculture with respiratory viruses or immune, fibroblast, or smooth muscle (mm) cells and assays are noted

system is included, the focus of this chapter is the manipulation and analysis of the culture system relevant to asthma. The reader is strongly encouraged to review detailed versions of the basic protocol [14].

1.2 Manipulation of mTEC and Coculture Conditions

The essential factors used for proliferation and differentiation of mTEC are similar to those used to culture airway epithelial cells from human and other species [15–17]. The culture of mTEC is critically dependent on the isolation of an adequate number of cells and subsequent proliferation of an amplifying progenitor cell population [13]. The mouse trachea harbors pluripotent epithelial basal cells within the epithelium, and the paratracheal glands located at the most proximal region of the trachea [8, 18]. Proliferation of these basal cells ultimately results in a confluent layer of cells that can readily differentiate using air–liquid interface (ALI) conditions and growth factor-enriched media. These conditions favor the differentiation of ciliated epithelial cells and a smaller population of cells expressing the Clara cell marker, Scgb1a1 [10, 13]. If cells remain submerged, the undifferentiated basal cell population persists [19].

Increased numbers of mucous secretory cells (goblet cells) is a cardinal feature of airway remodeling in asthma. Goblet cells are uncommon in the normal laboratory mouse airway, and are rarely found in standard mTEC preparations [13]. Goblet cell metaplasia can be induced in the cultured mTEC system by the addition of specific cytokines. Prolonged treatment with IL-13 induces the differentiation and proliferation of mucin (MUC5AC)-filled goblet cells and increases mucus secretion [1, 12, 20]. Likewise, IL-6 and IL-17 increase MUC5AC expression in cultured mouse airway cells [21]. In each case, the cytokine dose and treatment timing relative to the stage of cell differentiation impacts the extent of mucous cell metaplasia.

Cultured mTEC are devoid of immune cells; however, the preparations can be supplemented to study the interaction of airway epithelial cells and immune cells such as lymphocytes, dendritic cells, or neutrophils [11, 22, 23]. mTEC are grown on supported membranes with apical and basal chambers allowing apical basolateral surface interaction to study cell–cell interaction using mouse syngeneic immune cells, smooth muscle cells, or fibroblasts with specific genetic deficiencies. The coculture system may also be used in the study of host-pathogen responses to infection by respiratory viruses or bacteria [2, 3].

mTEC may be genetically modified using recombinant viruses for gene transfer [19, 24, 25] or treated with drugs or bioactive agents on the apical or basal surfaces. Finally, mTEC on supported membranes are amenable to analysis using multiple approaches to easily characterize the status of differentiation, gene expression, and ultrastructural features.

1.3 Approach to Protocols for mTEC Cultures

A timeline of the mTEC preparation protocol is shown Fig. 1. Materials (*see* Subheading 2) and Methods (*see* Subheading 3) are organized to match this sequence. Media and reagents required should be prepared prior to harvest. Isolation of tracheal epithelial cells is accomplished over 2 days. Trachea are harvested and incubated in pronase overnight. The following day epithelial cells are released from the trachea then isolated by differential adhesion of fibroblasts on culture plates, leaving mTEC in suspension. mTEC are seeded on supported, semi-permeable membranes in a media favoring proliferation, called mTEC plus. At this time, transduction with viral vectors can be used. Once a confluent layer of cells is established, an ALI condition is created. Media are changed to one with lower concentrations of growth factors using mTEC/NS, containing a serum with proprietary additives (NuSerum™), or mTEC/SF, a serum-free, defined medium. At this time, cytokine treatment or other interventions can be used to manipulate subsequent differentiation that occurs within 3–14 days.

2 Materials

2.1 Stock Components for mTEC Media

1. Prepare stock components prior to cell isolation (*see* Table 1, **Note 1**).

2.2 Media (See Table 2)

1. Ham's F-12/Pen-Strep is used for the harvest of cells. Fetal bovine serum, 10 % is added in some cell isolation steps.
2. mTEC/Basic is the core medium used to prepare proliferation and differentiation media.
3. mTEC/Plus is used to proliferate cells.
4. mTEC/NS (serum-containing; 2 % Nuserum) or mTEC/SF (serum-free) are used to differentiate cells at ALI.
5. RA Stock B (10,000×) must be freshly added to aliquots of media prior to each use (*see* Table 1 and **Note 1**).

2.3 Trachea Harvest (Day 1)

1. Mice from wild type or genetic defined strains (C57Bl/6, SV129/J, C57Bl/6-SV129/J hybrid, Balb/c, FVB, and Swiss Webster backgrounds) (**Note 2**).
2. Ethanol, 70 % for cleansing and wetting euthanized mice prior to dissection.
3. Freshly prepared 0.15 % Pronase (Sigma-Aldrich), in Ham's F-12/Pen-Strep at 0.15 % (w/v). Make 2–5 mL in a 15 mL tube, rock to mix, then filter sterilize.

2.4 Tracheal Epithelial Cell Isolation (Day 2)

1. Plastic sterile Petri dishes, 100 mm, for resected tracheas.
2. Ham's F12/Pen-Strep, on ice.
3. Fetal bovine serum (FBS, 3–5 mL), warmed to 37 °C.
4. Primaria™ (BD Bioscience) tissue culture plates to enhance fibroblast adherence.
5. DNase solution: Crude pancreatic DNase I (Sigma-Aldrich) 0.5 mg/mL, with bovine serum albumin, 1 mg/mL, in Ham's F-12/Pen-Strep. Filter, aliquot, and store in 5 mL aliquots at -20 °C.

2.5 Tracheal Epithelial Cell Seeding and Proliferation

1. Supported semipermeable membranes ("inserts") and culture plates. To get multiple samples, use 6.5 mm, 0.33 cm^2 polycarbonate (Transwell®, Corning) or polyester (polyethylene terephthalate, Transwell®-Clear) membranes with 0.4 μm pores. These fit into a 24-well plate. Include at least one clear membrane in each plate for inspection of cells by microscopy.
2. Rat tail collagen (type I, BD Biosciences). Dilute at 50 μg/mL in 0.02 N acetic acid (in tissue culture grade water) and filter. Store at 4 °C up to 8 weeks.

Table 1
Stock components for mTEC media

Stock	Components	Concentration	Aliquot size for 250 mL	Comments
Retinoic acid (RA) Stock A	Retinoic acid (50 mg) in 100 % ethanol, 33.3 mL	5×10^{-3} M	500 μL	Sigma-Aldrich Protect from light, use glass pipettes Filter sterilize, Store −80 °C up to 12 months
Retinoic acid Stock B (10,000×)	RA stock A, 0.5 mL in 100 % ethanol, 4.5 mL	5×10^{-4} M	500 μL	Filter sterilize Protect from light, avoid freeze-thaw Store −80 °C up to 6 months
I	Insulin, 50 mg in HCl (4 mM), 25 mL	2 mg/mL	1,250 μL for mTEC/Plus; 625 μL for mTEC/SF	Sigma-Aldrich Filter sterilize Store −20 °C
T	Transferrin (human), 100 mg plus 200 μL BSA (100 mg/mL) in HBSS, 19.8 mL	5 mg/mL	250 μL for mTEC/Plus; 250 μL for mTEC/SF	Sigma-Aldrich Filter sterilize Store −20 °C
EGF	Epidermal growth factor (mouse), 100 μg plus 200 μL BSA (100 mg/mL) in HBSS, 19.8 mL	5 μg/mL	1,250 μL for mTEC/Plus; 250 μL for mTEC/SF	BD Biosciences Filter sterilize Store −20 °C
CT	Cholera toxin, 1 mg plus 200 μL BSA (100 mg/mL) in HBSS, 19.8 mL	100 μg/mL	250 μL for mTEC/plus; 62.5 μL for mTEC/SF	Sigma-Aldrich Filter sterilize Store −20 °C
BPE	Bovine pituitary extract, 7.5 mg total protein in HEPES buffered saline	Varies with preparation	Volume of 7.5 mg protein, for 250 mL of mTEC/Plus or mTEC/SF	Frozen bovine pituitaries (Pel-Freeze) [15], or use Pel-Freeze BPE 57136 Store −80 °C
BSA	BSA (Fraction V), 5 g in HBSS, 50 mL	100 mg/mL	2.5 mL for mTEC/SF	Fisher, Filter sterilize Store −20 °C
Nu-Serum	NuSerum (contains 25 % serum), 5 mL	NA	5 mL for mTEC/NS	BD Biosciences Store −20 °C

3. Cell proliferation medium mTEC/Plus (*see* Subheading 2.2, **item 3** and **Note 1**).
4. Hemocytometer and trypan blue (0.4 % w/v), to assess cell viability.

2.6 Tracheal Epithelial Ciliated Cell Differentiation Using the ALI Condition

1. Cell differentiation media, either serum-containing mTEC/NS or serum-free mTEC/SF with defined components (*see* Subheadings 2.1 and 2.2, **item 4**).

2.7 Induction of Mucous Cell Metaplasia

1. Recombinant mouse IL-13 (Peprotech), IL-6 (R&D Systems), and IL-17 (R&D Systems).

2.8 Genetic Modification of mTEC with Viral Vectors

1. Use recombinant adenovirus or lentivirus, each with a titer of at least 10^7 infectious units/mL. Generate virus using standard protocols. Handle according to biosafety guidelines at the user's institution (*see* **Note 3**).

2.9 Cell Coculture Systems

1. Isolate lymphocytes, neutrophils or other immune cells, fibroblasts or smooth muscle cells, or others using specialized protocols.

2.10 Pathogen Infection Models

1. Infectious agents (e.g., influenza virus, respiratory syncytial virus, and bacteria) used in a coculture system should be handled using standard protocols and biosafety guidelines (*see* **Note 3**).

2.11 Analysis of mTEC Differentiation by Immunofluorescence

1. Fixative 4 % paraformaldehyde (*see* **Note 3**) in PBS. Prepared fresh or freshly defrosted. Use PBS to wash cells on the inserts.
2. Scalpel (#22) to cut the membrane from the plastic supports and forceps to hold membranes.
3. A blocking solution of 5 % donkey serum (Sigma-Aldrich), 3 % BSA and Add detergent Tween 0.2 %. (Sigma-Aldrich) in PBS.
4. Antibodies: Mucous cell marker, mouse anti-Muc5AC (Abcam), cilia marker, mouse anti-acetylated α-tubulin (clone 6-11B-1, Sigma-Aldrich) and anti-mouse, fluorescent-labeled secondary antibodies.
5. Mounting medium containing nuclear DNA stain Hoechst or 4′, 6 diamidino-2-phenylindole (DAPI) such as Vectashield® (Vector, Burlingame, CA). DNA binding chemicals are potentially carcinogenic (*see* **Note 3**).
6. Glass microscope slides and large cover slips (24×50 mm) to cover several pieces of mTEC membranes on a single slide.

2.12 Additional Methods to Assess Gene Expression and Differentiation of mTECs

1. mTEC flow cytometry; use 0.1 % EDTA or 0.25 % trypsin with 0.1 % EDTA in Cell Dissociation Solution (Sigma) for releasing cells from membrane (*see* Subheading 3.11, **step 1**). Use 2 % FCS in PBS (2 % FCS/PBS) for re-suspending the cells and staining with antibodies. Use standard protocols for flow cytometry.
2. Mini Cell Scrapers (Biotium) or 200 μL pipette tips for scraping cells off membranes.

3. RNA isolation from mTEC: Qiagan RNA Easy® Microkit and Kontes Pellet Pestle®.
4. DMEM to collect mucus and ATPγS (Sigma) 100 μM to induce mucus secretion.

2.13 Assessment of Cell Physiology

1. Transepithelial electrical resistance (Rt) using a Voltohmmeter with electrode "chopstick" pair (EVOM, World Precision Instruments).
2. Cilia beat frequency (CBF) measurement using specialized automated software (e.g., Sisson-Ammons Video Analysis, Ammons Engineering) [26], and an inverted microscope with phase contrast filters and objectives (20×), and high-speed video camera.

3 Methods

3.1 Media preparation

1. Prepare all stock components for media as described in subheading 2.1.
2. Prepare media (see Table 2).

3.2 Preparation of Materials for mTEC Isolation and Initiation of Culture

1. Coat the apical surface of the Transwell® insert membrane with rat tail type I collagen solution in the hood. Incubate plates at room temperature for 18–24 h or for a minimum of 4 h at 37 °C. Rinse apical and basal surfaces with sterile PBS three times then dry for 5 min. Prepare three inserts per trachea harvested.
2. Cells may be cultured on standard tissue culture plastic when coated with rat tail collagen, but will not differentiate to ciliated types.

3.3 Trachea Harvest (Day 1)

1. In the tissue culture hood, prepare two 100 mm dishes (non-tissue culture) with 10 mL cold sterile Ham's F-12/Pen-Strep on ice, to hold resected tracheas.
2. Immerse the euthanized mouse in 70 % ethanol.
3. Expose the trachea. Incise the abdominal skin circumferentially, and then invert the entire layer of skin toward the head to reveal the neck. Separate the neck muscles and open the thoracic cavity to expose the trachea and mainstem bronchi.
4. Resect the trachea. Bluntly dissect the trachea from the posterior surface of the esophagus. Cut the trachea just distal to the larynx, leaving the larynx intact. Place the trachea in the dish of Ham's F-12/Pen-Strep on ice.
5. In the hood, strip off adherent tissues from trachea with a small forceps. Place each cleaned trachea in a dish of cold sterile Ham's F-12/Pen-Strep on ice.

Table 2
mTEC media

Media name	Components and amount (final concentration)		Comments
Ham's F-12/ Pen-Strep	Pen/Strep (1,000×) Ham's F-12	500 μL (100 U Penicillin 100 μg Streptomycin) Add to 500 mL final volume	Store at 4 °C
mTEC/basic	1 M HEPES Glutamine 200 mM $NaHCO_3$ 7.5 % Ampho B (250 μg/mL)[a] Pen/Strep (1,000×) DMEM/F-12	7.5 mL (15 mM) 10 mL (4 mM) 2.0 mL (3.6 mM) 500 μL (0.25 μg/mL) 500 μL (100 U Pen/100 μg Strep) Add to 500 mL final volume	Filter sterilize Store at 4 °C Stable up to 6 weeks
mTEC/Plus[b] (High concentration growth factors)	I T CT EGF BPE[c] FBS mTEC Basic medium	1,250 μL (10 μg/mL) 250 μL (5 μg/mL) 250 μL (0.1 μg/mL) 1,250 μL (25 ng/mL) TBD μL (7.5 mg protein/250 mL) 12.5 mL (5 % v/v) Add to 250 mL final volume	Filter sterilize Store at 4 °C Stable up to 6 weeks
mTEC/NS[b] (*NuSerum*)	NuSerum mTEC Basic medium	5.0 mL Add to 250 mL final volume	Store at 4 °C Stable up to 6 weeks
mTEC/SF[b] (*Serum-Free* media)	I T CT EGF BPE[c] BSA stock mTEC Basic medium	625 μL (5 μg/mL) 250 μL (5 μg/mL) 62.5 μL (0.025 μg/mL) 250 μL (5 ng/mL) TBD μL (7.5 mg protein/250 mL) 2.5 mL (1 mg/mL) Add to 250 mL final volume	Filter sterilize Store at 4 °C Stable up to 6 weeks

[a]Amphotericin B: do not filter
[b]RA, stock B 10,000×: add 1 μL to each 10 mL of mTEC/Plus, mTEC/NS, mTEC/SF immediately prior to adding media to cells
[c]BPE: TBD, to be determined, concentration varies with preparation. Use an amount to provide 7.5 mg protein/250 mL of medium

6. Cut each trachea lengthwise to open and submerge in freshly made pronase.
7. Incubate at 4 °C overnight (18–24 h).

3.4 Tracheal Epithelial Cell Isolation (Day 2)

1. Thaw the DNase solution on ice. Thaw and warm FBS to 37 °C in a water bath.
2. Gently invert the tube containing the tracheas in pronase about five times. Warm the tube to room temperature for 10 min and mix gently.

3. Add warmed FBS to a final concentration of 10 % and invert again gently 15–20 times (down and up is a single cycle) to dislodge epithelial cells.
4. Remove each trachea from the tube with a Pasteur pipette and place it in a new 15 mL tube with 3 mL of Ham's F-12/10 % FBS. Invert the tube 15 times.
5. Remove tracheas from the tube and place in a third 15 mL tube containing 3 mL of Ham's F-12/10 % FBS. Invert the tube 15 times.
6. Using a Pasteur pipette, remove and discard the tracheas.
7. Combine the contents of all three tubes containing the enzyme-released cells. Centrifuge at 500 × *g*, 4 °C, for 10 min.
8. Carefully aspirate the supernatant, and re-suspend the cells in DNase solution (~200 μL per trachea).
9. Put the tube on ice for 5 min, then collect the cells by centrifugation at 500 × *g*, 4 °C, for 5 min.
10. Resuspend the cells in mTEC/Basic medium containing 10 % FBS, using 2–3 mL per 10 tracheas. Plate the cells in a Primaria™ tissue culture dish. Incubate at 37 °C, 5 % CO_2 for 3–4 h. During this incubation, allow the fibroblasts to attach, while the epithelial cells remain nonadherent and suspended in the medium.
11. Gently swirl the medium in the culture dish. Carefully collect the supernatant containing the nonattached epithelial cells and place in a sterile tube.
12. Gently rinse the dish one or two times with warm mTEC Basic medium/10 % FBS to recover additional airway epithelial cells, collect the wash and add to a sterile cell collection tube (from **step 11**). Avoid excessive force that detaches fibroblasts.
13. Centrifuge at 500 × *g*, 4 °C, for 5 min.
14. Aspirate the supernatant and re-suspend the cell pellet in a small, measured volume (e.g., 100–200 μL/trachea) of mTEC/Plus medium with fresh RA. Do not try to pipette the cell clumps vigorously to form a single cell suspension.
15. Calculate the number of viable cells with a hemocytometer. Cells viability by trypan blue exclusion should be greater than 90 %. Single cells and clumps will be present. Do not overestimate cell numbers within clumps, or include red blood cells. Yields are $1–2 \times 10^5$ cells per trachea.

3.5 Tracheal Epithelial Cell Seeding and Proliferation

1. Seed cells at 1.0×10^5 cells/cm^2. Density is critical for proliferation and differentiation. Higher seeding density may be required if cultures are manipulated by cytokine treatment or gene transfer.

2. Add the cell suspension to the apical chamber and gently move the plate to distribute the cells on the membrane. Add mTEC/Plus with RA to the basal compartment. This is culture day 0.
3. On Day 3, change the medium in apical and basal compartments. Adherent cells should appear elongated and in islands.
4. On Day 5, the cells are typically confluent, but may require 7 days. Transepithelial cell resistance is typically greater than 1,000 Ω cm^2 (*see* **Note 4**).

3.6 Induction or Inhibition of Ciliogenesis

1. Confluent cells can be differentiated to induce ciliated cells using ALI conditions and either mTEC/NS or mTEC/SF. This time point is ALI day 0. Aspirate media from the apical chamber and supply fresh medium only to the basal chamber. The apical surface should remain dry (*see* **Note 4**).
2. Change the medium every other day, including freshly added RA.
3. Follow cells by inspection and microscopy. The apical surface should remain dry or have a small ring of mucus that can be washed with warm media or PBS. Cells develop a cobblestone appearance. Beating cilia may be seen by microscope as early as ALI day 5. Ciliated cells gradually increase in number, to over 30 % of the surface by ALI day 14.
4. The cells can be maintained at ALI for over 2 months without loss of differentiation.
5. Inhibition of differentiation. To maintain basal cells in a polarized state, block ciliogenesis and minimize proliferation, culture the cells with mTEC/Plus until confluent, then change the media to mTEC/NS or mTEC/SF with RA and keep cells submerged by applying media to the apical compartment. Reversion to the air–liquid interface condition can induce differentiation.
6. Absence of retinoic acid in the media prevents normal airway differentiation in both submerged and ALI conditions.

3.7 Induction of Mucous Cell Metaplasia

1. Seed the cells at $1 \times 10^5/cm^2$ or higher. The extent of mucous cell metaplasia will increase when seeding cells at $1.5 \times 10^5/cm^2$.
2. Add 10 ng/mL of mouse IL-13 to mTEC/Plus media at seeding day 3, which is 2 days prior to establishing ALI. Titrate the dose of IL-13 for the desired degree of mucus cell metaplasia, using a range of 1–100 ng/mL.
3. Upon creation of ALI, add fresh IL-13 to the mTEC/NS or mTEC/SF media in the basal compartment and provide fresh IL-13 with each media change. Wash the cell surface to remove mucus.

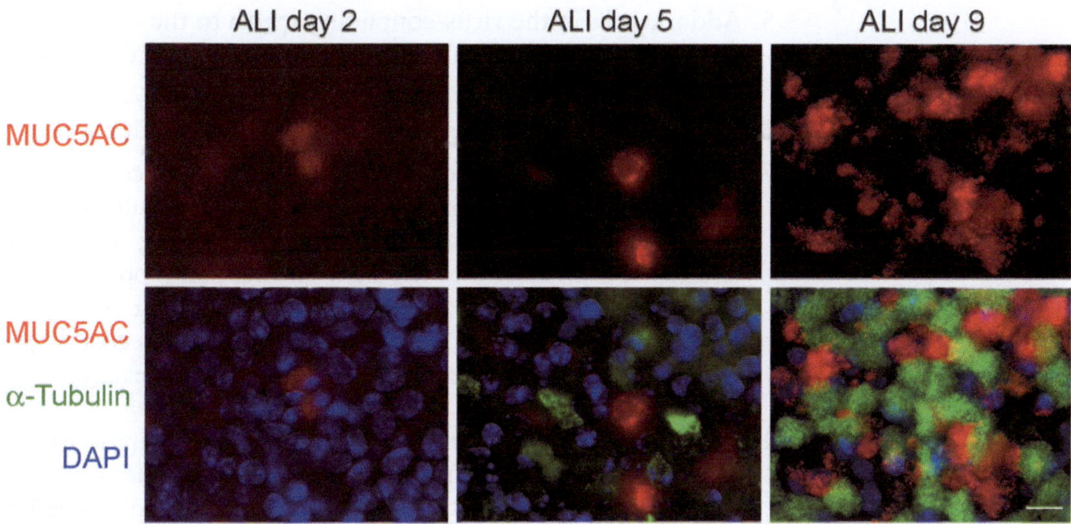

Fig. 2 Induction of mucous cells in mTEC models the asthmatic airway. mTEC were treat with IL-13 (10 ng/mL, in mTEC/NS medium) at ALI day 0 and immunostained at indicated times for the mucous marker MUC5AC (*red*) and cilia marker acetylated α-tubulin (α-tubulin, *green*). DNA is stained with DAPI (*blue*). Photomicrographs, en face of fixed membranes mounted on glass slides. Bar = 10 μm

4. Harvest cells after 3–21 days to assay for mucous cell markers, such as MUC5AC, using quantitative real time PCR, immunostaining, or ELISA (*see* Subheadings 3.11 and 3.12 and Fig. 2).
5. Treatment of well-differentiated mTEC at ALI with 10 ng/mL of IL-13 for 3–14 days will result in mucous cell metaplasia. This metaplasia will be less abundant than levels observed following earlier treatments with the cytokine.
6. 10 ng/mL of IL-6 or IL-17 (the dose can range from 1 to 200 ng/mL) may also be used to induce mucous cell metaplasia using a protocol that is similar to the IL-13 treatment.

3.8 Genetic Modification of mTEC with Viral Vectors

1. Generate viral particles using the desired recombinant adenovirus or lentivirus vectors for over expression or gene silencing using established methods.
2. Lentivirus generated by the producer cell line in culture should be collected in mTEC/Plus medium. Dilute adenovirus into mTEC/Plus medium.
3. Resuspend freshly isolated mTEC cells in virus media using a multiplicity of infection of 25–200. Adenovirus should be titered in the mTEC medium.
4. To achieve a high percentage of adenovirus transfected cells at the time of establishing ALI, seed cells at $1.5–2.0 \times 10^5/cm^2$. This speeds the time of reaching ALI. Alternatively, mTEC can be transfected with adenovirus 2 days prior to establishing ALI.

5. Add the cells in the virus-containing media to the apical chambers. The basalateral chamber should be filled with the same infection media.
6. Change the basolateral media 16–18 h after transduction.
7. If the lentivirus also codes for an antibiotic resistance gene (i.e., puromycin), the antibiotic can be added to the culture media approximately 48 h after infection. When using a selection strategy, it is important to use a g high viral titer (approximately 1×10^7 infectious particles/mL) and a high seeding density. An infection of at least 50 % of the cells will allow recovery of a confluent layer so that an ALI condition can be created.

3.9 Cell Coculture Systems

1. Proliferate or differentiate mTEC to desired status, *see* Protocols 3.6–3.8. Transwell membrane pore density varies depending on composition and manufacturer and may affect immune cell migration. mTEC culture is less successful on membranes with pores greater than 0.4 μm. However, this pore size will accommodate neutrophil migration [22].
2. Tissue culture plates containing wells with cultured smooth muscle cells, fibroblasts, or other types may be prepared to receive inserts with mTEC.
3. If mTEC are well differentiated (older than ALI day 7) or undifferentiated and submerged, then the immune cell culture media can be used without concern for significant loss of mTEC differentiation over a 5–7 day period.
4. Apply immune cells, such as lymphocytes or neutrophils, or other cell types directly on the apical surface of mTEC or add to the lower chamber.
5. If immune cell contact with the basolateral aspect of the mTEC is desired, then the Transwell insert with confluent mTEC is inverted and set into the well of a tissue culture plate. Immune cells are then applied to the basal surface of the membrane, held in place by surface tension or if necessary a collar of ethanol rinsed Parafilm®. The plate must be covered to avoid evaporation of media on the basal surface.
6. Immune cells can be recovered from either compartment by gentle aspiration and the immune cells can be collected with the mTEC by scraping the surface to release cells. The immune cells can then be assayed as desired by experimental method such as flow cytometry.

3.10 Pathogen Infection Models

1. Proliferate or differentiate mTEC to desired status, *see* Protocols 3.6–3.8. Antibiotics may be removed from mTEC media as needed.
2. Apply viruses or bacteria directly on the apical surface of mTEC. Initial multiplicity of infection is 0.01–10 infectious

particles/cell for respiratory viruses. Titrate exposure time and multiplicity of infection to the desired effect. mTEC can support some viruses over many weeks.

3. If contact of pathogen interaction with the basolateral aspect of mTECs are desired, assemble inserts as described in Protocol 3.9, **step 5**.
4. Collect cells on whole membranes for immunostaining, as cell suspensions, lysates or as required for assay, *see* Protocols 3.11 and 3.12.

3.11 Analysis of mTEC Differentiation and Mucus Cell Metaplasia by Immunofluorescent Staining

1. Fix the cells. Wash the cells gently with PBS, aspirate the PBS, and then fill the chambers with 4 % paraformaldehyde to cover the membranes (this chemical is toxic, *see* **Note 3**). Incubate at room temperature for 10 min without rocking. Remove and properly discard the paraformaldehyde. Wash the cells on the membrane three times for 5 min each, by adding PBS to both chambers and slowly rocking the plate.
2. Cut the membrane from the plastic support. Do not allow the membrane to dry. Invert the insert and with a scalpel, cut the membrane from the plastic ring support. Prepare a wet surface for delivery of the membrane by adding 1 mL of PBS to a tissue culture dish. Position the insert, with the basal surface on the plate, and use fine forceps to release the membrane. To produce multiple samples from one membrane, cut into quarters by rocking the scalpel blade across the membrane. Notch the outer bottom corner of each quarter to orient to the cell surface. Handle the membrane at the edge with fine forceps. Fixed cells on membranes can be stored in sterile PBS at 4 °C in a Parafilm® sealed plate for several months.
3. Block nonspecific antibody binding on the cells (*see* Subheading 2.12, **item 3**). Transfer the membrane pieces to a 24- or 96-well plate. Cover the membrane with blocking solution and slowly rock at room temperature for 30–60 min.
4. Immunostain cells with an anti-cilia (acetylated α-tubulin) or anti-mucous (MUC5AC) antibody (*see* Fig. 2). Simultaneous use of two mouse primary antibodies can be achieved using Fab labeling of one antibody (e.g., Zenon, Life Technologies). Dilute primary antibody in the blocking solution (*see* Subheading 2.12, **item 3**). Use an isotype-matched antibody as a control. Incubate with cells on a piece of membrane for 1 h at room temperature or overnight at 4 °C. Wash membrane with PBS three times for 5 min each. Add a fluorescent-labeled secondary antibody for 30 min, and wash three times.
5. Mount immunostained membranes on slides. Transfer the membrane to a glass microscope slide and apply 10–20 μL of

mounting medium containing DAPI. Inspect the membrane under the fluorescence microscope if the membrane orientation is not certain. Apply the coverslip and seal the edges with nail polish. Examine by fluorescent microscopy.

3.12 Additional Methods to Assess Differentiation and Gene Expression in mTEC

1. Flow cytometry of mTEC. To obtain a cell suspension use 0.1 % EDTA in Cell Dissociation Solution. To detect an intracellular protein, use 0.25 % trypsin with 0.1 % EDTA in Cell Dissociation Solution. Put the appropriate solution in both chambers, place in the tissue culture incubator for 5–20 min. Aspirate the basal compartment. Release the cells from the apical compartment by mixing with a mini cell scraper or a pipette tip. Transfer the cells to a tube. Add 2 % FCS/PBS, 200 μL ($0.33\ cm^2$ membrane) to the apical chamber, pipette to recover additional cells. Repeat this twice more and pool all washes. Pass the cell suspension through a 70 μM cell strainer to obtain a single cell suspension. Centrifuge the cells at $500 \times g$, 4 °C, for 5 min. Resuspend the cell pellet in 2 % FCS/PBS. The typical yield is 2×10^5 cells per $0.33\ cm^2$ insert. Proceed using relevant flow cytometry protocols.
2. Protein blot analysis of mTEC. Put the plate with the inserts on ice, wash the cells twice with ice cold PBS. Add 25–30 μL of the appropriate lysis buffer on the apical surface of a $0.33\ cm^2$ of membrane. Incubate at 4 °C, rocking slowly. After 20 min, pipette and gently scrape the surface to release cells. Transfer the lysate solution to a microcentrifuge tube on ice and process using standard protocols. Typical yield of protein is 25–40 μg per $0.33\ cm^2$ membrane.
3. RNA isolation. Collect cells in the Qiagan RNA Easy® Microkit. Freeze at −80 °C then break cells with the Kontes Pellet Pestle® for 90 s. Continue according to the manufactures' instructions. The typical RNA yield is 6–10 μg per cm^2 membrane. Analyze expression by real time PCR.
4. Collection of mucus secretions [27]. Gently wash the apical insert surface with 100 μL of warm DMEM, incubate 10 min and repeat three more times. Determine the period of baseline secretion to be sampled (e.g., 1–24 h). Then add 100 μL of warm DMEM, incubate at 37 °C for 10 min, repeat three times and pool washings as baseline readings. Then stimulate with 100 μM ATPγS, and repeat collection after 30–60 min. A conventional ELISA assay with a monoclonal antibody for MUC5AC can then be used to measure the amount of a secreted mucin.
5. Electron microscopy for SEM or TEM. Wash cells with cold PBS. Fix the cells in 2.5 % glutaraldehyde in sodium cacodylate buffer at 4 °C overnight on the membrane. Consultation with the EM facility should guide sample preparation.

3.13 Physiologic Measurements of Cell Function

1. Transepithelial Electrical Resistance (Rt). Use a voltohmmeter to assess junction integrity and maturation. A typical Rt for a confluent membrane is greater than 1,000 Ω cm^2. It is highest early in ALI and decreases with differentiation.
2. Immerse the probe in 70 % ethanol, air dry, and rinse with sterile water or PBS.
3. Add medium to both chambers for the measurement of Rt. A coated membrane without cells is used to a obtain baseline Rt. The baseline value is subtracted from the observed Rt from the membrane with cells to obtain the Rt.
4. Cilia beat frequency. Wash the apical surface with warm PBS at least 1 h prior to measuring cilia beat frequency measurement. Image at least five fields (*see* Subheading 2.13, **item 2**).

4 Notes

1. Media preparation
   Reagents and components for cell isolation should be filter sterilized using a 0.22 μM syringe filter with low protein binding (e.g., Pall PN 4602). Aliquot stock components in volumes appropriate for preparing 250 mL of media. Retinoic acid (RA, stock B 10,000×) should be freshly added to media at a final concentration of 5×10^{-8} M. RA supplemented media should be used within 48 h. If prior fungal contamination has occurred, 0.25 μg/mL of Amphotericin B should be added to media without filtering and should be used until the cells are changed to ALI conditions. Sustained use of Amphotericin B over several weeks should be avoided due to toxicity.
2. Mice
   The growth and differentiation of mTEC from mice ages 4 weeks to over 18 months is similar. Isolation of cells from younger and smaller mice is more technically challenging and the total cell number recovered is diminished. Some strain-dependent differences (e.g., SV129, FVB) in proliferative populations can be overcome by increasing the seeding density.
3. Cautions regarding potentially toxic materials
   The fixatives paraformaldehyde and glutaraldehyde are toxic. The DNA binding compounds Hoechst, DAPI, and sodium cacodylate are potentially carcinogenic. These reagents and viruses used for gene transfer or pathogen studies should be handled according to biosafety guidelines at the user's institution.
4. Troubleshooting mTEC preparations
   Failure of cells to proliferate to confluence or differentiate may have several causes including the following: (1) not resecting the entire trachea, especially that containing the paratracheal

glands (so that basal cell numbers are insufficient); (2) inadequate pronase activity; (3) fibroblast contamination; or (4) infection. To correct these issues, assure proper dissection of the complete length of the trachea (but avoid the larynx), increase the number and force of "shakes" of tracheas in pronase, assure the pronase is fresh, and increase the pronase concentration (e.g., to 0.20 %). Increasing the time of pronase digestion does not significantly improve cell yield; however, pronase activity varies with supplier and lot. To minimize the fibroblast contamination, allow adequate time for adherence of fibroblast in the culture dish and avoid over-washing the culture dish after fibroblast adherence. Low levels of fungal contamination may inhibit cell growth. The addition of Amphotericin B 0.25 μg/mL to stock media or antifungal/antibiotic, Primocin™ 50 mg/mL (InvivoGen) may be helpful.

Acknowledgments

This work was supported by awards to S.L.B. from the National Institute of Health and the Children's Discovery Institute of Saint Louis Children's Hospital and Washington University.

References

1. Lankford SM, Macchione M, Crews AL, McKane SA, Akley NJ, Martin LD (2005) Modeling the airway epithelium in allergic asthma: interleukin-13-induced effects in differentiated murine tracheal epithelial cells. In Vitro Cell Dev Biol Anim 41:217–224
2. Ibricevic A, Pekosz A, Walter MJ, Newby C, Battaile JT, Brown EG, Holtzman MJ, Brody SL (2006) Influenza virus receptor specificity and cell tropism in mouse and human airway epithelial cells. J Virol 80:7469–7480
3. Brockman-Schneider RA, Amineva SP, Bulat MV, Gern JE (2008) Serial culture of murine primary airway epithelial cells and ex vivo replication of human rhinoviruses. J Immunol Methods 339:264–269
4. Mebratu YA, Dickey BF, Evans C, Tesfaigzi Y (2008) The BH3-only protein Bik/Blk/Nbk inhibits nuclear translocation of activated ERK1/2 to mediate IFNgamma-induced cell death. J Cell Biol 183:429–439
5. Nakagami Y, Favoreto S Jr, Zhen G, Park SW, Nguyenvu LT, Kuperman DA, Dolganov GM, Huang X, Boushey HA, Avila PC, Erle DJ (2008) The epithelial anion transporter pendrin is induced by allergy and rhinovirus infection, regulates airway surface liquid, and increases airway reactivity and inflammation in an asthma model. J Immunol 181:2203–2210
6. Sel S, Rost BR, Yildirim AO, Sel B, Kalwa H, Fehrenbach H, Renz H, Gudermann T, Dietrich A (2008) Loss of classical transient receptor potential 6 channel reduces allergic airway response. Clin Exp Allergy 38: 1548–1558
7. Tachdjian R, Mathias C, Al Khatib S, Bryce PJ, Kim HS, Blaeser F, O'Connor BD, Rzymkiewicz D, Chen A, Holtzman MJ, Hershey GK, Garn H, Harb H, Renz H, Oettgen HC, Chatila TA (2009) Pathogenicity of a disease-associated human IL-4 receptor allele in experimental asthma. J Exp Med 206: 2191–2204
8. Rock JR, Onaitis MW, Rawlins EL, Lu Y, Clark CP, Xue Y, Randell SH, Hogan BL (2009) Basal cells as stem cells of the mouse trachea and human airway epithelium. Proc Natl Acad Sci USA 106:12771–12775
9. Wong AP, Keating A, Lu WY, Duchesneau P, Wang X, Sacher A, Hu J, Waddell TK (2009) Identification of a bone marrow-derived epithelial-like population capable of repopulating injured mouse airway epithelium. J Clin Invest 119:336–348
10. Ghosh M, Brechbuhl HM, Smith RW, Li B, Hicks DA, Titchner T, Runkle CM, Reynolds SD (2011) Context-dependent differentiation of multipotential keratin 14-expressing

tracheal basal cells. Am J Respir Cell Mol Biol 45:403–410

11. Deppong CM, Xu J, Brody SL, Green JM (2012) Airway epithelial cells suppress T cell proliferation by an IFNgamma/STAT1/TGFbeta-dependent mechanism. Am J Physiol Lung Cell Mol Physiol 302:L167–L173
12. Zeki AA, Thai P, Kenyon NJ, Wu R (2012) Differential effects of simvastatin on IL-13-induced cytokine gene expression in primary mouse tracheal epithelial cells. Respir Res 13:38
13. You Y, Richer EJ, Huang T, Brody SL (2002) Growth and differentiation of mouse tracheal epithelial cells: selection of a proliferative population. Am J Physiol Lung Cell Mol Physiol 283:L1315–L1321
14. You Y, Brody SL (2013) Culture and differentiation of mouse tracheal epithelial cells. In: Randell SH, Fulcher M L (eds) Epithelial cell culture protocols, 2nd edn. Humana Press, New York, pp 123–143
15. Lechner J, LaVeck M (1985) A serum-free method for culturing normal human bronchial epithelial cells at clonal density. J Tissue Cult Meth 9:43–48
16. Whitcutt MJ, Adler KB, Wu R (1988) A biphasic chamber system for maintaining polarity of differentiation of cultured respiratory tract epithelial cells. In Vitro Cell Dev Biol 24: 420–428
17. Wu R (1997) Growth and differentiation of tracheobronchial epithelial cells. In: MacDonald J (ed) Growth and development of the lung. Deckker, New York, pp 211–241
18. Borthwick DW, Shahbazian M, Krantz QT, Dorin JR, Randell SH (2001) Evidence for stem-cell niches in the tracheal epithelium. Am J Respir Cell Mol Biol 24:662–670
19. You Y, Huang T, Richer EJ, Schmidt JE, Zabner J, Borok Z, Brody SL (2004) Role of f-box factor foxj1 in differentiation of ciliated airway epithelial cells. Am J Physiol Lung Cell Mol Physiol 286:L650–L657
20. Tyner JW, Kim EY, Ide K, Pelletier MR, Roswit WT, Morton JD, Battaile JT, Patel AC, Patterson GA, Castro M, Spoor MS, You Y, Brody SL, Holtzman MJ (2006) Blocking airway mucous cell metaplasia by inhibiting EGFR antiapoptosis and IL-13 transdifferentiation signals. J Clin Invest 116:309–321
21. Chen Y, Thai P, Zhao YH, Ho YS, DeSouza MM, Wu R (2003) Stimulation of airway mucin gene expression by interleukin (IL)-17 through IL-6 paracrine/autocrine loop. J Biol Chem 278:17036–17043
22. Farberman MM, Ibricevic A, Joseph TD, Akers KT, Garcia-Medina R, Crosby S, Clarke LL, Brody SL, Ferkol TW (2011) Effect of polarized release of CXC-chemokines from wild-type and cystic fibrosis murine airway epithelial cells. Am J Respir Cell Mol Biol 45:221–228
23. Kreisel D, Lai J, Richardson SB, Ibricevic A, Nava RG, Lin X, Li W, Kornfeld CG, Miller MJ, Brody SL, Gelman AE, Krupnick AS (2011) Polarized alloantigen presentation by airway epithelial cells contributes to direct CD8+ T cell activation in the airway. Am J Respir Cell Mol Biol 44:749–754
24. Schmid A, Bai G, Schmid N, Zaccolo M, Ostrowski LE, Conner GE, Fregien N, Salathe M (2006) Real-time analysis of cAMP-mediated regulation of ciliary motility in single primary human airway epithelial cells. J Cell Sci 119:4176–4186
25. Pan J, You Y, Huang T, Brody SL (2007) RhoA-mediated apical actin enrichment is required for ciliogenesis and promoted by Foxj1. J Cell Sci 120:1868–1876
26. Sisson JH, Stoner JA, Ammons BA, Wyatt TA (2003) All-digital image capture and whole-field analysis of ciliary beat frequency. J Microsc 211:103–111
27. Abdullah LH, Wolber C, Kesimer M, Sheehan JK, Davis CW (2012) Studying mucin secretion from human bronchial epithelial cell primary cultures. Methods Mol Biol 842: 259–277

Chapter 8

Isolation and Characterization of Mast Cells in Mouse Models of Allergic Diseases

Martina Kovarova

Abstract

After their activation, mast cells release a variety of bioactive mediators that contribute to characteristic symptoms of allergic reactions. Ex vivo analysis of mast cells derived from their progenitors or isolated from mice is an indispensable tool for the development of newer and more effective therapies of allergic syndromes. Here, we describe the differentiation and isolation of mouse mast cells from different sources including differentiation from bone marrow, differentiation from fetal liver, and isolation of residential connective tissue-type mast cells from the peritoneum. These techniques are valuable tools for the study of mast cell function and their contribution to allergic reactions.

Key words Mast cells, Allergy, Peritoneum, Bone marrow, Fetal liver

1 Introduction

Mast cells play a central role in allergic reactions. Their response to an allergen underlies the symptoms seen in acute and chronic allergic disease. In allergic disease, mast cells are most frequently activated by an allergen-specific IgE, which is produced by B cells during a Th2 response to allergen exposure. FcεRI on the mast cell surface binds the allergen-specific IgE with high affinity. This high-affinity binding results in a half-life of cell-bound IgE that is on the order of days [1, 2]. Therefore sensitization of mast cells is persistent when serum IgE levels are increased. Cross-linking of the FcεRI-bound IgE with the specific allergen activates mast cells and leads to the release of histamine, serotonin, and a variety of other biologically active mediators that are stored in preformed granules. This process is called degranulation, and elicits the immediate hypersensitivity. Mast cells also produce a variety of cytokines and lipid mediators, such as leukotrienes and prostaglandins that are major contributors to the late or chronic phase of allergic disease [3].

Mast cells have essential roles in mediating allergic diseases and have been studied with a focus on understanding the molecular

Irving C. Allen (ed.), *Mouse Models of Allergic Disease: Methods and Protocols*, Methods in Molecular Biology, vol. 1032, DOI 10.1007/978-1-62703-496-8_8, © Springer Science+Business Media, LLC 2013

mechanism of their activation. Likewise, mast cells are often sought-after target for the development of treatments and management of allergic diseases.

Ex vivo studies using mast cells mainly depend on a reliable source of large numbers of cells. Mast cells are tissue-resident cells that are present only in small numbers. In the mouse system, protocols were developed to allow differentiation and culture of mast cells from bone marrow mast cell progenitors using mast cell growth factors and cytokines. This approach is especially useful when combined with the availability of mouse lines carrying mutations in virtually all known genes. By culturing bone marrow from these animals, using established protocols described in this chapter, mast cells lacking a specific gene or carrying a specific mutation could be obtained and the impact of the mutation on mast cell function can be easily determined. However, in some cases, the mutation of interest results in an embryonic lethal phenotype or death early after birth, making isolation of bone marrow progenitors from those mice inaccessible. In these cases, two alternatives can be used: (1) derivation of mast cells from embryonic stem cells [4], or (2) to obtain progenitors for mast cell differentiation from fetal or neonatal liver, if available [5, 6].

Although bone marrow-derived mast cells are a useful model for mast cell studies, they are phenotypically different from residential mast cell populations, including differences associated with the level of maturation and the level of mast cell protease expression. For example, bone marrow-derived mast cells are similar to mucosal mast cells in vivo and stain by alcian blue due to the high expression of chondroitin sulfate. However, peritoneal mast cells have a phenotype that is more consistent with connective tissue mast cells. The peritoneal mast cells express high amounts of heparin and stain with safranin, but not alcian blue [7]. In vivo, mast cells derive from a distinct precursor in the bone marrow and mature under local tissue microenvironmental factors [8], which make each population unique and hard to model in vitro. Resident mast cells can be relatively easy to isolate from the peritoneal cavity using a Percoll gradient. Although this isolation technique provides only a small amount of mast cells, the recovered cells are a valuable source of fully differentiated connective tissue mast cells that matured in a specific tissue microenvironment.

The characterization of mast cells is essential for the evaluation of mast cell differentiation or isolation. Expression of FcεRI on the cell surface is not only crucial for mast cell function in allergic reactions, but it can also be used together with c-Kit expression as a landmark for successful differentiation and maturation of bone marrow-derived mast cell cultures. In rodents, expression of the FcεRI receptor is limited to mast cells and basophils. Thus, this receptor can be used as a marker for the quality of mast cells isolated from the peritoneal cavity. Another important aspect of mast cell culture and isolation is the quality of the granules. This can be assessed either by their specific staining or by functional assays that test the cells' ability to degranulate. Together, this chapter provides protocols allowing for the efficient differentiation, isolation, and characterization of mast cells for studies evaluating the molecular mechanisms of mast cell activation.

2 Materials

2.1 Mast Cell Differentiation from Bone Marrow or Fetal Liver

1. Surgical tools: Two forceps and two scissors.
2. 70 μm cell strainer.
3. Low-linting paper wipers.
4. 15 ml conical tube.
5. 1× PBS.
6. 70% EtOH.
7. 25 G needle.
8. 5 cc syringe.
9. Tissue culture plates (6-well, 3 cm, and 10 cm).
10. Centrifuge.
11. Laminar flow hood.
12. CO_2-humidified incubator.
13. Mast cell medium: 500 ml of Iscove's modified Dulbecco's medium (IMDM), 6 ml of 100× penicillin–streptomycin–glutamine, 6 ml of 1 M HEPES buffer, 6 ml of 100× nonessential amino acids, 6 ml of 100 mM sodium pyruvate, 2 μl of 2-mercaptoethanol, 60 ml of heat-inactivated fetal bovine serum, 5 ng/ml of mouse recombinant IL-3, and 10 ng/ml of mouse recombinant SCF (*see* **Note 1**).

2.2 Peritoneal Mast Cell Isolation

1. Surgical tools: Two forceps and two scissors.
2. 1× PBS.
3. 70% EtOH.
4. 25 G needle.
5. 5 cc syringe.
6. Disposable transfer pipettes (5 ml).
7. Centrifuge.
8. 50 ml of Peritoneal mast cell medium: 46.5 ml of Dulbecco's modified Eagle medium (DMEM), 2.5 ml of fetal bovine serum (final concentration of 5% v/v), and 1.0 ml of 1 M HEPES (final concentration of 20 mM) (*see* **Note 1**).

Table 1
Antibodies for staining FcεRI and c-kit on mast cells differentiated

Sample number	Type of staining	Antibody used (clone)
1.	Isotype control for FITC and PE	Mouse IgG1-FITC (P3.6.2.8.1.); rat IgG2b-PE (A95-1)
2.	FITC IgE specific + PE isotype	Anti-mouse FcεRI alpha (MAR-1); rat IgG2b-PE (A95-1)
3.	PE c-Kit specific + FITC isotype	Anti c-Kit-PE (2B8); mouse IgG1-FITC (P3.6.2.8.1)
4.	FITC and PE specific	Anti-mouse FcεRI alpha (MAR-1); anti c-Kit-PE (2B8)

9. 70% Percoll solution: 7 ml of Percoll, 1 ml of 10× PBS, 0.1 ml of heat-inactivated fetal bovine serum, and 1.9 ml of H_2O (*see* **Note 1**).
10. 1 L of 10× Phosphate-buffered saline (PBS): 80.0 g of NaCl, 11.6 g of Na_2HPO_4, 2.0 g of KH_2PO_4, 2.0 g of KCl, bring the volume up to 1 L with H_2O, and pH to 7.0.

2.3 Material for Characterization of Mast Cells

1. Mouse IgE (monoclonal, clone SPE-7).
2. FACS staining buffer (1% BSA in PBS).
3. HBSS buffer with calcium and magnesium.
4. Blocking antibody (anti-mouse FcγIII/II).
5. Specific antibodies to c-Kit and FcεRI, fluorescently labeled (Table 1).
6. Centrifuge.
7. Fluorescence-activated cell sorting instrument.
8. 5-ml polypropylene tubes.
9. Cytospin.
10. Microscopic slides.
11. Xylene.
12. Permount mounting solution.
13. Toluidine working solution: Mix 0.5 ml of toluidine blue stock solution (0.5 g toluidine blue O in 50 ml of 70% EtOH) in 4.5 ml of 1% sodium chloride (0.5 g NaCl in 50 ml ddH_2O).
14. Alcian blue staining solution (0.5% of Alcian blue in 0.3% of acetic acid): Dissolve 50 mg of Alcian blue 8 GX in 10 ml of ddH_2O with 30 μl of glacial acetic acid.

15. Safranin staining solution (0.1% safranin O in 0.1% acetic acid): Dissolve 10 mg of safranin O in 10 ml of ddH_2O with 10 μl of glacial acetic acid.
16. Glycine/carbonate buffer (0.2 M glycine, 0.1 M Na_2CO_3, pH 10.0): 1.06 g of Na_2CO_3, 1.50 g of glycine, and bring the volume up to 100 ml with H_2O.
17. Citrate buffer (0.1 M sodium citrate, 0.1 M citric acid, pH 4.5): Dissolve 2.94 g of sodium citrate in 100 ml H_2O. Dissolve 2.10 g of citric acid in 100 ml of H_2O. Mix 25 ml of 0.1 M citric acid and 20 ml of 0.1 M sodium citrate to get 45 ml of citrate buffer.
18. p-NAG solution (2.5 mM s *p*-nitrophenyl *N*-acetyl-β-d-glucosaminide in citrate buffer): 38.7 mg in 45 ml of citrate buffer.

3 Methods

3.1 Isolation and Differentiation of Bone Marrow-Derived Mast Cells from Mast Cell Progenitors

1. Euthanize mice 6–12 weeks of age by CO_2 inhalation and saturate the mouse with 70% ethanol.
2. Clip the abdominal skin below the sternum, grab on both sides of the incision with forceps, and remove the skin from the lower part of the body including the legs. Dissect the legs away from body with scissors.
3. Remove muscle from the legs with scissors and cut off the fibula. Clean the remaining tissue from a tibia using low-linting paper wipers. It is important to remove all the tissue to prevent contamination of the bone marrow preparation.
4. Separate the tibia from the femoral bone at the knee joint. Ensure that the tibia is intact to prevent contamination of the bone marrow. Saturate the tibia with 70% ethanol and place it on a 3 cm plastic plate with sterile ice-cold PBS. From this point, it is necessary that all procedures are carried out in a laminar flow hood with sterile tools, material, and solutions.
5. Grip the tibia with sterile forceps and cut off each end of bone.
6. Using a 25 G needle and a 5 cc syringe filled with mast cell medium (*see* **Note 2**), expel the bone marrow from both ends of the bone with a jet of medium directed into a 15 ml conical tube.
7. Centrifuge at 300 × *g* for 10 min at 4 °C and resuspend cells in 4 ml of mast cell medium.
8. Culture mast cells in 1 well of a 6-well tissue culture plate. Incubate cells at 37 °C in a humidified incubator under 5% (v/v) CO_2 for 4 weeks (*see* **Note 3**).

9. Change medium every 5–7 days or any time the medium changes color to orange or yellow. Regularly remove adherent cells from the culture by transferring the mast cell culture to a new plate. Remove excess mast cells or split the cell culture into bigger tissue culture plates if necessary (*see* **Note 3**).

3.2 Isolation and Differentiation of Mast Cell Progenitors from Newborn Liver

1. Isolate the liver and keep it on ice in IMDM medium.
2. Immediately after isolation, cut the liver into small pieces and pass them through the 70 μm nylon cell strainer by mincing with the tip of a 10 ml pipette containing mast cell medium.
3. Spin the cell suspension at 300×*g* for 10 min at room temperature.
4. Wash cells once with 5 ml of mast cell medium.
5. Resuspend cells in mast cell medium and transfer them to a 10 cm tissue culture plate with 20 ml of complete media.
6. Change medium every 5–7 days or any time the medium changes color to orange or yellow for 4 weeks. Regularly remove adherent cells from the culture by transferring the cells in suspension to a new plate.

3.3 Isolation of Peritoneal Mast Cells

1. Prepare a 5 ml syringe fitted with a 25 G short needle and filled with 3 ml of PBS. Leave approximately 1 ml of air in the syringe (*see* **Note 4**).
2. Euthanize mice by CO_2 inhalation.
3. Make an incision into the abdominal skin below the sternum, taking care not to clip the peritoneal wall.
4. Grab the two sides of the cut using forceps and gently pull apart the abdominal skin, exposing the sternum and the pelvis.
5. Hold the peritoneum with forceps and gently fill the abdominal cavity with PBS and the air without disturbing blood vessels. The peritoneum should self-seal after removal of the needle.
6. Shake the mouse body gently about 20 times to increase the yield of cells in the peritoneal fluid.
7. Hold the peritoneal wall with forceps and make a small hole using scissors to insert a transfer plastic pipette into the air pocket in the peritoneal cavity. The previously injected air minimizes the loss of fluid in this step (*see* **Note 5**).
8. Express the air from the pipette in the cavity and aspirate the medium and the peritoneal cells.
9. While still holding the peritoneum, longitudinally open the abdominal wall using scissors. Collect the remaining peritoneal fluid.

10. Collect peritoneal cells from five mice (*see* **Note 6**).
11. Centrifuge the cell suspension for 5 min at 300 × *g* at room temperature and remove supernatant.
12. Resuspend the pellet in 8 ml of 70% isotonic Percoll solution and transfer to a 15 ml conical tube (*see* **Note 7**).
13. Gently overlay the 70% Percoll solution with 2 ml of peritoneal mast cell (PMC) medium and centrifuge for 15 min at 700 × *g* at room temperature. Mast cells and red blood cells (RBC) will form a pellet, while other cells will form a layer on the Percoll/PMC medium interface.
14. Carefully remove and discard the top layer and Percoll gradient without disturbing the mast cell pellet at the bottom of the tube.
15. Resuspend the mast cell pellet with 0.5 ml of PMC medium and transfer to a clean 15 ml conical tube with 10 ml of PMC medium (*see* **Note 8**).
16. Centrifuge for 5 min at 400 × *g* and resuspend the pellet in 1 ml of PMC medium (*see* **Note 9**).

3.4 Characterization of Mast Cells Based on FcεRI and c-Kit Receptor Expression Using Fluorescence-Activated Cell Sorting (See Fig. 1)

1. Harvest 2×10^6 cells from each tested culture of mast cells.
2. Centrifuge cells for 5 min at 300 × *g* at room temperature, and resuspend the cell pellet in 4 ml of fluorescence-activated cell sorting (FACS) staining buffer.
3. Separate cells into four 5 ml polypropylene tubes, each of which will contain 1 ml of cell suspension (5×10^5 cells).
4. Centrifuge the cells for 5 min at 300 × *g* at room temperature, resuspend the cells in 250 μl of 1:100 diluted blocking antibody

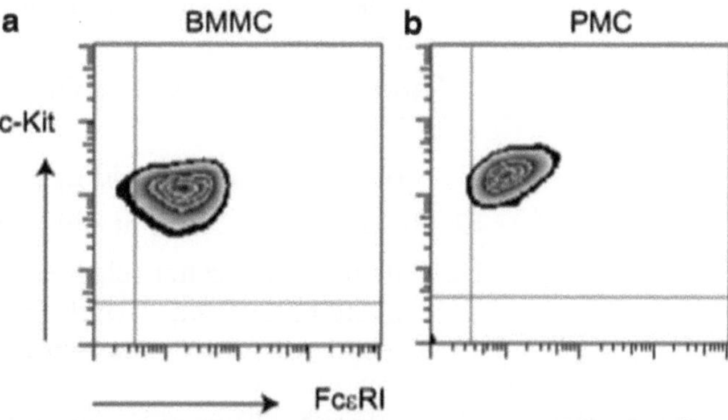

Fig. 1 Analysis of FcεRI and c-Kit expression on the surface of mast cells using fluorescence-activated cell sorting. Mast cells were differentiated from bone marrow (**a**) or isolated from mouse peritoneal cells (**b**). Cells were stained with fluorescently labeled specific antibodies and analyzed on a FACS Cyan (Beckman Coulter). Surface expression of FcεRI and c-Kit is similar in both types of mast cells

(anti-mouse FcγIII/II) in FACS staining buffer, and incubate for at least 5 min at room temperature.

5. Add 250 μl of 1:100 dilution of appropriate specific Ab in FACS staining buffer into each tube, as shown in Table 1 (*see* **Note 10**).
6. Incubate for at least 30 min at room temperature.
7. Wash once with 2 ml of FACS staining buffer.
8. Resuspend the cells in 0.5 ml of FACS staining buffer and measure fluorescence using a FACS instrument. More than 95% of mast cells in culture should be positive for both c-Kit and FcεRI in order to be ready for experiments.

3.5 Characterization of Mast Cells Based on Hexosaminidase Release

1. Incubate 3×10^6 mast cells with 1 μg of IgE overnight.
2. Wash cells two times in HBSS buffer with calcium and magnesium and 0.1% bovine serum albumin (BSA).
3. Resuspend cells in 2.0 ml of HBSS buffer.
4. Dilute antigen (HSA–BSA) by twofold serial dilution in HBSS buffer with calcium and magnesium and 0.1% BSA. The highest concentration recommended is 100 ng/ml. Prepare 0.2% Triton X-100 by mixing 40 μl of Triton 10% solution in 2 ml of PBS.
5. Pre-warm the cell suspension at 37 °C and transfer 100 μl of the cell suspension (150,000 cells) to each well of a 96-well plate.
6. Add 100 μl of diluted antigen, 0.2% Triton X-100 for positive control, or HBSS buffer for negative (basal release) control.
7. Incubate at 37 °C for 30 min.
8. Spin the plate in a centrifuge at $300 \times g$ for 3 min.
9. Transfer 10 μl of supernatant from each sample to a new 96-well plate.
10. Add 50 μl of p-NAG solution and incubate for 90 min at 37 °C.
11. Stop the reaction by adding 200 μl glycine/carbonate buffer.
12. Read the absorbance at 405 nm.
13. Calculation: For net release, subtract the basal release of non-activated cells from all of the results. The release in 0.2% Triton X-100 equals 100% (*see* **Note 11**).

3.6 Staining Mast Cell Granules Using a Cytospin Preparation

1. Wash 10^5 cells from the mast cell cultures or isolations in cold 1% BSA/PBS once and resuspend in 100 μl of cold 1% BSA/PBS.
2. Place marked slides and filters into appropriate slots in the cytospin with filters facing the center of the cytospin.

3. Aliquot 100 μl of each sample into the appropriate wells of the cytospin.
4. Place the cytospin lid over the samples and spin at 300 × *g* for 3 min.
5. Remove the filters and slides.
6. Examine each slide under the microscope to ensure that the cells are reasonably dispersed.
7. Air-dry the slides overnight. Do not fix the cells for toluidine and alcian blue/safranin staining.

3.7 Characterization of Mast Cells Based on Alcian Blue: Safranin O Staining

1. Incubate the air-dried cytospin for 10 min with a solution of 0.5% alcian blue in 0.3% acetic acid (pH 3).
2. Wash slides in PBS two times.
3. Incubate slides for 10 min with a solution of 0.1% safranin O in 0.1% acetic acid (pH 4).
4. Wash with PBS.
5. Air-dry.
6. Mount with mounting medium.

3.8 Characterization of Mast Cells Based on Toluidine Blue Staining (See Fig. 2)

1. Stain air-dry cytospins in toluidine blue working solution for 5 min.
2. Wash in PBS three times.
3. Dehydrate quickly in 100% EtOH.
4. To further clear slides, wash slides in xylene three times.
5. Air-dry in a chemical hood.
6. Mount with mounting medium.

4 Notes

1. Media are prepared under sterile conditions in a laminar flow hood to prevent contamination. After mixing all components, medium must be filtered through a 0.22 μm filter to sterilize and store up to 1 month at 2–8 °C.
2. This protocol is using mast cell medium based on IMDM. Alternatively, RPMI can be used. However, to reach the same efficiency of proliferation and differentiation of mast cell cultures as with IMDM, the concentrations of IL-3 in RPMI medium should be increased to 20 ng/ml.
3. Mast cell progenitors are expanding exponentially during differentiation. The amount of mast cells can be increased by transferring mast cell cultures to bigger tissue culture plates. Volume of culture medium can be increased at any time during

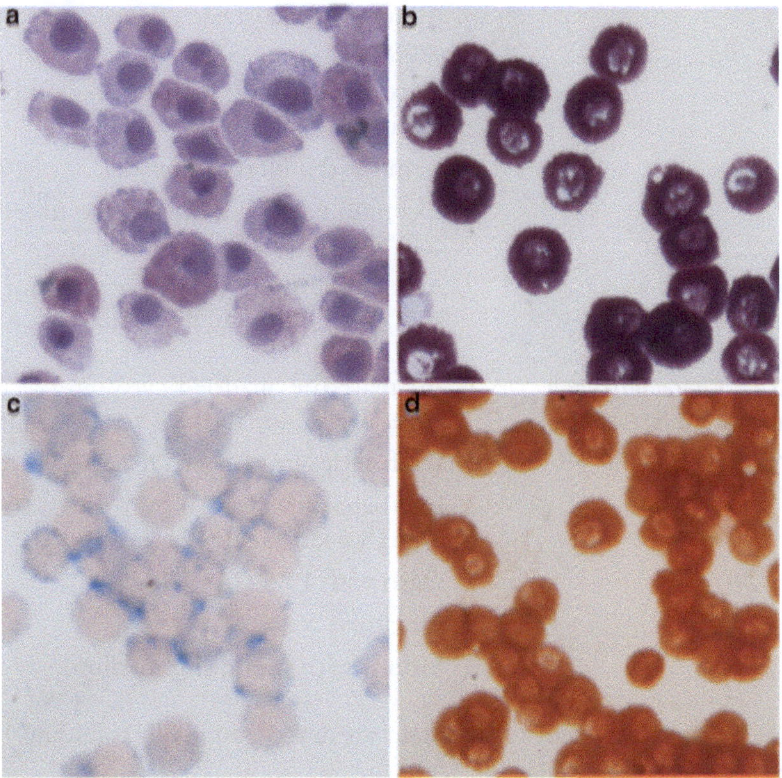

Fig. 2 Mast cell staining and evaluation of mast cell maturity and protease content in mast cell granules. Mast cells were obtained either by differentiation from bone marrow (**a**, **c**) or isolated from mouse peritoneal cells (**b**, **d**). Cells were stained with toluidine blue (**a**, **b**) or with alcian blue/safranin (**c**, **d**). Bone marrow-derived mast cells have only minimal amount of toluidine-stained granules compared to peritoneal mast cells. Bone marrow-derived mast cells stained with alcian blue, but not with safranin. Peritoneal mast cells have high heparin content and their granules can be stained with safranin

the culture process. For this reason, the protocol only uses the tibia for bone marrow isolation and 4 ml of medium for culture. This provides a sufficient amount of mast cells for most applications. For high-volume mast cell cultures, bone marrow from both femurs of the mouse and larger volumes of medium can be used at the beginning of differentiation.

4. Injected air makes collection of the fluid from the peritoneal cavity easier and minimizes fluid loss.
5. In this protocol, RBC are isolated together with mast cells. Thus, it is important to avoid any disturbance of blood vessels on the peritoneal wall during the isolation of peritoneal cells.
6. On average, the mouse peritoneal cavity contains only 10^5 mast cells. For effective isolation, five mice have to be pooled on one Percoll gradient.

7. The Percoll solution must be of room temperature during the cell separation for effective isolation of mast cells from the other peritoneal cells.
8. Mast cells are isolated together with RBC. RBC-lysis buffer can remove RBC. However, this treatment interferes with some applications (i.e., assessments of mast cell apoptosis). Small numbers of RBC do not affect most mast cell studies. Thus, for most applications RBC lysis is not necessary.
9. Isolated peritoneal mast cells can be immediately used for experiments; alternatively, PMC can be cultured in mast cell medium for several weeks. Their expansion, however, is minimal compared to mast cells derived from mast cell progenitors.
10. Samples 2 and 3 in Table 1 are not necessary for each culture tested. Those samples are needed only for compensation during the setup of the FACS instrument.
11. Mast cell degranulation typically ranges from 15 to 80% depending on many factors including the type of stimulation, mouse strain [9], and amount of cytokines in the culture medium [10].

References

1. Kovarova M, Rivera J (2004) A molecular understanding of mast cell activation and the promise of anti-allergic therapeutics. Curr Med Chem 11:2083–2091
2. Isersky C, Rivera J, Mims S, Triche TJ (1979) The fate of IgE bound to rat basophilic leukemia cells. J Immunol 122:1926–1936
3. Galli SJ, Tsai M (2012) IgE and mast cells in allergic disease. Nat Med 18:693–704
4. Kovarova M, Latour AM, Chanson KD, Tilley SL, Koller BH (2010) Human embryonic stem cells: a source of mast cells for the study of allergic and inflammatory diseases. Blood 115:3695–3703
5. Olivera A, Mizugishi K, Tikhonova A, Ciaccia L, Odom S, Proia RL, Rivera J (2007) The sphingosine kinase-sphingosine-1-phosphate axis is a determinant of mast cell function and anaphylaxis. Immunity 26:287–297
6. Kovarova M, Wassif CA, Odom S, Liao K, Porter FD, Rivera J (2006) Cholesterol deficiency in a mouse model of Smith-Lemli-Opitz syndrome reveals increased mast cell responsiveness. J Exp Med 203:1161–1171
7. Feyerabend TB, Hausser H, Tietz A, Blum C, Hellman L, Straus AH, Takahashi HK, Morgan ES, Dvorak AM, Fehling HJ, Rodewald HR (2005) Loss of histochemical identity in mast cells lacking carboxypeptidase A. Mol Cell Biol 25:6199–6210
8. Collington SJ, Williams TJ, Weller CL (2011) Mechanisms underlying the localisation of mast cells in tissues. Trends Immunol 32:478–485
9. Yamashita Y, Charles N, Furumoto Y, Odom S, Yamashita T, Gilfillan AM, Constant S, Bower MA, Ryan JJ, Rivera J (2007) Genetic variation influences Fc epsilonRI-induced mast cell activation and allergic responses. J Immunol 179:740–754
10. Ito T, Smrž D, Jung MY, Bandara G, Desai A, Smržová Š, Kuehn HS, Beaven MA, Metcalfe DD, Gilfillan AM (2012) Stem cell factor programs the mast cell activation phenotype. J Immunol 188:5428–5437

Chapter 9

Purifying and Measuring Immunoglobulin E (IgE) and Anti-IgE

Jamie L. Sturgill and Daniel H. Conrad

Abstract

Immunoglobulins (Igs) are a critical component of the adaptive immune system of both man and mouse. The ability to detect and characterize Igs is an invaluable technique for immunology in either a research or a clinical setting. The advent of enzyme-linked immunosorbent assays (ELISAs) and monoclonal antibody technology has proven instrumental for advancing the science of Ig biology. IgE is of interest as it is the primary Ig responsible for allergic reactions ranging from allergic rhinitis to anaphylaxis. Here, we describe the history behind the IgE discovery and the protocol for purifying IgE and anti-IgE in the mouse. This is followed by our ELISA protocol for mouse IgE detection.

Key words ELISA, Immunoglobulin, IgE, Hybridoma, Antibody purification

1 Introduction

Allergies are defined as the body's response to a normally innocuous substance, such as pollen. Allergic diseases occur in many forms, such as rhinitis, sinusitis, conjunctivitis, eczema, asthma, gastroenteral complications, or in severe cases anaphylaxis or even death. The World Health Organization (WHO) estimates that over 20 % of the world's population suffers from some type of allergic disease with about 150 million people having allergic asthma alone. In the United States, the National Institute of Allergy and Infectious Diseases (NIAID) approximates that between 40 and 50 million Americans suffer from these types of illnesses. With such widespread prevalence in the global population, allergic disease ranks as one of the highest causes of chronic illness and costs billions of dollars annually.

While the general public is all too familiar with the outward signs and symptoms, the underlying biological cause of allergic disease is due to a hypersensitivity reaction of the immune system to inherently harmless matter. Hypersensitivity reactions were classified

Irving C. Allen (ed.), *Mouse Models of Allergic Disease: Methods and Protocols*, Methods in Molecular Biology, vol. 1032, DOI 10.1007/978-1-62703-496-8_9,

into four distinct groups, or types, by Gell and Coombs in 1963 [1]. Allergic reactions are classified as type 1 because they are mediated by IgE. However at the time, Gell and Coombs referred to Type 1 simply as an "immediate hypersensitivity" because a reaction occurred in minutes. Furthermore, this temporal classification stood because IgE was not officially recognized as the fifth immunoglobulin subtype until 1968.

Although the immediate hypersensitivity phenomenon was officially classified in the 1960s, its existence had been reported since the early 1800s. In 1819, Dr. John Bostock reported the first case of pollen-induced hay fever to the Royal Medical and Chirurgical Society in London and the patient he presented was himself [2]. However, it would take almost another 100 years to link the symptoms of hay fever to a soluble serum factor. In the early 1900s, a French physiologist by the name Richet observed that "while a foreign substance might induce a mild reaction upon first exposure, it could produce severe hypersensitive symptoms and even death when re-introduced late." [3]. Richet observed that a repeated dose offered no protection, or phylaxis. Thus he coined the term, "anaphylaxis," meaning without protection. In 1919, Ramirez reported the first case of an asthma attack subsequent to a blood transfusion. In this case, a man by the name of "H.T.," who had no prior personal or family medical history of allergic disease, received a blood transfusion for anemia. Subsequently, after an encounter with a horse at Central Park, the man suffered a violet asthma attack [4]. While this was an observational report, the first experimental evidence was provided by Prausnitz and Küstner. Küstner, who was a German gynecologist, had previously noted that he developed allergic symptoms after consuming fish. Prausnitz, who was also a fellow German physician, decided to inject some of Küstner's serum into the skin of his abdomen. After eating some fish himself, Prausnitz's, who had no prior adverse reactions to fish, suffered from hot, red, swollen skin at the site of the serum injection, confirming their hypothesis that Küstner was indeed allergic to fish. The work of these two men led to the development of the passive transfer of a positive skin test, later coined the PK test [5].

Although these types of hypersensitivities had been described as allergies, a term coined by Clemens Peter Freiherr von Pirquet, two American physicians felt that the "allergy" label was too limiting. Thus, in 1923, Coca and Cooke introduced the word "atopy" into medical vernacular. They felt atopy, which was derived from the Greek word "άτοπία" meaning placelessness, was a more suitable term to cover all forms of immediate hypersensitivities [6]. They went on to add that atopy was a result of "bodies" they referred to as "reagins." However, ironically enough they recommended that the term "antibody" should be avoided as they determined that "no evidence of these bodies appear as the result of immunologic stimulation" [7].

It took the next 40 years and the work of two pioneering groups to determine that "reagin" was indeed an antibody. Two Swedish scientists by the name of Bennich and Johansson studied structure and function of immunoglobulins (Ig). Their primary source of human Ig was multiple myeloma serum. In the summer of 1965, they came across a serum of a patient, "N.D.," whose serum contained an atypical Ig subtype. When compared to IgA, IgM, IgG, or even the newly identified IgD, they saw no similarities. They called this new protein IgX, for the unknown Ig. After further investigation, they discovered that IgX had unique biochemical properties, which were distinct from the other four types. They went on to develop very sensitive assays for the detection of IgX and noted that the normal serum concentration of IgX as compared to IgG was about 200,000-fold less. After collaborating with D.R. Stanworth, it was shown that IgX could block the PK test. Thus, all evidence was pointing to a new class of Ig. Eventually IgX was renamed IgND after the initial patient from which it was isolated. Because of the finding that IgND could inhibit the PK test, Bennich and Johansson began to look at IgND in the context of atopic disease and ultimately went on to develop the radioallergosorbent test (RAST) [8].

Meanwhile in Denver CO, a husband and wife team were approaching a similar problem, but from a different angle. Kimishige and Teruka Ishizaka were interested in identifying the biological cause of the reagin-mediated histamine release reaction. In 1964, they first reported that the antibody responsible for this was a type of IgA, which they initially called γA [9]. While this was not widely accepted in the field, they persevered and ultimately identified an antiserum capable of precipitating a serum fraction that could block the PK reaction [10]. This activity did not appear to be similar to any of the other known four Ig types; thus they called it γE-globulin because it had the ability to cause an erythema reaction. However, despite all their hard work, the Ishizakas were never able to make a purified preparation of γE-globulin from normal human serum. However, given its extremely low concentration in normal serum, this observation is not too surprising. In early 1967, a fruitful collaboration between the Ishizakas and the Swedish took place. They decided to swap reagents and it was indeed found that IgND and γE-globulin were one in the same. In February of 1968 at a workshop at the WHO, it was agreed upon that IgE would be the new nomenclature for the newly identified fifth Ig subclass [11].

Like all immunoglobulins, IgE comprises two identical light chains, either κ or λ, and two identical heavy chains, the ε chains, which are held together by disulfide bonds. Both light and heavy chains each contain a variable and constant domain. This basic chemical structure of Igs was solved by the work of Edelman and Porter for which they received the Nobel Prize in 1972 [12]. The variable regions of IgE are responsible for antigen binding specificity, whereas the heavy chain determines effector function. The characteristics that make IgE unique from the other subclasses reside in the ε heavy-chain component. IgE has a molecular weight of about 190 kDa, which when resolved under reducing conditions yields two light chains and two heavy chains of about 23 and 72 kDa, respectively [13]. IgE is slightly larger than the monomeric forms of IgG, IgA, and IgD because it has an additional domain in the heavy ε chain called Cε4 and it is more heavily glycosylated. Studies with tunicamycin have shown that the glycosylation of IgE is N-linked; however, these additional sugar moieties are not critical for IgE binding to its receptors on mast cells [14].

In addition to its unique structure, IgE has biological activities that are much different than its other Ig counterparts. IgE fails to neutralize, opsonize, participate in antibody-directed cellular cytotoxicity (ADCC), or fix complement. IgE also fails to transport across epithelial surfaces or the placenta and only under instances of widespread inflammation can IgE diffuse into extravascular sites. Serum IgE has a half-life of approximately 3 days, whereas IgG is stable for up to 3 weeks. The reported mean serum levels of IgE are approximately $0.5–3 \times 10^{-5}$ mg/ml, which is much less than 1.5, 9, or 2.1 mg/ml as seen with IgM, IgG1, or IgA, respectively [15].

Although most equated with unwanted reactions of the immune system, IgE serves a very important evolutionary role in the defense against parasitic disease. Elevated levels of IgE are observed in both man and mouse during parasite infections. Capron et al. have shown a critical role for IgE in the clearance of *Schistosoma mansoni* [16] and it has been reported that IgE-deficient mice have increased worm burden following infection with *S. mansoni* [17], *Brugia malayi* [18], and *Trichinella spiralis* [19]. This protective effect of IgE in the context of microbial pathogens is the basis for the hygiene hypothesis. This theory, originally proposed by the epidemiologist Strachan in the 1980s, states that the declining microbial exposure in industrialized countries is a major causative factor in the increased rise in atopic disease [20].

In this review, we summarize newer methodologies to grow and isolate large amounts of monoclonal mouse IgE and anti-IgE. The use of the purified anti-IgE to measure mouse IgE is also given.

2 Materials

2.1 Antibody Purification

1. The anti-mouse IgE hybridomas B1E3 [21] and R1E4 (kindly provided by M. Kehry) and the mouse IgE anti-DNP hybridoma [22] (kindly provided by F-T. Liu) were all maintained in our laboratory.

2. If needed, antibodies were biotinylated using a 100-fold molar excess of EZ-link Sulfo-NHS-biotin (Pierce, Rockford IL) as per the manufacturer's protocol and dialyzed against 1× PBS.
3. All antibodies were prepared from hybridoma cell culture supernatant using the CL-1000 Adhere CELLine flasks (Integra Biosciences, Switzerland).
4. Cells were grown in complete RPMI-1640 containing 10 % heat-inactivated fetal bovine serum, 2 mMl-glutamine, 50 μg/ml penicillin, 50 μg/ml streptomycin, 1 mM sodium pyruvate, 50 μg/ml amphotericin B, 50 μM 2-mercaptoethanol, 2 μg/ml gentamicin, 100 μM NEAA, and 20 mM HEPES buffer.
5. Cell viability is always measured via Trypan Blue exclusion and if this falls below 50 %, dead cells are removed by density centrifugation over Ficoll-Hypaque.
6. All antibodies were purified by hydrophobic charge induction chromatography using the MEP HypeCel sorbert (Pall Life Sciences, East Hills, NY).
7. Antibody purification is done on a Bio-Rad BioLogic DuoFLow FPLC system.
8. Elution is performed using a series of pH buffers (*see* Table 1).

Table 1
Full eluotropic series

	Buffer/sample	Concentration and amount
1	PBS	25 ml
2	Sample	50–200 ml
3	PBS	Until OD280 < 0.05
4	Water	40 ml
5	2-(*N*-Morpholino)ethanesulfonic acid (MES)	0.05 M, pH 5.5
6	MES	0.05 M, pH 5.2–50 ml
7	Sodium acetate	0.05 M, pH 4.9–50 ml
8	Sodium acetate	0.05 M, pH 4.6–50 ml
9	Sodium acetate	0.05 M, pH 4.4–50 ml
10	Sodium acetate	0.05 M, pH 4.0–50 ml
11	Sodium acetate	0.05 M, pH 3.0–50 ml
12	PBS	50 ml

PBS is 0.01 M Na phosphate, 0.14 M NaCl, pH 7.4

9. After chromatography was complete, fractions were separated on a 10 % Bis–Tris gel (Invitrogen) by SDS-PAGE under reduced conditions.
10. To visualize proteins, gels were stained with SDS-PAGE stain (2.5 g Commassie Blue Brilliant Blue R-250, 100 ml glacial acetic acid, 450 ml methanol, and 450 ml dH_2O) for 30 min during continual motion.
11. Gels were then subsequently destained with SDS-PAGE Destain (30 % methanol, 10 % acetic acid, 60 % dH_2O).
12. Protein was concentrated by ultrafiltration with an Amicon filtration unit (Millipore Corporation, Bedford, MA) and dialyzed against 1× PBS.

2.2 ELISA

1. All coating steps are done with borate-buffered saline (0.17 M boric acid, 0.125 M NaCl, pH 8.5, and filter sterilized). Do not attempt to make a 10× stock of BBS as the solution will become saturated.
2. ELISA wash, when indicated, is 1× PBS with 0.02 % Tween-20.
3. Mouse IgE block is 5 ml of 10 mM Hepes, 2 % FBS, up to 500 ml with PBS. Filter sterilize and add 0.02 % Tween-20.
4. Streptavidin AP antibody is purchased from Southern Biotech.
5. Substrate tablets are pNPP substrate tablets (Sigma).
6. Substrate buffer is made by adding to 300 ml water 0.1 g $MgCl_2 \cdot 6H_2O$, 0.2 g NaN_3, 50 ml diethanolamine, pH to 9.8, up to 500 ml. It is important to keep this solution away from light.

3 Methods

3.1 Antibody Purification (See Notes 1 and 2)

1. The integra flasks have an outer compartment which holds 1 L of serum-free media and cells are seeded into the inner chamber, which contains 15 ml of the same media plus 10 % heat-inactivated FBS. Flasks were initially seeded with 100×10^6 cells.
2. Two times per week, the outside media is replaced and the cells removed from the inner chamber. The inner chamber supernatant is collected and frozen and 1/3 of the cells are returned to the inner chamber with fresh media.
3. Cell viability is always measured via Trypan Blue exclusion and if this falls below 50 %, dead cells are removed by density centrifugation over Ficoll-Hypaque.
4. When supernatants were harvested, they were centrifuged at $400 \times g$ for 5 min and stored at −20 °C until purification.

5. When at least 200 ml has been collected, just prior to purification, supernatants were pooled and further clarified by centrifugation at 2,400 × *g* for 30 min.
6. All antibodies from hybridomas were purified by hydrophobic charge induction chromatography using the MEP HypeCel sorbert, which is immunoglobulin selective and binds a broad range of Ig subtypes as previously described both due to hydrophobic and affinity reasons, virtually all immunoglobulin classes bind to this absorbent [23] (*see* **Note 3**).
7. This purification is done on a Bio-Rad BioLogic DuoFLow FPLC system and the program is adjusted so as to wash with PBS until OD from applied supernatant (up to 200 ml can be applied at a time—the flow rate is maintained at 2/ml/min) drops below 0.05 OD280 (*see* **Note 4**).
8. The column is then washed for 10 min with water, which helps elute bound albumin—then the protein is eluted with a low pH buffer. If using a new monoclonal and the eluting pH is not known, then a series of pH buffers are applied (*see* Table 1) and the pH at which the monoclonal Ig elutes is recorded.
9. Subsequent purifications can then use the eluting pH plus the pH 3.0 buffer. The latter elutes bound light chain, which is a common contaminant in monoclonal supernatants. An example of the FPLC purification of mouse IgE anti-DNP is shown in Fig. 1 and IgG anti-mouse IgE (R1E4) [24] in Fig. 2.
10. After chromatography was complete, fractions were separated on a 10 % Bis–Tris gel by SDS-PAGE under reduced conditions (*see* **Note 5**).
11. To visualize proteins, gels were stained with SDS-PAGE stain for 30 min during continual motion.
12. Gels were then subsequently destained with SDS-PAGE Destain.
13. After the fractions which were determined to contain purified antibody were pooled together, protein was concentrated by ultrafiltration with an Amicon filtration unit and dialyzed against 1× PBS.
14. In each case the insert shows the SDS-PAGE analysis of the purified protein and as can be seen, a purity of about 95 % is accomplished in just this single step. The mouse IgE anti-DNP yield, as well as most monoclonal IgG yields, is about 50–75 mg per 200 ml of Integra supernatant.

3.2 ELISA for IgE Detection

1. Coat a Maxisorp ELISA plate with 100 μL/well of the 10 μg/ml of the rat anti-mouse IgE mab clone B1E3 in borate-buffered saline (*see* **Note 6**).
2. Incubate either for 1 h at 37 °C or O/N at 4 °C (*see* **Note 7**).

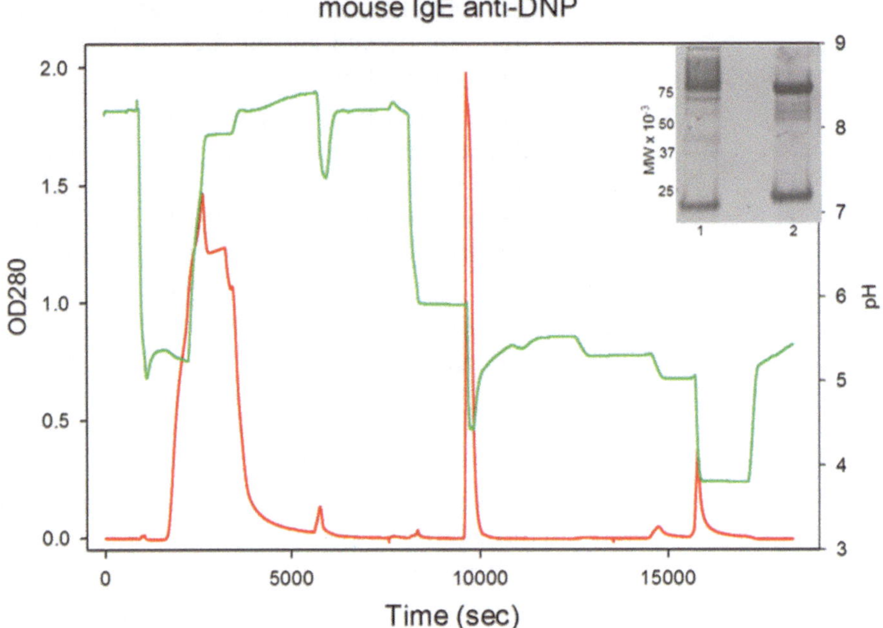

Fig. 1 Mouse IgE anti-DNP purification on MEP-Hypercel. 200 ml of Integra collected sample is applied to a 20 ml MEP-Hypercel column ((red solid line) OD280, (green solid line) pH. The column is then washed with PBS until the OD280 is less than 0.05. 50 ml of distilled water is followed by 50 ml of PBS and then the IgE is eluted using 0.05 M Na acetate, pH 4.9. After the IgE peak is completely off the column, residual light chain is eluted using the Na acetate buffer at pH 3.0. The MEP-Hypercel is then washed with 50 ml of PBS and reused for additional IgE purifications as needed. The *insert* shows (*Lane 1*) rat IgE, IR162, purified by conventional chromatography (*ref*) and (*Lane 2*) the mouse IgE anti-DNP after pooling the peak and concentrating. 10 μg of protein was applied per lane

3. Wash the plate twice with diH_2O.
4. Block the plate with mouse IgE block 200 μL/well.
5. Incubate either for 2 h at 37 °C or O/N at 4 °C (*see* **Note 7**).
6. Wash the plate twice with diH_2O.
7. Add 100 μL/well of the samples, blanks, and standards. Standard curves were generated with mouse IgE anti-DNP beginning at a concentration of 1,000 ng/ml and diluted 1:2 across the plate.
8. Incubate either for 1 h at 37 °C or O/N at 4 °C (*see* **Note 7**).
9. Wash plates 2× with diH_2O, 2× with ELISA wash, and 2× with diH_2O.
10. Detection is done by incubation of the plates with 100 μL/well of the biotinylated rat anti-mouse IgE mab R1E4. We purify from hybridoma in house and use at a concentration of 1:4,000.
11. Incubate for 1–2 h at 37 °C.

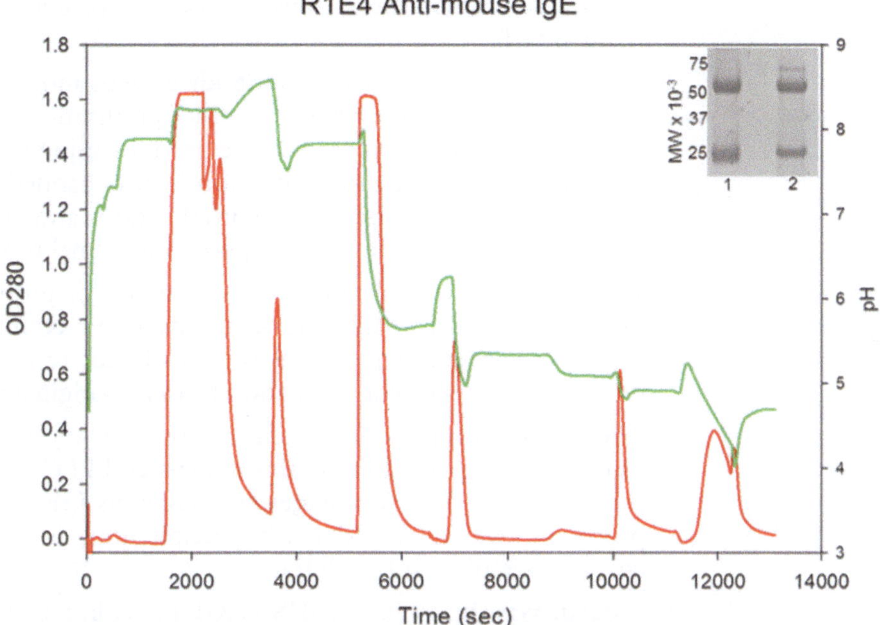

Fig. 2 Monoclonal anti-mouse IgE (R1E4) purification on MEP-Hypercel. 200 ml of Integra collected sample is applied to a 20 ml MEP-Hypercel column as in Fig. 1; *lines* are also presented as in Fig. 1. The column is then washed with PBS, water, and PBS again. Following the second PBS wash, the R1E4 is eluted by using the 0.05 M MES, pH 5.2 buffer. Some additional R1E4 is eluted with the pH 4.9 buffer, the second peak is less pure (not shown). Residual light chain and other contaminants are eluted with the pH 3.0 buffer and washed with PBS. The *insert* shows commercial rat IgG (*Lane 1*) and the pH 5.2 R1E4 peak after pooling and concentrating (*Lane 2*). 10 μg of protein was applied per lane

12. Wash plates 2× with diH_2O, 2× with ELISA wash, and 2× with diH_2O.
13. Add 100 μL/well of streptavidin-AP at 1:400 for 1 h at 37 °C.
14. Wash plates 2× with diH_2O, 2× with ELISA wash, and 2× with diH_2O.
15. To develop plates add 100 μL/well of substrate. Substrate is pNPP substrate tablets diluted in substrate buffer. Add one tablet for every 5 ml of substrate buffer.
16. Read at OD 405 nm.

4 Notes

1. Given the relatively low concentration of IgE in serum and the fact that IgE is only made after multiple rounds of cellular division in vitro, detection of IgE needs to be specific and sensitive. This protocol has been used in our previous publications

and the source of the various monoclonal proteins is noted there as well.

2. This strategy for monoclonal antibody growth and purification has considerable advantages over other purification strategies. Use of the Integra flasks avoids the need for using animals for ascite production. Ascite production is now banned in many areas due to animal discomfort considerations and even when allowed, strict regulations are required for animal monitoring.
3. We reuse the MEP-hypercel multiple times for purifying the same monoclonal. While the same adsorbent could also be used for different monoclonal Igs, this is not recommended due to low levels of contamination from the original protein.
4. The final Ig product is free from any contamination by normal mouse or rat Ig. In addition, this single-step FPLC purification procedure has clear advantages over previous IgE purification protocols, which required salt precipitation, ion exchange chromatography, and gel filtration.
5. Indeed, as is shown in the SDS-PAGE insert in Fig. 1, the IgE purity is superior to the multistep protocol [24] that was used for the IR162 rat myeloma IgE.
6. The ELISA plates we utilize are the Nunc Maxisorp Plates which ensure high protein binding.
7. This step in the ELISA protocol can be done overnight.

References

1. Gell P, Coombs R (1963) Clinical aspects of immunology. In: Blackwell K (ed) 1st edn. Oxford, England
2. Hurwitz SH (1929) The lure of medical history: John Bostock (1773–1846): author of the first clinical description of hay fever. Cal West Med 31(2):137–138
3. Tan SY, Yamanuha J (2010) Charles Robert Richet (1850–1935): discoverer of anaphylaxis. Singapore Med J 51(3):184–185
4. Ramirez M (1919) Horse asthma following blood transfusion: report on a case. J Am Med Assoc 73(13):984–985
5. Prausnitz D, Kustner H (1921) Studien uber die Ueberempfindlichkeit. Zentrabl Bakteriol [A] 86:160–175
6. Coca A, Cooke R (1923) On the classification of the phenomena of hypersensitiveness. J Immunol 8:163–182
7. Johansson SG (2006) The discovery of immunoglobulin E. Allergy Asthma Proc 27(2 Suppl 1):S3–S6
8. Stanworth DR, Humphrey JH, Bennich H, Johansson SGO (1968) Inhibition of Prausnitz-Kustner reaction by proteolytic-cleavage fragments of a human myeloma protein of immunoglobulin class E. Lancet 2:17–18
9. Ishizaka K, Ishizaka T, Hathorn EM (1964) Blocking of Prausnitz-Kuestner sensitization with reagin by 'A Chain' of human gamma1A-globulin. Immunochemistry 1:197–207
10. Ishizaka K, Ishizaka T (1967) Identification of gamma-E-antibodies as a carrier of reaginic activity. J Immunol 99(6):1187–1198
11. Bennich HH, Ishizaka K, Johansson SG, Rowe DS, Stanworth DR, Terry WD (1968) Immunoglobulin E: a new class of human immunoglobulin. Immunology 15(3):323–324
12. (2010) Nobel Prize. http://www.nobelprize.org
13. Bennich H, Johansson SGO (1971) Structure and function of human immunoglobulin E. Adv Immunol 13:1–55
14. Conrad DH (1985) Structure and synthesis of IgE. In: Kaplan AP (ed) Allergy. Churchill Livingstone, New York, pp 3–21
15. Janeway CA, Travers P (1996) Immunobiology: the immune system in health and disease, 2nd edn. Current Biology Ltd., New York

16. Capron M, Capron A (1994) Immunoglobulin E and effector cells in schistosomiasis. Science 264:1876–1877
17. Conrad DH, Tinnell SB, Kelly AE (1998) Immunoglobulin E. In: Kaliner MA (ed) Current review of allergic disease. Blackwell Science, Philadelphia, pp 39–50
18. Spencer LA, Porte P, Zetoff C, Rajan TV (2003) Mice genetically deficient in immunoglobulin E are more permissive hosts than wild-type mice to a primary, but not secondary, infection with the filarial nematode Brugia malayi. Infect Immun 71(5):2462–2467
19. Gurish MF, Bryce PJ, Tao H, Kisselgof AB, Thornton EM, Miller HR, Friend DS, Oettgen HC (2004) IgE enhances parasite clearance and regulates mast cell responses in mice infected with Trichinella spiralis. J Immunol 172(2):1139–1145
20. Strachan DP (1989) Hay fever, hygiene and household size. Br Med J 229:1259–1260
21. Keegan AD, Fratazzi C, Shopes B, Baird B, Conrad DH (1991) Characterization of new rat anti-mouse IgE monoclonals and their use along with chimeric IgE to further define the site that interacts with $Fc_{\varepsilon}RII$ and $Fc_{\varepsilon}RI$. Mol Immunol 28:1149–1154
22. Liu F-T, Bohn JW, Ferry EL, Yamamoto H, Molinaro CA, Sherman LA, Klinman NR, Katz DH (1980) Monoclonal dinitrophenyl-specific murine IgE antibody: preparation, isolation, and characterization. J Immunol 124(6):2728–2737
23. Schwartz W, Jiao J, Ford J, Conrad D, Hamel JF, Santanbien P, Bradbury L, Robin T (2004) Application of chemically-stable immunoglobulin-selective sorbents: harvest and purification of antibodies with resolution of aggregate. BioProcess J 3(5):53–62
24. Isersky C, Kulczycki A Jr, Metzger H (1974) Isolation of IgE from reaginic rat serum. J Immunol 112:1909–1919

Chapter 10

Protocols for the Induction and Evaluation of Systemic Anaphylaxis in Mice

Elizabeth Doyle, Julia Trosien, and Martin Metz

Abstract

Mouse models of systemic anaphylaxis are important tools for the study of mast cell function, for the elucidation of the pathomechanisms of anaphylaxis, and for identifying and characterizing potential therapies for anaphylaxis. Here, we describe two murine models of systemic anaphylaxis that have been a key part of research in these areas. In a passive model, mice are sensitized with antigen-specific IgE antibody 24 h prior to antigen challenge. In an active model, mice are instead sensitized with antigen 18–21 days prior to challenge. Hypothermia serves as the primary quantifiable indicator of anaphylaxis in these models.

Key words Anaphylaxis, Anaphylactic shock, Active systemic anaphylaxis, Passive systemic anaphylaxis, Mast cell, IgE receptor, DNP–HSA, Ovalbumin, Pertussis toxin

1 Introduction

Those who have ever experienced and survived anaphylactic shock know about the dramatic nature of this reaction. Without warning, a life-threatening, systemic allergic reaction can occur within minutes after contact with an otherwise relatively innocuous substance like peanuts or venom from a wasp sting.

There are many open questions about anaphylaxis that still need to be addressed, for example: Why do only some people experience anaphylactic shock while others do not? It is well known that many allergic patients exhibit high levels of circulating antigen-specific IgE without ever experiencing anaphylaxis, whereas other subjects with low concentrations of specific IgE in the blood can suffer anaphylactic shock [1]. It must be inferred that other factors, in addition to antigen-specific IgE, also contribute to the occurrence or the severity of anaphylaxis.

Various candidates have emerged in the clinic and at the bench. For example, clinical observations have identified certain

Irving C. Allen (ed.), *Mouse Models of Allergic Disease: Methods and Protocols*, Methods in Molecular Biology, vol. 1032,
DOI 10.1007/978-1-62703-496-8_10, © Springer Science+Business Media, LLC 2013

drugs or vitamin D deficiency as non-IgE factors involved in occurrence and severity of anaphylaxis [2, 3]. In mouse models, we have identified a role for endothelin-1, a vasoconstrictive peptide that is up-regulated in some bacterial infections, in enhancing mast cell activation and thus likely contributing to the severity of an anaphylactic shock in mice [4]. Furthermore, there are continuing discussions about which cells and mediators are involved in anaphylaxis. While the importance of mast cells, the IgE receptor, and histamine are generally acknowledged, other cells, receptors, and mediators are also hypothesized to potentially affect an anaphylactic reaction [3, 5–7]. Additional cells and mediators include natural killer T cells, basophils, eosinophils, TRP proteins, IL-33, or PAF.

The use of mouse models of anaphylaxis is crucial to increasing our understanding of the pathomechanisms in anaphylaxis, and to identifying and characterizing potential therapeutic strategies for the treatment or the prevention of anaphylaxis. Because of the sudden and rapid reaction in the patient, the onset and course of an anaphylactic reaction can rarely be monitored, and provocation of anaphylaxis in a patient for scientific purposes is unethical.

Additionally, mouse models of systemic anaphylaxis can be utilized as model systems for in vivo analysis specifically of mast cell function. They offer unique opportunities to identify and characterize specific receptors on the mast cell surface or substances released by mast cells which might play a role in the many physiological or pathophysiological processes in which mast cells are involved.

Many different protocols for mouse models of systemic anaphylaxis have been reported in the literature. The main differences in these models are the experimental allergens (usually DNP–HSA, TNP–OVA, OVA, or BSA), the route of sensitization and challenge (i.p. or i.v.), and most importantly the method of sensitization of the mice. Passive sensitization, i.e., injection of antigen-specific IgE prior to challenge with the antigen, leads to the classical pathway of anaphylaxis involving IgE, mast cells, and histamine. Active sensitization in contrast is performed by sensitization with an allergen and adjuvant and involves IgG, macrophages, and PAF [8]. Here, we describe protocols for both passive and active systemic anaphylaxis.

It is important to note that the relevance of mouse models of systemic anaphylaxis to human anaphylaxis is not entirely clear. Therefore, as is always the case in work with mouse models, care should be taken when extrapolating experimental data to the human system.

2 Materials (*See* Note 1)

2.1 Passive Systemic Anaphylaxis

1. Mice at 6–12 weeks of age (*see* **Note 2**).
2. Monoclonal mouse anti-DNP IgE antibody (Sigma-Aldrich) (*see* **Note 3**).
3. Dinitrophenyl–human serum albumin (DNP–HSA; Sigma-Aldrich).
4. Needles and syringes for i.p. and i.v. injections (27G needles; 1 ml syringes).
5. Microprobe thermometer with a rectal probe for mice (Physitemp Instruments) (*see* **Note 4**).
6. Needles and syringes for peritoneal lavage (27G and 22G needles; 10 ml syringes).
7. May-Grünwald Stain (Sigma-Aldrich).
8. Giemsa Stain, Modified (Sigma-Aldrich).
9. McJunkin-Hayden Buffer (6.63 g of KH_2PO_4, 2.56 g of Na_2HPO_4, and double-distilled water to 1 L).
10. Cytocentrifuge or centrifuge with cytospin attachments.
11. Cytospin cuvette.
12. Cytospin paper.
13. Glass slides.
14. Phosphate-buffered saline with calcium and magnesium (PBS w/Ca & Mg) (*see* **Note 5**).

2.2 Active Systemic Anaphylaxis (ASA)

15. Mice at 6–8 weeks of age (*see* **Note 2**).
16. Ovalbumin from chicken egg white (OVA; Sigma-Aldrich).
17. Pertussis toxin from *Bordetella pertussis* (Sigma-Aldrich).
18. Aluminum potassium sulfate dodecahydrate (Sigma-Aldrich).
19. Needles and syringes for i.p. and i.v. injections (27G Needle; 1 ml syringes).
20. Microprobe thermometer with a rectal probe for mice (Physitemp Instruments) (*see* **Note 4**).

3 Methods

3.1 Passive Systemic Anaphylaxis [9] Sensitization

1. Prepare 100 μg/ml of monoclonal mouse anti-DNP IgE antibody in 0.9 % NaCl (*see* **Note 6**).
2. Sensitize mice by intraperitoneal injection (*see* **Note 7**) with 200 μl of IgE solution (the mice will receive a total of 20 μg of IgE anti-DNP). Inject control mice with 200 μl of 0.9 % NaCl.
3. Wait 24 h before challenge.

3.2 PSA Challenge

1. Prepare 10 mg/ml of DNP–HSA in 0.9 % NaCl.
2. Measure baseline temperature using a rectal probe for mice (*see* **Note 8**).
3. Immediately challenge mice by intravenous injection with 100 μl of DNP–HSA solution (*see* **Note 9**).
4. Measure rectal temperature at 10-min intervals for the first hour, and then at 90 and 120 min following the challenge.
5. After 2 h, euthanize mice and disinfect the abdominal skin.
6. Perform a 2 cm midline abdominal incision, expose the peritoneum, and slowly inject 2 ml of 0.9 % NaCl (or medium) and 8 ml of air into the peritoneal cavity (*see* **Note 10**) using a 27G needle.
7. Gently massage the abdomen for 3 min and recover the peritoneal fluid using a 22G needle.
8. Wash the recovered cells in PBS w/Ca & Mg and resuspend at a concentration of $1–2 \times 10^6$ cells/ml PBS w/Ca & Mg.
9. Prepare cytospins following standard procedures and stain with May-Grünwald-Giemsa for analysis of mast cell degranulation [10].
10. For additional assessment of mast cell mediator release, repeat the passive systemic anaphylaxis (PSA) (**steps 1–4**) and sacrifice the mice after the first temperature measurement (10 min after induction of anaphylaxis). Collect whole blood (for example by cardiac puncture) and peritoneal lavage fluid (PLF). Leave blood sample for at least 1 h to clot, centrifuge the sample at (1,000–2,000 × *g*) for 20 min, and remove the serum from the clot by gently pipetting off into a clean tube. To assess mast cell activation, measure mMCP-1 and/or histamine by ELISA in serum and PLF.

3.3 Active Systemic Anaphylaxis (ASA) Sensitization

1. Prepare a solution of 1 mg/ml of OVA with 1 μg/ml of Pertussis toxin and 10 mg/ml of aluminum potassium sulfate as adjuvants in saline solution. Prepare control solution identically, but without OVA.
2. Actively sensitize mice by injecting 100 μl of OVA solution intraperitoneally.
3. Wait for 18–21 days before challenge.
4. One day before challenge collect tail vein blood in 1.5 ml polypropylene tubes for measurement of OVA-specific IgG_1 and OVA-specific IgE to verify proper sensitization (*see* **Note 11**). If not used on the same day, store serum at −80 °C.

3.4 ASA Challenge

1. Measure the baseline rectal temperature (*see* **Note 8**).
2. Prepare 10 mg/ml of OVA solution in 0.9 % saline.

3. Inject 50 μl of OVA solution (500 μg of OVA) intraperitoneally or intravenously.
4. Monitor rectal temperature and signs of morbidity at regular intervals until death or until 30 min following challenge, whichever is first. Morbidity (shivering, reduced activity) should be closely monitored and documented according to the respective regulations. Mice should be sacrificed immediately if they reach or surpass the previously defined humane endpoint.

4 Notes

1. Prepare all solutions using sterile 0.9 % NaCl. Prepare and store all reagents at 2–8 °C unless indicated otherwise. Diligently follow all waste disposal regulations. Perform all animal work in accordance with the national guidelines on the care and use of animals for scientific purposes.
2. The number of mast cells differs between mouse strains and increases with age of mice. Higher mast cell numbers lead to a more pronounced temperature drop.
3. Prepare a stock solution in NaCl. Store aliquots for long-term storage at −20 °C and do not refreeze after thawing. IgE working solutions should be discarded if not used within 12 h.
4. Alternatively, subcutaneously implanted transponders (e.g., BMDS-Bio Medic Data Systems) can be used to monitor temperature.
5. The use of PBS w/Ca & Mg improves cell adhesion to slides.
6. Our preferred model of PSA uses monoclonal mouse anti-DNP IgE antibodies and DNP–HSA. However, a variety of substances have been used in other models.
7. Sensitization and challenge can be i.p. or i.v., with similar results. In the case of i.p. injections, be careful not to inject into the intestine as the sensitization will fail. This will be noticeable only after the mice have been challenged the next day and may lead to false-negative results.
8. Because the change in temperature can be quite small, it is important to carefully control for factors that might affect body temperature, such as the number of mice per cage, the time of day they are tested, and the amount of handling and stress each mouse experiences during the procedures.
9. Like the sensitization, the challenge can be performed by i.v. or i.p. injection. If the effect of a substance on the outcome of the anaphylactic reaction is to be tested, the site of the antigen injection should differ from the route of administration of the test substance. For example, if the substance in question is

injected i.p., DNP–HSA should be injected i.v. into the tail vein and vice versa.

10. Always place needles in the lateral side through the abdominal muscles.

11. This is of special importance if different genotypes are compared. Any difference observed in the biological response could be either due to differences in the challenge phase and the respective cells and mediators involved during challenge, or in the sensitization phase, for example by effects on immunoglobulin levels.

References

1. Summers CW, Pumphrey RS, Woods CN et al (2008) Factors predicting anaphylaxis to peanuts and tree nuts in patients referred to a specialist center. J Allergy Clin Immunol 121:632–638.e632
2. Lee JK, Vadas P (2011) Anaphylaxis: mechanisms and management. Clin Exp Allergy 41:923–938
3. Sicherer SH, Leung DY (2012) Advances in allergic skin disease, anaphylaxis, and hypersensitivity reactions to foods, drugs, and insects in 2011. J Allergy Clin Immunol 129:76–85
4. Metz M, Schäfer B, Tsai M et al (2011) Evidence that the endothelin A receptor can enhance IgE-dependent anaphylaxis in mice. J Allergy Clin Immunol 128:424–426.e1
5. Freichel M, Almering J, Tsvilovskyy V (2012) The role of TRP proteins in mast cells. Front Immunol 3:150
6. Khan BQ, Kemp SF (2011) Pathophysiology of anaphylaxis. Curr Opin Allergy Clin Immunol 11:319–325
7. Vöhringer D (2011) Basophils in allergic immune responses. Curr Opin Immunol 23:789–793
8. Finkelman FD (2007) Anaphylaxis: lessons from mouse models. J Allergy Clin Immunol 120:506–515
9. Ando A, Martin TR, Galli SJ (1993) Effects of chronic treatment with the c-kit ligand, stem cell factor, on immunoglobulin E-dependent anaphylaxis in mice. Genetically mast cell-deficient Sl/Sld mice acquire anaphylactic responsiveness, but the congenic normal mice do not exhibit augmented responses. J Clin Invest 92:1639–1649
10. Metz M, Piliponsky AM, Chen CC et al (2006) Mast cells can enhance resistance to snake and honeybee venoms. Science 313:526–530

Chapter 11

Contact Hypersensitivity Models in Mice

Irving C. Allen

Abstract

The contact hypersensitivity (CHS) reaction is commonly utilized to study cell-mediated host immune responses to epicutaneously applied allergens. This reaction is divided into two distinct phases, the afferent phase and the efferent phase. During the afferent phase of this model, mice are exposed to a contact allergen, which is typically a hapten that is applied to a location distal to the site of elicitation. Following a brief intermission, mice are reexposed to the contact allergen during the elicitation phase at a site proximal to the location of sensitization. In mice, the pinna of the ear is typically utilized to evaluate the elicitation phase. While the CHS reaction is typically utilized to study Th1-mediated immune responses, it is now evident that Th2 and Th17 cells also contribute during the elicitation phase of the model. Likewise, in humans, elevated immune responses to contact allergens are associated with a variety of atopic diseases. Here, we describe a common protocol for the induction and assessment of the CHS reaction in mice.

Key words CHS, Delayed-type hypersensitivity, DTH, Chemical-induced hypersensitivity, Skin allergy, In vivo, Oxazolone, Th1, Th2, Th17

1 Introduction

The contact hypersensitivity (CHS) reaction is a common in vivo assay to study cell-mediated host immune responses to contact allergens. The CHS reaction consists of two distinct stages, the afferent phase and the efferent phase. During the afferent or the sensitization phase, animals are epicutaneously exposed to contact allergens, which are typically exogenously applied haptens. Once exposed, dermal dendritic cells and Langerhans cells migrate from the skin to the draining lymph nodes, where they present haptene-major histocompatibility complex (MHC) moieties to T lymphocytes [1–4]. During the efferent or the elicitation phase, animals are reexposed to the contact allergen used for sensitization, which results in the trafficking of haptene-specific T lymphocytes to the site of antigen deposition and the subsequent production of proinflammatory cytokines [4]. Two types of T helper cells have been described to participate in this response, the Th1 and Th2 cells.

Irving C. Allen (ed.), *Mouse Models of Allergic Disease: Methods and Protocols*, Methods in Molecular Biology, vol. 1032,
DOI 10.1007/978-1-62703-496-8_11, © Springer Science+Business Media, LLC 2013

Traditionally, laboratories have utilized CHS reactions and the related delayed-type hypersensitivity (DTH) reactions to study Th1-mediated T-cell responses. Indeed, it is clear that many aspects of both the CHS and DTH reactions are mediated by $CD4^+$ T lymphocytes and the production of interferon-γ. However, recent studies have revealed a role for Th2 cells during the elicitation phase of the CHS reaction. Specifically, studies utilizing *Il-4*$^{-/-}$ and *Il-13*$^{-/-}$ mice have revealed that these proinflammatory mediators are necessary for the CHS reaction to specific epicutaneously applied allergens [4–10]. Epicutaneous exposure to antigen is associated with the development of contact dermatitis in humans and has been associated with atopic disease progression. Thus, it is essential to understand the basic mechanisms associated with allergic sensitization through the skin. In this chapter, we describe the detailed protocols for the induction and evaluation of CHS in mice.

2 Materials

2.1 Mice

1. Adult female mice (*see* **Note 1**), 6–12 weeks old (*see* **Note 2**) that have been bred (*see* **Note 3**) and housed under specific pathogen-free conditions (*see* **Note 4**).

2.2 Reagents and Solutions

1. 100 % Ethanol (EtOH).
2. 4-Ethoxymethylene-2-phenyl-2-oxazolin-5-one (oxazolone) (*see* **Note 5**).
3. 3 % Oxazolone in EtOH (prepared fresh immediately prior to use).
4. Nair™ Chemical Hair Removal Product (*see* **Note 6**) (commercially available).
5. 10 % Neutral buffered formalin.

2.3 Materials and Equipment

1. Cotton-tipped applicator swabs.
2. Pipette (p200).
3. Forceps.
4. Scissors.
5. 8 mm leather hole punch.
6. Cork board.
7. Analytical balance.
8. Calipers (dial thickness gauge, 0.01–12.5 mm).
9. Indelible marking pen.
10. 24-well tissue culture plates.

3 Methods

3.1 Contact Hypersensitivity (Sensitization)

1. While securely holding the mouse, thoroughly remove the hair from the ventral side at the posterior of the mouse using Nair™ (*see* **Notes 7** and **8**).
2. Using a pipette, epicutaneously apply 100 μl of the 3 % oxazolone solution to the belly of the mouse (*see* **Note 9**). Continue to restrain the animal for an additional 3–5 s to allow the solution to dry.

3.2 Contact Hypersensitivity (Elicitation)

1. Five days post allergen sensitization, measure baseline pinna thickness for both ears using calipers (*see* **Note 10**).
2. Immediately following pinna thickness assessments, using a pipette, epicutaneously apply 10 μl of the 3 % oxazolone solution to each side of the right pinna (20 μl total). Apply 10 μl of 100 % ethanol (vehicle) epicutaneously to each side of the left pinna (20 μl total) (*see* **Note 11**). Additional controls should also include sensitized but unchallenged mice and mice that were challenged on the pinna, but never sensitized. Naïve mice should also be included for reference (*see* **Note 12**).
3. Identify each animal using tail marks with the indelible pen for temporary identification.

3.3 Pinna Harvest

1. Twenty-four hours post elicitation, measure pinna thickness using calipers.
2. Calculate the change in pinna thickness (ΔT):

$$\Delta T = (\text{pinna thickness 24 h following elicitation}) - (\text{baseline pinna thickness})$$

   Calculate ΔT for both the right (challenged pinna) and left (unchallenged pinna) and show as either ΔT or percent change.
3. Euthanize the mice following appropriate institutional guidelines (*see* **Note 4**).
4. Optional: If systemic assessments of circulating cytokines or immunoglobulins are desired, whole blood can be collected utilizing cardiac puncture immediately following euthanasia for serum evaluation.
5. Remove the left and right pinna, taking care to keep the hapten-treated and vehicle control ears separate (*see* **Note 13**).
6. Once all of the pinna are removed from the mice, place each individual pinna on a cork board and use the 8 mm leather punch to remove the central most portion of the ear. The punch should include the majority of the pinna and be located in the same area for all animals, taking care to avoid the thicker cartilage at the base of the pinna (*see* **Note 13**).

7. Weigh each 8 mm pinna punch using an analytical scale.
8. Calculate the change in pinna weight (ΔW) between the challenged pinna and the unchallenged pinna:

$$\Delta W = (\text{pinna weight of the hapten-challenged ear}) - (\text{pinna weight of the vehicle-treated ear})$$

Show as either ΔW or percent change.

9. Following weight assessments, each pinna punch should be fixed in 10 % neutral buffered formalin, paraffin embedded, sectioned, and H&E stained for histology (*see* **Note 14**). Immune cell infiltration and histopathology can then be evaluated [11].

4 Notes

1. Female mice are preferred in these assays due to their more docile nature. There is an increased probability that adult male animals will become aggressive during the course of this type of experiment, which can lead to fight wounds and ear damage. If male mice are to be utilized, consider individual housing.
2. We have successfully utilized 6–12-week-old C57Bl/6, 129SvEv, and BALB/c mice in these assays. If strain is not a limiting factor, BALB/c mice are preferred due to their robust response in the ear swelling assays. It is possible that some aspects of this protocol may need to be adjusted and further optimized when using mice from different genetic backgrounds.
3. When breeding and identifying mice by ear punch or ear tag, all attempts should be made to limit excessive damage to the ears and preserve the tissue integrity. If possible, avoid using ear punch or ear tags to identify mice directed to CHS studies.
4. All studies should be conducted in accordance with the local and institutional animal care and use guidelines and in accord with the prevailing national regulations.
5. There are a variety of other commonly utilized allergen for the CHS reaction, including FITC, 2,4-dinitro-1-fluorobenzene (DNFB), and 2,4,6-trinitrochlorobenzene (TNCB; picryl chloride). In fact, many older protocols utilize TNCB as their model allergen for CHS studies. However, due to human safety concerns, TNCB is currently difficult to obtain in many countries and requires additional safety precautions during handling and use. Many peptides that are commonly utilized in allergy studies, such as ovalbumin (OVA), can also be utilized in the CHS reaction with slightly modified protocols for

sensitization and elicitation. Each allergen listed here utilizes a specific solvent; thus, protocols utilizing alternative allergens must adjust the solvent.

6. It is essential that the hair on the abdomen be removed prior to oxazolone administration. We have had the best success utilizing chemical hair removal products, such as Nair™. However, many protocols utilize a small animal hair clipper/trimmer as an alternative approach. Do not remove the hair on the ear.
7. If large numbers of mice will be sensitized, animal can be anesthetized either using drop method isoflurane or by an approved anesthetic.
8. The Nair™ should be applied to an area that is approximately 2–3 cm in diameter on the belly of the animals with cotton-tipped applicators. For best results, apply the Nair™ in 5–10 concentric circles in a clockwise motion, followed by 5–10 concentric circles in a counterclockwise motion. Allow the Nair™ to remain in contact with the skin and fur for approximately 30 s. Remove the fur using the back of a pair of forceps or another hard, flat, and thin surface. The fur should be easily and completely removed from the animal. Small areas of partially removed fur are acceptable. However, if the majority of fur is not removed by the Nair™, then repeat the procedure.
9. The ethanol and the residual Nair™ may produce a colorimetric reaction, where the oxazolone solution will turn pink or red in color. This will temporarily dye the skin of the mouse's abdomen and is normal.
10. The caliper assessments of ear thickness are the most likely source of error in this procedure. Thus, it is essential that individuals be trained and practice using calipers to assess ear thickness prior to the start of this procedure. As an alternative to calipers or to confirm the caliper findings, ear thickness can be assessed using digital imaging [11].
11. One of the strengths of this model is the ability to evaluate the CHS reaction using experimental and control ears from the same animal.
12. In general, there will be a high level of variability in this model due to the complex nature of the CHS response. Therefore, large groups of mice should be used. We typically prefer >7 animals per group. Likewise, the health and age of the animals can dramatically influence the CHS response.
13. We have found that placing the pinna in individual wells in a labeled 24-well tissue culture plate is ideal.
14. As an alternative to histology evaluation, the 8 mm pinna punches can also be frozen on dry ice or by liquid nitrogen and manually homogenized for protein or RNA extraction using standard protocols and reagents.

References

1. Hemmi H, Yoshino M, Yamazaki H, Naito M, Iyoda T, Omatsu Y, Shimoyama S, Letterio JJ, Nakabayashi T, Tagaya H, Yamane T, Ogawa M, Nishikawa S, Ryoke K, Inaba K, Hayashi S, Kunisada T (2001) Skin antigens in the steady state are trafficked to regional lymph nodes by transforming growth factor-beta1-dependent cells. Int Immunol 13:695–704
2. Yoshino M, Yamazaki H, Nakano H, Kakiuchi T, Ryoke K, Kunisada T, Hayashi S (2003) Distinct antigen trafficking from skin in the steady and active states. Int Immunol 15:773–779
3. Yoshino M, Yamazaki H, Shultz LD, Hayashi S (2006) Constant rate of steady-state self antigen trafficking from skin to regional lymph nodes. Int Immunol 18:1541–1548
4. Dieli F, Sireci G, Salerno A, Bellavia A (1999) Impaired contact hypersensitivity to trinitrochlorobenzene in interleukin-4-deficient mice. Immunology 98:71–79
5. Berg DJ, Leach MW, Kuhn R, Rajewsky K, Müller W, Davidson NJ, Rennick D (1995) IL-10 but not IL-4 is a natural suppressant of cutaneous inflammatory response. J Exp Med 182:99
6. Weigmann B, Schwing J, Huber H, Ross R, Mossmann H, Knop J, Reske-Kunz AB (1997) Diminished CHS in IL-4 deficient mice at a late phase of the elicitation reaction. Scand J Immunol 45:308
7. Dieli F, Asherson GL, Colonna RG, Sirechi G, Gervasi F, Salerno A (1994) IL-4 is essential for the systemic transfer of DTH by T cells. Role of gama/delta cells. J Immunol 152:2698
8. Salerno A, Dieli F, Sireci G, Bellavia A, Asherson GL (1995) IL-4 is a critical cytokine in contact sensitivity. Immunology 84:404
9. Nieuwenhuizen N, Herbert DR, Brombacher F, Lopata AL (2009) Differential requirements for interleukin (IL)-4 and IL-13 in protein contact dermatitis induced by Anisakis. Allergy 64(9):1309–1318
10. Herrick CA, Xu L, McKenzie AN, Tigelaar RE, Bottomly K (2003) IL-13 is necessary, not simply sufficient, for epicutaneously induced Th2 responses to soluble protein antigen. J Immunol 170(5):2488–2495
11. Arthur JC, Lich JD, Ye Z, Allen IC, Gris D, Schneider M, Roney KE, O'Connor BP, Moore CB, Morrison A, Sutterwala FS, Koller BH, Bertin J, Liu Z, Ting JPY (2010) Cutting edge NLRP12 controls dendritic and myeloid cell migration to affect contact hypersensitivity. J Immunol 185(8):4515–4519

Chapter 12

Induction of Allergic Rhinitis in Mice

Virginia McMillan Carr and Alan M. Robinson

Abstract

We describe a method for allergic rhinitis (AR) induction in mice. Methodology involves nasal infusions of small volumes of ovalbumin for both initial sensitization and challenges. The latter are frequent and carried out over several weeks. This methodology more closely resembles natural AR induction than does the common use of systemic sensitization, often with adjuvants, followed by nasal challenges with relatively large allergen volumes. Also described are methodologies for collection of cardiac blood and perfusion for preparation of histological samples, both essential in verifying AR induction in individual animals.

Key words Allergic rhinitis induction, Murine allergic rhinitis model, Nasal tissues, Cardiac blood collection, Mouse perfusion, Nasal sinuses, Ovalbumin, Olfactory epithelium, Respiratory epithelium, Eosinophils

1 Introduction

Allergic rhinitis (AR) is the most common atopic disease [1] and can often cause seriously compromised olfactory function [2, 3]. It is induced by repeated nasal exposure to low levels of allergenic material. Mice provide convenient models in which to study the onset, progression, termination, and amelioration of AR. However, to date, in efforts to guarantee robust immune responses in relatively short experimental periods, most murine AR studies have used models that involve subcutaneous or intraperitoneal systemic initial sensitization, with only the subsequent challenges being delivered nasally. Moreover, adjuvant is often used in conjunction with sensitization; and the nasal challenges often involve relatively large, rather than small, infusate volumes and high allergen concentrations (e.g., [4–8]).

In contrast, McCusker and colleagues, in investigations of murine upper and lower airway allergic diseases [1], recognized the unnaturalness of such induction methods. McCusker et al. noted that the use of the nasal route for both sensitization and challenge and the use of both low allergen doses and numerous

Irving C. Allen (ed.), *Mouse Models of Allergic Disease: Methods and Protocols*, Methods in Molecular Biology, vol. 1032,
DOI 10.1007/978-1-62703-496-8_12, © Springer Science+Business Media, LLC 2013

small exposures over a period of several weeks more closely reflect natural allergic induction than do the other models. They also used the non-microbially derived protein ovalbumin (OVA) as their allergen. This avoids induction of additional innate, non-AR immune responses to microbe-associated molecular patterns of microbial antigens (e.g., [9–11]). Using their consequently developed protocol [1], McCusker et al. were able to show induction of pronounced allergic reactions as measured by the standard indicators of OVA-specific IgE and IgG serum levels, pronounced upper and lower airway eosinophil infiltration, and increased IL-5 and polymorphonuclear leukocyte presence in postchallenge bronchoalveolar lavage fluid.

Our own interests concerned AR effects on olfactory capabilities in affected animals. To investigate these capabilities, it was first necessary to demonstrate the induction of allergic responses in the nasal cavity itself, using slight modifications of the McCusker protocol [12]. Our protocol is detailed below. Induction of AR was verified by high OVA-specific serum IgE levels in ELISA blots and by pronounced nasal cavity eosinophil infiltration. These two AR indicators were highly correlated in all study animals.

Our study further examined the effects of extended allergen exposure, such as would occur with chronic or perennial seasonal allergen exposure. This extended OVA exposure was found to cause noticeably more pronounced nasal histological changes [12]. Interestingly, nasal responses appeared complicated, with olfactory epithelial histological changes being secondary to respiratory epithelial responses. That intriguing issue, along with analysis of numerous other histological and molecular components of the observed responses, still awaits examination, as do the effects on olfactory function itself. Distinct nasal sinus responses were also noted, but these were not further investigated.

2 Materials

2.1 Animals

1. Virus-free 7–11-week-old BALB/c mice (*see* **Note 1**), housed under conventional conditions in the institutional animal facility and treated strictly according to the NIH and institutional animal care protocol requirements throughout the duration of the entire experiment.

2.2 Reagents (See Note 2)

1. Phosphate-buffered saline (PBS), pH 7.4, prepared from a commercial concentrate solution by dilution with H_2O (*see* **Note 3**).
2. Allergen: 1.0 % (wt/vol) OVA in PBS (*see* **Note 4**). Make this in 10 ml batches: Add 0.1 g OVA to 10 ml PBS; vortex to dissolve. Filter sterilize (0.02 μm pore size), and aliquot into sterile plastic vials, 40–50 μl/vial. Store at −20 °C. Thaw as needed on the day of use.

3. PBS controls: Dilute from the 10× concentrate above and then filter sterilize, aliquot, and store in the same manner as the OVA.
4. Anesthetics for blood collection and perfusion: Ketamine and xylazine (0.65 and 0.035 mg, respectively, *per* g b.wt. for each mouse; *see* **Note 5**).
5. Fixative for histological preparation: Paraformaldehyde (PFA) in PBS (*see* **Note 6**), 1 N sodium hydroxide (NaOH) for titration to solubilize the PFA. PFA is made and stored as 16 % in H_2O and on the day of perfusion is then diluted to 4 % with PBS and H_2O (*see* Subheading 3).

2.3 Additional Materials

1. For blood collection and perfusion: ½–1 in. 22 G disposable needles and thin polyethylene tubing, cut into 1.5–2.5 cm and 20–25 cm lengths. Internal tubing diameter should be just wide enough to tightly fit over the needles.
2. Metal file and wire/metal cutters for cutting disposable needle tips.
3. Nail polish.
4. Perfusion pump.
5. Various sized syringes for anesthetization; blood collection; and perfusion, if fluid delivery by syringe is preferred to a perfusion pump.
6. Various surgical scissors and tweezers for tissue isolation.
7. Small centrifuge tubes for blood; jars for collected specimens; and Pasteur pipettes.

3 Methods

3.1 Nasal Infusions

1. Nasal infusions are carried out in a procedure hood in the animal facilities following institutional guidelines.
2. Wipe the hood and work spaces with disinfectant.
3. Mice are housed at a maximum of five per cage. Animals receiving allergen (OVA) or control buffered saline (PBS) should be housed separately. Before beginning infusions prepare a fresh cage for each cage of animals to be infused. Infuse all animals from the same cage sequentially, and transfer each to the same clean cage immediately after infusion (*see* **Note 7**).
4. Before removing an animal from its cage for infusion, have ready for use two pipettors, one for each naris, fitted with sterile 10 μl tips and each filled with 7.5 μl (*see* **Note 8**) of the appropriate solution (allergen or buffer). This avoids having to change and fill pipette tips between the infusions into each side while still holding a mouse. Do not allow the pipette tips to touch any surfaces.

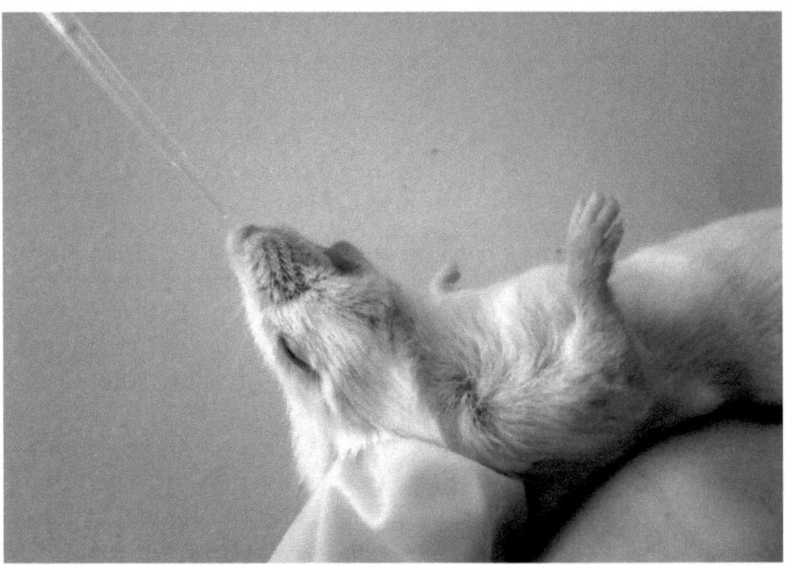

Fig. 1 Image of mouse being held for nasal fluid infusion. The head and neck are held firmly between the thumb and forefinger of the nondominant hand. The trunk and hind legs are held firmly but gently with the remaining free fingers of that hand (not pictured). The pipettor is held in the dominant hand, with the pipette tip placed just above and slightly to the outer side of the naris opening so that the infusion fluid is dispensed right over the naris

5. Remove an animal to be infused from its cage (*see* **Note 9**). With the thumb and first finger of the nondominant hand grasp the animal's neck and neck skin quite firmly behind the ears and along the neck. Firmly but gently anchor the hind legs and trunk with the remaining fingers of that hand. Tip the mouse back so that its nose points upwards, and bring the tip of the first pipette to one of the nares. Holding the pipette tip over the naris from the side, infuse the solution onto the naris opening (Fig. 1). To maximize the amount of fluid reaching the posterior-most nasal regions, hold the mouse on its back for several seconds until it stops struggling. Mice are obligate nose breathers, so the fluid will be inhaled. Repeat for the second naris using the second prepared pipette. Place the infused mouse into the fresh cage, and then prepare the set of pipettes for the next mouse. When finished infusing all mice from a given cage, remove the old and fresh cages from the hood and wipe down the hood surface with disinfectant before starting the next cage of mice (*see* **Notes 10–14**).
6. The infusion schedule is given in Fig. 2. Chronically exposed mice are treated for either 6 or 11 weeks with either the sterile 1 % OVA or PBS (PBS chronic controls) solutions above. For the 6-week exposures, mice receive daily infusions for 5 days

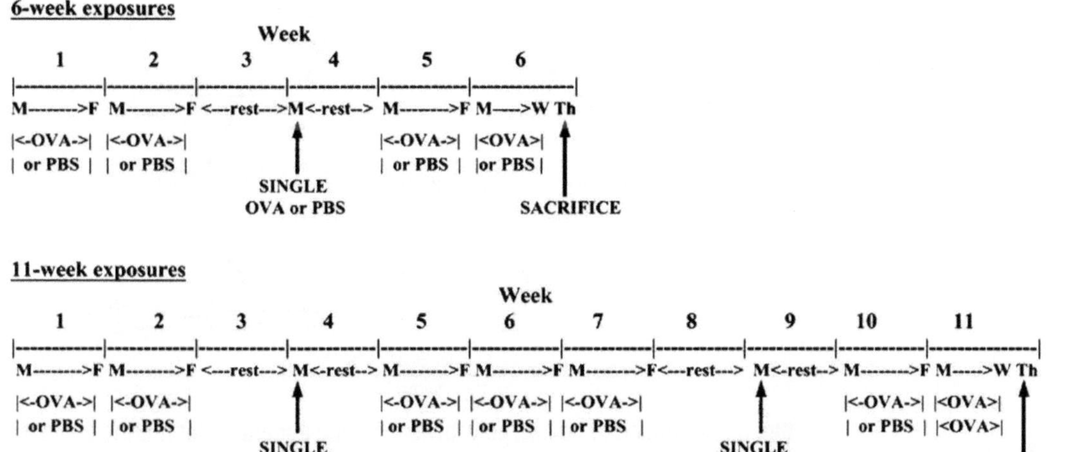

Fig. 2 Nasal infusion protocols for 6- and 11-week chronic exposure regimens for murine allergic rhinitis induction. Ovalbumin (OVA) is the allergenic infusate and phosphate-buffered saline (PBS) the control. Infusions occur on weekdays (*see* **Note 15**). For the 6-week chronic exposures, infusions occur Monday (M)–Friday (F) of weeks 1–2. A 2-week rest period follows in weeks 3–4 with single infusions on Monday of week 4 (*see* **Note 16**). Daily infusions are then resumed for the 5 days of week 5 and the first 3 days of week 6. Animals are sacrificed on the Thursday (Th) of week 6. For 11-week chronic exposures, this pattern is modified so that daily nasal infusions occur on the 5 weekdays in weeks 1–2, 5–7, and 10 and on the first 3 days of week 11. There are also two break periods, in weeks 3–4 and 8–9, with single infusions occurring on the Mondays of weeks 4 and 9. The specific days of the week on which infusion is performed can be altered to suit researchers' needs as long as the temporal pattern is maintained

for weeks 1 and 2 (*see* **Note 15**). Week 3 is a rest week, with no infusions. This is followed by single bilateral infusions on the first day of week 4 (*see* **Note 16**). The daily infusion pattern is then resumed for the 5 days of week 5 and the first 3 days of week 6. The mice are then sacrificed on the fourth day of week 6, 1 day after their final infusion. For the 11-week exposure animals, daily infusions occur in weeks 1–2 and 5–7. Rest periods similar to that of weeks 3–4 of the 6-week exposure schedule occur in weeks 3–4 and 8–9 (*see* **Note 16**), with single bilateral infusions occurring on the first day of both weeks 4 and 9. Daily nasal infusions then resume for the 5 days of week 10 and the first 3 days of week 11. The mice are sacrificed on the fourth day of week 11. Acutely treated animals receive single bilateral 7.5 μl infusions of OVA or PBS 1 day prior to sacrifice. Untreated controls receive neither OVA nor PBS prior to sacrifice (*see* **Note 17**).

7. It is essential to verify that AR has indeed been induced in any animal included in the subsequent analyses. We utilize both ELISA of blood serum OVA-specific IgE levels and the Luna stain [13] for histological verification of nasal epithelial

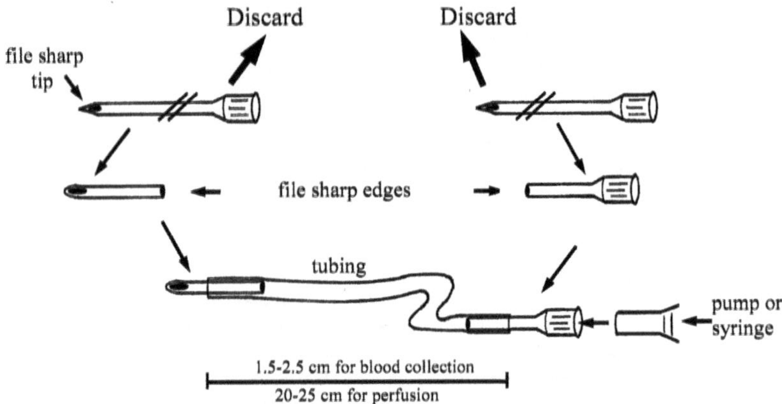

Fig. 3 Preparation of needle/polyethylene tubing apparatus for murine blood collection and perfusion. The dispensing end of the apparatus (*left*) is prepared by cutting a ½–1 in. 22 G disposable needle close to its plastic adaptor end. The sharp tip and the rough cut edges are blunted using a metal file. The blunted cut end is threaded into thin polyethylene tubing just wide enough to tightly hold the cut needle. The adaptor end of the apparatus (*right*) is prepared from a second disposable needle cut close to its pointed tip. The cut end of this needle is also blunted and fitted into the free end of the polyethylene tubing. Polyethylene tubing should be 1.5–2.5 cm long for blood collection apparatus and 20–25 cm for perfusion apparatus. Additionally, for the perfusion tubing a small drop of nail polish should be added just below the needle opening to prevent the needle from slipping out of the ventricle (not shown)

eosinophil infiltration [12] (*see* **Note 18**). It is also highly advisable that investigators of AR familiarize themselves with the morphology and tissue distribution through the entire extent of the mouse nasal cavity. Consequently, anesthetization, collection of cardiac blood, and fixation by transcardial perfusion are described below. For molecular and biochemical analysis for which unfixed tissue is required, only the ELISA would be possible.

3.2 Preparation of Cardiac Insertion Needles for Blood Collection and Perfusion (Fig. 3)

1. Prior to of the day of perfusion prepare needles for blood collection and perfusion. Slightly blunt the tips of ½–1 in. 22 G disposable needles with a metal file. Cut off and discard the plastic adaptor ends. Blunt the rough cut edges of the remaining needle tubes (*see* **Note 19**). Carefully thread one of these blunted top ends into a piece of thin polyethylene tubing just wide enough to hold the needle tightly. For blood collection the polyethylene tubing should be 1.5–2.5 cm long; for perfusion the tubing should be 20–25 cm long. The shorter length for blood collection provides less volume for loss or coagulation of drawn blood while still being long enough to provide some flexibility during blood collection. The longer length for

perfusion allows for maximum flexibility and maneuverability, but is not so long as to add to the clutter of instruments, perfusion fluids, and fluid waste containers that fill the hood during perfusion.

2. Trim off the pointed tips of a second set of needles, leaving most of the needle length (~0.5–1 cm) still attached to the plastic adaptor tops. Blunt the cut edges. Thread these cut ends into the free ends of the polyethylene tubing prepared above. The finished adapted needles are essentially thin polyethylene tubes that can be inserted into a mouse ventricle at their tips and attached to the nipple of a syringe or perfusion pump tubing via their plastic adaptor ends.
3. Additionally, for the needles to be used for perfusion, place a small drop of nail polish just below the opening of the needle tip and allow it to dry. This will serve to anchor the tip of the needle in the ventricle during perfusion.

3.3 Animal Anesthetization

1. After the allergen and PBS exposure period, animals are sacrificed according to institutional protocols and the requirements of subsequent procedures. Anesthetization is required. All procedures that follow should be carried out in a hood using gloves and proper eye cover.
2. On the day animals are to be perfused or otherwise sacrificed, weigh the animals, and calculate the combined total weight.
3. Cover the work space with plastic-backed absorbent paper.
4. Animals are deeply anesthetized by intraperitoneal injection of their individual weight-based calculated volumes of ketamine and xylazine. These are used in a combined "cocktail" solution with final drug concentrations of 9.8 mg of ketamine and 0.49 mg of xylazine/1.0 ml of anesthetic, with PBS as the diluent (*see* **Note 5**). These ketamine and xylazine concentrations work out to 0.65 ml of the "cocktail" for each 25–30 g mouse (0.022–0.026 ml of "cocktail"/g b.wt.). Allow an additional 0.1 ml/mouse in case extra anesthetic is needed to fully anesthetize any individual mice.
5. Each animal is anesthetized just prior to the start of the blood collection, perfusion, or other procedure being carried out. Deep anesthesia is indicated by the absence of an eye blink and/or tail pinch response, depending on individual institutional regulations. This usually requires 5–10 min. If the animal is not completely anesthetized in this time, administer additional anesthetic in 0.05 ml increments. Once deep anesthetization is achieved, subsequent procedures can be initiated.

3.4 Blood Collection by Cardiac Puncture for ELISA

1. Place the fully anesthetized animal on its back in a container large enough to ultimately hold all of the perfusion buffer and fixative but small enough to allow ready access to the animal.
2. With small scissors and surgical tweezers cut open the abdominal skin, cut through the diaphragm from the abdominal cavity into the thoracic cavity, and gently lift the ribs out of the way or remove them.
3. Rapidly insert a needle apparatus prepared for blood collection, with a 0.5–1.0 ml disposable syringe attached, into the base of the left ventricle. Gently draw as much blood as possible into the syringe from the heart.
4. Quickly but gently remove the needle from the ventricle. Be careful not to enlarge the needle penetration hole if the animal is to be subsequently perfused.
5. Dispense the blood into a small plastic centrifuge tube and immediately place this in the cold and store upright overnight so that the serum collects on the top. The next morning spin down the blood samples (13,800 × *g* on a tabletop centrifuge for 5 min), carefully collect the serum from the top layer of each, and store that in individual vials or containers at −80 °C until used for allergen-specific ELISA.
6. If the nasal tissues are to be used for molecular or biochemical studies and no perfusion is to be carried out, cut the head from the remainder of the body. Trim off the skin and lower jaw, and carefully remove the palate to expose the nasal cavity. Isolate the nasal septum and store as appropriate for subsequent procedures. The nasal turbinates and nasal sinuses can also be removed as needed. If desired, the olfactory and respiratory epithelia can be further isolated from the septal epithelium using a dissecting microscope.

3.5 Transcardial Perfusion of Animals for Histological Examination

1. Several days before perfusion, prepare a stock solution of 16 % PFA (*see* **Note 20**). For each 100 ml of 16 % PFA, add 16 g of PFA powder to a beaker containing 100 ml of H_2O and a spinning magnetic stir bar on a stirring/hot plate set at a moderate spin speed. Carefully heat the mixture to 60 °C. The fluid will be cloudy. Slowly add 12 drops of 1 N NaOH with a Pasteur pipette and continue stirring until the PFA dissolves and the fluid clears. A small amount of additional NaOH may be necessary to fully clear the solution. Do this slowly, using a lower concentration of NaOH (e.g., 0.1 N). Turn off the heat, and let the stirring continue until the solution cools to room temperature. To hasten cooling move the beaker to an unheated stir plate and continue stirring. If making large volumes of PFA, the beaker can also be placed in an ice bath on this unheated stir plate. Store the 16 % PFA at 4–8 °C for up to a month.

2. On the day of perfusion, prior to anesthetization of any mice, prepare a solution of 4 % PFA in PBS. Note that the PBS final concentration should be 1×. Allow 60–80 ml/mouse for perfusion with a perfusion pump. Thus, for each mouse to be perfused, mix 20 ml of 16 % PFA, 8 ml of PBS 10× concentrate, and 52 ml of H_2O.
3. Perfusion can be carried out using a perfusion pump [12] or by manually perfusing using 50 ml syringes. If manually perfusing, fill one syringe with PBS and the other with fixative (*see* **Note 21**). If a perfusion pump is used, it should be set up according to the manufacturer's directions. Connect two pieces of polyethylene tubing (2–3 mm internal diameter) to the pump input tubing via a 3-way adaptor. Immerse the free end of one piece of this tubing into a container of the 4 % PFA and that of the other into a container of PBS (*see* **Note 22**). Attach one of the needles prepared previously for perfusion to the pump output tubing. Check to make sure that no air bubbles remain in the tubing prior to starting perfusion.
4. After completion of blood collection (Section 3.4), carefully replace the blood collection needle in the ventricle with one prepared for perfusion and attached to the pump or syringe. Do not enlarge the existing hole or make a new one. That can lead to loss of perfusion fluid through the original hole and reduced perfusion fluid pressure through the body, resulting in a less than optimal perfusion. The dried nail polish drop will help to hold the perfusion needle in place in the ventricle during perfusion.
5. If no cardiac blood collection was carried out, anesthetize the animal, expose the heart, and insert the perfusion apparatus-attached needle into the left ventricle as described above.
6. With the perfusion needle inserted into the ventricle, begin the flow of PBS at a rate of 10–15 ml/min (*see* **Note 23**). *Immediately* clip the right atrium with sharp scissors so that the perfusate will exit from there after transiting through the entire body. Initial fluid will be pink due to blood carried from the body. Once the exiting fluid is clear in color (*see* **Note 24**) and the animal thoroughly exsanguinated, quickly switch to the fixative (*see* **Note 25**). Perfuse the animal with fixative until it or, in the case of a fluid block below the heart, its head, jaws, and neck are completely stiff. This should take 3–5 min, but can sometimes take longer. During both PBS and fixative delivery, the animal should be checked periodically to make sure that the needle remains inserted into the ventricle.
7. Turn off the pump.
8. Cut the head from the body. Since AR involves the nasal cavity and associated tissues, only the head above the palate needs to be kept. Trim off the skin and lower jaws (*see* **Note 26**).

Immerse the trimmed head in a jar containing sufficient fixative to cover it, and using a Pasteur pipette, force a gentle stream of fixative through the nostrils to flush out any trapped air (*see* **Note 20**). Store the head in fixative overnight at 4–8 °C. The next morning thoroughly wash out the fixative by immersion in running water for 15 min followed by several additional changes of water for up to an hour (*see* **Notes 27** and **28**).

9. Follow all institutional guidelines for disposal of animal carcasses, parts, and tissues as well as fixative wastes.

4 Notes

1. BALB/c mice are preferable because this strain had been found to give more robust AR responses than either C57BL/6 or CBA/J mice in studies using the *Schistosoma mansoni* egg antigen as the allergen [10]. However, given that that allergen may also be inducing innate, non-AR responses to microbe-associated molecular patterns, in a truly thorough investigation other strains should ultimately be examined as well.
2. For all solutions use reagent-grade reagents and either deionized or distilled water (H_2O). Use protective gloves when working with anesthetics, fixatives, and animals. Follow all institutional usage and waste disposal requirements.
3. PBS can also be prepared de novo from powdered ingredients following readily available directions. However, to prevent microbial growth, all preparations should be made and stored as 10× concentrations and then subsequently diluted as needed. Other isotonic physiological buffers could also be used as controls and allergen diluent.
4. Ovalbumin was used as the allergen because it is not an inducer of toll-like receptors and the innate immune response, which could greatly complicate any analysis of AR. Other non-microbially derived allergens could also be used as long as they do not induce innate responses.
5. To minimize injection trauma to the mice, xylazine and ketamine are administered in an anesthetic "cocktail." Using 100 mg/ml of ketamine and 20 mg/ml of xylazine commercial preparations, the "cocktail" represents a vol/vol ratio of 87.5 % PBS, 9.8 % ketamine, and 2.4 % xylazine. This anesthetic "cocktail" should not be prepared more than a few hours prior to use. Strictly follow all institutional and governmental regulations for drug storage, use, and disposal.
6. We used 4 % PFA. However, investigators should use whatever fixative that best suits their own subsequent histological, molecular, or biochemical needs.

7. Maintaining this pattern for infusion avoids any confusion as to whether a particular animal has been infused. To avoid accidental infusate errors, infuse all animals receiving the same infusate before starting the animals receiving the other infusate solution and have tubes of only the appropriate infusate in the hood. Any exposure to the wrong infusate solution could induce an unintended immune response, invalidating the results from that particular mouse.
8. McCusker et al. [1] used 5 μl of infusate/naris. We have used 7.5 μl instead to guarantee that at least 5 μl gets into each side. Given animal squirming, we found that in our hands 7.5 μl was a more reliable volume to use. However, to insure that resulting immune responses do indeed induce only AR and not additional immune responses, much larger infusate volumes should be avoided.
9. Mice move very quickly. Thus, rather than completely uncovering the cage, slide the cage top back just enough to grab any mouse in the cage (since all in the cage will be receiving the same infusate).
10. Mice should be infused bilaterally rather than trying to use one side as a control. It is very difficult to completely guarantee that infusate from one side will not spill onto the other naris. Moreover, side-to-side and inter-animal histological differences readily occur [12]. For this reason each nasal cavity also must be analyzed separately for histological investigations.
11. It is helpful to relax one's arms during infusion procedures so that pipettes will be held as steady as possible. This also helps confine the infusate to the side being infused. Practice infusions may be useful.
12. When infusing many mice, it helps to routinely infuse either the right or the left naris first for each mouse. This avoids the possibility of infusing one naris twice and the other not at all. Not discarding pipette tips until both nares have been infused also helps to verify that both nares have indeed been infused.
13. To clearly see the nares it is helpful to wear magnifying reading glasses. If the reading glasses will be worn over regular glasses, purchase a pair large enough to fit over the regular glasses but not so large as to slip down. If additional magnification is still required, a magnifying glass such as used in crafts projects with a flexible stem and clamp holder that allows it to be clamped to the edge of the hood cover is invaluable.
14. To help insure that fluid indeed is reaching the olfactory regions in these experiments, test infusions should be carried out with a vital dye (e.g., Evan's Blue [1]) and the extent of dye dispersal determined histologically.

15. In addition to its convenience, the 5-day-per-week pattern for nasal infusion is reflective of often intermittent AR-inducing allergen exposure (C. McCusker, personal communication).
16. The weeks 3–4 rest period, including the single intranasal challenge on the first day of week 4, was found essential for maximizing the serum IgE responses in the McCusker site-specific nasal sensitization and challenge regimen ([1], and McCusker, personal communication). For the same reason, a similar break from daily infusions was included in weeks 8–9 of the 11-week extended exposure studies [12]. We assume that any further extensions of exposure periods should include additional similar breaks as appropriate, but always including one in the 4th and 3rd weeks prior to animal sacrifice.
17. It is essential to include chronic PBS control animals. Our study [12] found that both chronic and acute PBS, as well as acute OVA exposure, cause *non*allergic swelling of the respiratory epithelia, which must be considered in the overall conclusions.
18. It is highly advisable that investigators of AR familiarize themselves with the morphology, histology, and tissue distribution through the entire extent of the mouse nasal cavity. This includes the turbinates, sinuses, septal organ, vomeronasal organ, and relative distribution of olfactory versus respiratory epithelia. All are nasal cavity spatial landmarks and important in determining the degree of AR-induced epithelial disruption. Thorough familiarity should be gained for both unexposed normal morphology as well as for AR-induced changes. It was our experience that important points found in our AR study [12] had been previously overlooked or dismissed because many earlier investigators lacked a thorough nasal cavity familiarity. This includes our findings of nasal epithelial type-specific effects of AR, with the implication that nasal effects of AR are unexpectedly more complex than previously suspected. Readers are referred to that study [12].
19. Blunting the pointed tips of the needles lessens the chance of piercing through the back side of the heart during blood collection and perfusion; blunting the cut edges lessens the likelihood of tearing the polyethylene tubing.
20. All preparation and use of PFA should be carried out in a ventilated laboratory hood using gloves and goggles. Institutional regulations for its usage and disposal should be strictly followed.
21. The perfusate solutions can be chilled depending on subsequent needs.
22. Mark the tubing for PBS and for the fixative with different colors of lab tape near their insertion into the 3-way adaptor so that the different fluids they contain can be readily identified.

23. This flow rate is based on an optimum fixative delivery of approximately 1 ml/gb.wt./min for perfusion of an entire mouse (Dr. E. Weiler, personal communication). Perfusion can also be carried out using handheld syringes as long as care is taken to maintain an even fluid pressure and flow rate. In our experience a flow rate of 2.5 ml/min is acceptable for mice when using a handheld syringe. In either case, flow must be low enough to avoid damage to the nasal epithelia.
24. This can be tested by holding the corner of a piece of lab tissue wipe to the cut right atrium.
25. Failure to completely exsanguinate an animal can result in formation of blood clots on exposure to fixative within blood vessels and subsequently poor fixation due to limited fixative access to trans-clot regions.
26. If using a perfusion pump, the time during specimen isolation and trimming is a convenient time in which to flush pump tubing with PBS for several minutes to clear the fixative in preparation for exsanguination of the next animal or to fully clear it after the conclusion of all perfusions. Soiled instruments can also be immersed in a beaker of distilled water with soft toweling at the bottom during this time and then wiped clean of coagulated blood so as to have them clean before proceeding to the next animal.
27. In our experience the total time required *per* mouse is about 30 min: 5–10 min for anesthetization, 5–6 min for PBS exsanguination, 5–7 min for fixation, and time for trimming the head. Time can be saved by using the anesthetization time of a mouse to clean up the instruments and work space from the previous perfusion.
28. Alternatively, multiple changes of PBS can be used in place of water depending on the specific experimental requirements. However, it is absolutely essential to completely wash out all fixative from the dissected tissues as it can interfere with subsequent procedures.

Acknowledgments

The authors express appreciation to Dr. Robert Kern for his advice and support. This research was supported by the Department of Otolaryngology—Head and Neck Surgery, Northwestern University from in-house funds.

References

1. McCusker C, Chicoine M, Hamid Q, Mazer B (2002) Site-specific sensitization in a murine model of allergic rhinitis: role of the upper airway in lower airways disease. J Allergy Clin Immunol 110:891–898
2. Baroody FM, Naclerio RM (1991) Allergic rhinitis. In: Getchell TV, Doty RL, Bartoshuk LM, Snow JB Jr (eds) Smell and taste in health and disease. Raven, New York, pp 529–552
3. Apter AJ, Mott AE, Frank ME, Cline JM (1995) Allergic rhinitis and olfactory loss. Ann Allergy Asthma Immunol 75:311–316
4. Sato J, Asakura K, Murakami M, Uede T, Kaaura A (1999) Topical CTLA4-Ig suppresses ongoing mucosal immune responses in presensitized murine model of allergic rhinitis. Int Arch Allergy Immunol 119:197–204
5. Saito H, Howie K, Waattie J, Denberg A, Ellis R, Inman MD, Denberg JA (2001) Allergen-induced murine upper airway inflammation: local and systemic changes in murine experimental allergic rhinitis. Immunology 104:226–234
6. Martin P, Villares R, Rodriguez-Mascarenhas S, Zaballos A, Leitges M, Kovac J, Sizing I, Rennert P, Marquez G, Marinez-A C, Diaz-Meco MT, Moscat J (2005) Control of T helper 2 cell function and allergic airway inflammation by PKCε. Proc Natl Acad Sci USA 102:9866–9871
7. Rahman A, Yatsuzuka R, Jiang S, Ueda Y, Kamei C (2006) Involvement of cyclooxygenase-2 in allergic inflammation in rats. Int Immunopharmacol 6:1736–1742
8. Ozaki S, Toida K, Suzuki M, Nakamura Y, Ohno N, Ohasi T, Nakayama M, Hamajima Y, Ingaki A, Kitaoka K, Sei H, Marakami S (2010) Impaired olfactory function in mice with allergic rhinitis. Auris Nasus Larynx 37:575–583
9. van de Rijn M, Mehlhop PD, Judkins A, Rothenberg ME, Luster AD, Oettgen HC (1998) A murine model of allergic rhinitis: studies on the role of IgE in the pathogenesis and analysis of the eosinophil influx elicited by allergen and eotaxin. J Allergy Clin Immunol 74:65–74
10. Okano M, Nishizaki K, Abe M, Wang M-M, Yoshino T, Satoskar AR, Masuda Y, Harn DA Jr (1999) Strain-dependent induction of allergic rhinitis without adjuvant in mice. Allergy 54:593–601
11. Epstein VA, Bryce PJ, Conley DB, Robinson AM (2008) Intranasal *Aspergillus fumigatus* exposure induces eosinophilic inflammation and olfactory sensory neuron cell death in mice. Otolaryngol Head Neck Surg 138:334–339
12. Carr VMCM, Robinson AM, Kern RC (2012) Tissue-specific effects of allergic rhinitis in mouse nasal epithelia. Chem Senses 37:655–668
13. Luna LG (1968) Manual of histologic staining methods of the armed forces institute of pathology, 3rd edn. McGraw-Hill, New York, pp 111–112

Chapter 13

Induction of Allergic Airway Disease Using House Dust Mite Allergen

Irving C. Allen

Abstract

Mouse models of allergic airway inflammation have proven essential in understanding the mechanisms and pathophysiology underling human asthma. There is a diverse range of mouse models described in the literature that typically vary slightly by allergen, duration of exposure, and route of sensitization. In general, each of these models has proven to be acceptable surrogates for studying specific aspects of the human disease, including airway inflammation, airway hyperresponsiveness (AHR), and airway remodeling. Here, we describe a highly versatile model based on nasal sensitization with house dust mite antigen (DMA). Mice receive multiple intranasal inoculations with DMA each week for a period of 4–16 weeks, which results in increased Th2-mediated airway inflammation and AHR. However, an added feature of the long-term exposures described here is the ability to more accurately evaluate the impact of chronic inflammation on airway remodeling and lung pathophysiology in response to a clinically relevant allergen.

Key words Asthma, House dust mite, HDM, DerP, DerF, Airway inflammation, Airway hyperresponsiveness, AHR, Airway remodeling, Eosinophil, Th2

1 Introduction

Asthma is a complex genetic disease that is influenced by a diverse repertoire of environmental stimuli. The complex nature and broad spectrum of symptoms in humans have led experts to propose that asthma is not a single disease, but is actually a syndrome of related diseases [1]. Together, these issues can significantly hinder the development of animal models. While the underlying cause and severity of asthma vary greatly between patients, the disease can be characterized by the presence of three cardinal symptoms: chronic airway inflammation; airway hyperresponsiveness (AHR); and reversible airflow obstruction. These symptoms distinguish asthma from other forms of obstructive airway disease, such as cystic fibrosis, emphysema, and chronic obstructive airway disease [2]. The chronic airway inflammation associated with asthma is characterized by an influx of eosinophils into the lungs and airway and is

Irving C. Allen (ed.), *Mouse Models of Allergic Disease: Methods and Protocols*, Methods in Molecular Biology, vol. 1032, DOI 10.1007/978-1-62703-496-8_13, © Springer Science+Business Media, LLC 2013

predominately driven by the production of proinflammatory cytokines, such as IL-13, IL-4, and IL-5. This chronic inflammation is thought to underlie the airway remodeling that is often observed in patients and is characterized by mucus hyperproduction, airway smooth muscle hypertrophy, and collagen deposition [3]. In addition to airway inflammation, asthma is also characterized by AHR and airway smooth muscle (ASM) constriction, which both contribute to the reversible airflow obstruction that defines the disease. In the case of AHR, the presence and severity of the increased sensitivity to aerosolized stimuli is typically utilized as a surrogate marker for asthma disease progression [4]. Likewise, ASM hyperplasia and hypertrophy have both been shown to contribute to characteristics associated with asthma, including airway inflammation, airway wall remodeling, and airflow obstruction [5].

Due to the complex nature of asthma in humans, laboratory animal models have played pivotal roles in characterizing the pathophysiological mechanisms associated with this disease. Specifically, mouse models have proven to be highly relevant in deciphering the underlying genetic and environmental factors that are associated with airway inflammation and AHR. Mice are an ideal model organism for the study of simple physiological processes associated with allergic airway inflammation due to the ease of genetic manipulation and the availability of ample resources and novel techniques that have been optimized in the mouse that allow for accurate in vivo assessments of airflow obstruction and hyperresponsiveness. However, there are several disadvantages associated with the utilization of mice in asthma research. For example, the human airway has several structural, physiological, and neuronal changes that are associated with AHR, which are not fully recapitulated in mice [6]. Likewise, unlike humans, mice do not spontaneously develop asthma or any other asthma-like disease [7–9]. Thus, all mouse models require artificial induction of allergic airway disease using an exogenous allergen.

The vast majority of allergic airway disease models utilize short-term, acute exposures to simple protein antigens (such as ovalbumin) or complex microorganisms (such as *Aspergillus*). These models commonly evaluate antigen-specific IgE levels, increased T-helper cell 2 (Th2) cytokine production (including IL-4, IL-5, and IL-13), eosinophilic mediated lung inflammation, goblet cell metaplasia, and AHR [10]. However, while these models have been incredibly useful in understanding disease progression, the acute nature of these models does not fully recapitulate several distinct characteristics of human asthma. For example, the inflammation characteristics between these mouse models and human asthma are significantly different. In mice, the inflammation is characterized by acute peribronchiolar and perivascular inflammation in the lung parenchyma, rather than airway wall inflammation in humans [11]. Likewise, allergic airway disease in mice appears to occur through a mast cell-independent mechanism, whereas the mast cells are a critical component of the human disease [12]. The airway eosinophilia is also significantly different in mouse models. In mice, the eosinophils appear to lack activation, degranulation, and intraepithelial accumulation, which are all observed in humans [11]. Finally, the short-term, acute nature of the majority of allergic airway disease models in mice does not allow a thorough evaluation of the structural changes associated with airway remodeling that is characteristic of the human condition. While each of these differences between allergic airway inflammation in mice and asthma in humans represents a limitation of the current models, we believe that many of these limitations can be overcome by redesigning the models to focus on long-term, chronic inflammation rather than acute inflammation.

Here, we describe a model of allergic airway inflammation that is based on chronic house dust mite exposure. In our hands, this model successfully recapitulates many physiologically relevant aspects of human asthma and is preferred over the acute OVA models typically utilized for these types of studies. The protocols presented here are designed to maximize the data generated from individual mice and minimize the number of animals required to complete studies. In addition, we also present alternative protocols to evaluate specific aspects of allergic airway disease that are often overlooked by typical studies.

2 Materials

2.1 Mice

1. Adult female mice (*see* **Note 1**), 6–12 weeks old (*see* **Note 2**), that have been bred and housed under specific pathogen-free conditions (*see* **Note 3**).
2. Mice should be acclimated to the housing facility for at least 5 days prior to the beginning of the experiment.

2.2 Reagents and Solutions

1. Dust Mite Extract (Stock Solution of 5,000 AU/ml DerP and 5,000 AU/ml DerF mixed 50:50) (Greer Laboratories, Lenoir, NC) (*see* **Note 4**).
2. 1× Hank's buffered saline solution (HBSS).
3. 10× Phosphate-buffered saline (PBS).
4. Sterile water.
5. Isoflurane (Baxter Healthcare Corporation) (*see* **Note 5**).
6. Evans blue dye (EBD).
7. 10× Buffered formalin.
8. Trypan Blue.
9. Formamide.
10. Diff-Quick Staining Kit (Solutions 1, 2, and 3).

11. Permount.
12. ELISA Kits for IgE and IL-13.
13. O.C.T. Compound (Tissue-Tek).
14. Dry ice.
15. Liquid nitrogen.
16. Study-specific and/or standard reagents for RNA extraction, cDNA amplification, and real-time PCR analysis.
17. Study-specific and/or standard reagents for protein extraction and Western blot analysis.

2.3 Materials and Equipment

1. 1 ml Syringe (with 27 gage needle).
2. 1.5 ml microcentrifuge tubes.
3. Microcentrifuge.
4. p1000, p200, and p20 pipettes.
5. 10 ml Syringe (with 27 gage needle).
6. 1 ml Syringes (without needles).
7. 15 ml Conical tubes.
8. Tracheal Cannula (*see* **Note 6**) (Harvard Apparatus).
9. 4-0, Silk Surgical Suture.
10. Refrigerated benchtop centrifuge (with rotor to accommodate 15 ml conical tubes).
11. Hemacytometer.
12. Microscope (10× and 20× objectives).
13. Cytospin.
14. Microscope slides.
15. Coverslips.
16. Coplin jars.
17. 20 ml Disposable glass scintillation vials with lids.
18. 500 ml Beaker.
19. Clear plastic or glass plate (~7 in. × 7 in.).
20. Absorbent paper towels.
21. Tissue-embedding molds (at least 22 mm × 22 mm × 20 mm deep).
22. Ice bucket.
23. Cryostat.
24. Portable liquid nitrogen container or bucket.
25. Fine-tipped indelible marker.
26. 2 ml Screw cap cryo tubes.

27. Mouse necropsy tools: One pair of large blunt scissors to open the chest; one pair of straight forceps; one pair of blunt 90°-angled forceps; one pair of sharp 90°-angled scissors; one pair of slightly curved blunt scissors.

3 Methods

3.1 Induction of Allergic Airway Inflammation (See Notes 7 and 8)

1. Determine the required volume of HDM extract and generate working solutions. The stock solution is supplied as a 5,000 AU/ml mixture of both DerP and DerF extract. Dilute stock to a working concentration of 0.05 AU/ml. The animals will receive 50 μl of the 0.05 AU/ml solution per day.
2. Anesthetize mice using drop method isoflurane in the 500 ml beaker with a glass cover (*see* **Notes 9** and **10**).
3. Sensitization will occur for 5 consecutive days with 2 days of recovery per week for 4–16 weeks (Fig. 1) (*see* **Note 11**).

3.2 Tissue Collection

1. Twenty-four hours following the last DMA exposure, euthanize the mice following appropriate institutional guidelines (*see* **Note 12**).
2. For systemic assessments of circulating cytokines and immunoglobulins, whole blood should be collected utilizing cardiac puncture immediately following euthanasia (*see* **Note 13**). The whole blood should be allowed to coagulate at room temperature for at least 30 min prior to serum isolation.
3. The animals should be perfused using 1× HBSS. Carefully open the peritoneal cavity and cut the portal vein leading to the kidney (either side). This will allow the remaining blood to drain from the animal during the perfusion. Without opening

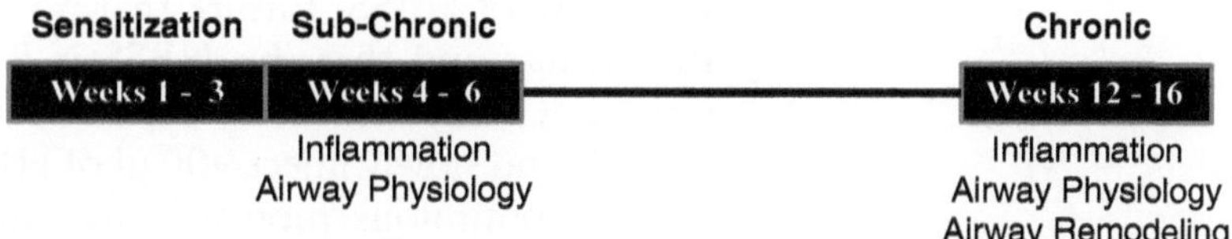

Fig. 1 Schematic depicting typical time courses associated with the induction of allergic airway inflammation in mice. Most models utilize a sensitization phase that lasts 1–3 weeks, based on multiple i.p. or i.n. administrations of a specific allergen. Acute and sub-chronic models typically induce allergic airway inflammation via multiple i.n. exposures to the allergen during weeks 4–6. Common assessments for these short-term models include the evaluation of airway inflammation and airway physiology. Chronic models typically induce allergic airway inflammation via multiple weekly i.n. exposures to the allergen during weeks 4 through 16. The chronic nature of these long-term models improves the evaluation of features associated with airway remodeling

the chest, carefully move the liver to expose the diaphragm. The lungs and heart should be visible behind the translucent diaphragm. Carefully clip the diaphragm at the point of contact with the sternum, making a small nick to access the chest. Once the nick is generated, the lungs and tissues should resend into the chest cavity. The bottom of the heart should now be visible. Using a 10 ml syringe with 27 gage needle attached, slowly and carefully inject the heart and gently perfuse 1–3 ml of HBSS. The lungs should begin to change color from red to pinkish/white and the liquid flowing from the excised kidney should change from red to clear. Caution: If too much pressure is applied to the syringe, saline can be forced into the airways and compromise additional data collection.

4. Once the animal has been perfused, the chest cavity can be exposed. Using a pair of blunt scissors, carefully open the chest cavity and remove each side of the rib cage as completely as possible and without damaging the lungs. Next, carefully remove the collar bones, taking care not to damage the underlying trachea. Using blunt-tipped forceps, separate the salivary glands and remove the thin layer of muscle that lies overtop of the trachea in the mouse's neck. The trachea should now be exposed from the lungs to the larynx.
5. Using the 90°-angled sharp scissors, make a small incision in the trachea 1–3 tracheal rings below the larynx. The incision should be just large enough to insert and secure the tracheal cannula. Caution: Do not sever the trachea as this will cause the trachea to retract into the chest cavity. Insert the tracheal cannula into the incision. Brace the trachea with the straight blunt forceps. Using the 90°-angled blunt forceps, thread the suture directly under the trachea and securely tie the cannula into place.
6. To collect the BALF, fill three 1 ml syringes (without needles) with 1 ml of HBSS. Ensure that no air bubbles are present in the syringe and that the HBSS is flush with the end of the syringe. Gently attach the hub of the syringe to the tracheal cannula and slowly inject 900 μl of HBSS into the mouse lungs in one continuous motion. The lungs should visibly inflate with no obvious leaks. Immediately withdraw the fluid in one slow and continuous motion. Deposit BALF into a 15 ml conical tube on ice. Repeat this process with the other two syringes. However, subsequent lavages should utilize the full 1 ml of HBSS per lavage. Record the final volume of BALF collected for each animal (this volume should be approximately 3 ml total). Keep the BALF on ice until ready to count.
7. To inflate and fix the lungs for histopathology, fill a 1 ml syringe with 10 % buffered formalin. Brace the trachea with the straight blunt forceps. Using the 90°-angled blunt forceps, thread a

second suture directly under the trachea and below the end of the cannula. Loop the suture in a half-tightened knot. Do not completely tie the second suture. Insert the 1 ml syringe into the cannula. Gently inflate the lungs with approximately 1 ml of 10 % buffered formalin. Do not overinflate the lungs as this will result in distortions in the lung histopathology. Once the lungs are inflated, secure the knot on the half-tied suture.

8. To remove the fixed and inflated lungs, remove the syringe and cannula from the trachea. Grasp the excess suture thread with the forceps and gently lift the trachea. Using the curved blunt scissors, slowly sever the trachea while lifting the inflated lungs out of the chest cavity. Carefully excise the lungs (with the heart still attached) without cutting them. Gently remove the inflated lungs from the mouse. Place the inflated lungs in a 20 ml disposable glass scintillation vial containing approximately 10 ml of 10 % buffered formalin. Place a lid on the vial and label with an indelible pen.
9. Properly dispose of the remaining mouse carcass.
10. For many applications, formalin fixation may yield suboptimal results or is incompatible with subsequent procedures (such as IHC or ISH). In these cases, it is preferable to freeze the lungs to generate frozen lung sections for subsequent histology. To generate frozen lung sections, fill a 1 ml syringe with O.C.T. compound. Fill an ice bucket with dry ice. Label a tissue-embedding mold using an indelible pen and place the mold in the dry ice, taking care to maximize contact with the dry ice. Harvest the whole blood, cannulate the animal, and collect the BALF as previously described. Insert the syringe containing the O.C.T. compound into the cannula. Apply gentle pressure to the syringe plunger and inflate the lungs with O.C.T. (*see* **Note 14**). Tie off the lungs as described above for the formalin fixation protocol.
11. To embed the O.C.T. inflated lungs for histology, place a small amount of O.C.T. compound in the bottom of the tissue mold. This initial layer of O.C.T. should completely cover the bottom of the mold. Carefully remove the lungs from the chest cavity, as described above for the formalin fixation protocol. Place the lungs in the tissue mold and carefully hold in place until the initial layer of O.C.T. thickens enough to secure the bottom of the lungs to the tissue mold. The excess suture thread should not be inserted in the mold. Immediately begin filling the remaining tissue mold with O.C.T. by adding the compound in a circular motion while gently balancing the top of the lungs with the forceps to ensure that they remain vertical and centered in the mold. Once the tissue mold is filled, cut the excess suture thread with scissors. The O.C.T. compound

should completely freeze within 10 min and samples can be stored at −80 °C until ready for use.

12. Histology sections should be prepared using a cryostat. It is also important that the lungs be prepared in either a dorsal or a ventral orientation to maximize visualization of the airway.
13. For studies evaluating gene expression and/or protein levels, it may be preferable to harvest the lungs for RNA or protein extraction rather than for histology. Fill an ice bucket, or other approved container, with liquid nitrogen. For each sample, label a cryotube with an indelible pen. Harvest the whole blood and BALF as described above. Remove the cannula and sutures. Remove the lungs, one lobe at a time, with the curved blunted scissors without inflating. Special care should be taken to remove any additional material from the chest cavity to avoid contaminating material (i.e., ensure that the lung sections do not also include pieces of heart, thymus, lymph node, or esophagus). Place each lung lobe into the cryotube and drop the tube in the liquid nitrogen to flash freeze the tissue. Store the tissue in liquid nitrogen until ready for homogenization.

3.3 Sample Preparation for Analysis

1. Collect the serum from the whole blood. After allowing the whole blood to coagulate at room temperature for at least 30 min, spin the samples in a microcentrifuge at maximum speed (~17,000 × *g*) for 5 min. Label a 1.5 ml microcentrifuge tube for serum collection with the indelible pen, one tube for each serum sample. Carefully remove the tubes containing the now separated whole blood from the centrifuge. Note the separation of the blood into two distinct phases. The serum is isolated in the top layer. Carefully remove the serum from the tube using a p1000 pipette and transfer the serum to the newly labeled microcentrifuge tube. Keep the tubes on ice until ready for storage. The recovered volume of serum should be approximately equivalent to 20 % of the total volume of whole blood. Store the serum at −80 °C until ready for use.
2. For cytokine and immunoglobulin analysis by ELISA, the serum should be diluted 1:5–1:20 depending on the assay. These dilutions should be empirically determined prior to running the bulk of the samples. Due to the low volume of serum collected, most sample volumes can be reduced by half for loading on the ELISA plate. For example, most commercial ELISAs utilize 100 μl volumes of standards and samples; for serum, load 50 μl of standards and diluted samples. Common ELISAs for serum include IL-13, IgE, and antigen-specific IgE.
3. Collect cell-free BALF from the BAL for cytokine analysis. Spin the BALF that was collected in the 15 ml conical tubes in a refrigerated tabletop centrifuge at 1,530 × *g* for 5 min to

pellet the cells. Label two 1.5 ml microcentrifuge tubes with the indelible pen. Carefully remove the 15 ml tubes from the centrifuge without disturbing the cell pellet. Carefully transfer the BALF supernatant to the 1.5 ml microcentrifuge tubes and keep on ice. Store the BALF at −80 °C until ready for use.

4. For cytokine and immunoglobulin analysis by ELISA, the BALF should be used neat or diluted 1:5 depending on the assay. These dilutions should be empirically determined prior to running the bulk of the samples. Unlike the serum, the BALF should yield ample volume for ELISA and western blot analysis. However, most sample volumes can also be reduced by half for loading on the ELISA plate, as discussed for the serum. Common ELISAs for the BALF include IL-13, IL-4, and IL-5.
5. Collect the cells from the BALF for cellular composition analysis. Lyse the red blood cells by hypotonic saline (*see* **Note 15**). Resuspend the cells in 900 μl of distilled water. Immediately add 100 μl of 10× PBS. Samples should be lysed one at a time. If samples contain excessive amounts of red blood cells, the cells can be spun down in the tabletop centrifuge at 2,040 × *g* for 5 min and repeat the lysis procedures described above.
6. Determine the total BALF cellularity in the 1 ml suspension using a hemacytometer under 10–20× magnification with Trypan Blue staining. These data can be evaluated by either showing as cells/ml or multiplying with the volume of BALF collected and shown as cells/mouse.
7. Collect cells for differential staining (*see* **Note 16**). Label standard microscope slides using a pencil or a solvent-resistant pen. Secure the slides into the holder and funnel for the cytospin. Remove 150 μl of BALF and cytospin at 1,020 × *g* for 5 min. Allow the slides to air-dry overnight. Differential stain the slides following the manufacturer's protocols. Allow the slides to air-dry overnight. Coverslip the slides using permount. Evaluate the slides using a microscope equipped with a 20× and 40× objective.
8. Harvest the remaining cells for subsequent analysis, such as FACS, electron microscopy, confocal microscopy, RNA extraction for gene expression evaluation, and/or protein extraction for Western Blot. In general, these subsequent assays, such as flow cytometry, will be limited by the number of cells collected by the lavage. For most protocols, the cells can be collected by centrifugation at 1,530 × *g* for 5 min, the supernatant removed, and samples stored at −80 °C until ready for use.
9. Prepare the lungs for histopathology evaluation. After 24–48 h of formalin fixation, the whole inflated lungs should be ventrally orientated and embedded in paraffin. The resultant blocks

should be cut to expose the main airway. Increased scoring accuracy can be achieved by orientating the lungs in the same position and cut to the same depth. Five micron serial sections of the lungs should be cut and stained with hematoxylin and eosin (H&E), Masson's Trichrome, and Alcian-blue/periodic acid-schiff reaction (AB/PAS). Additional sections can be cut and prepared for in situ hybridization using standard protocols.

10. Utilize H&E staining and scoring to evaluate overall lung inflammation. The most efficient technique to evaluate H&E staining in these types of assays is through semiquantitative inflammation scoring of the left lung lobe. Sections of the left lobe should be cut to yield the maximum longitudinal visualization of the intrapulmonary main axial airway. Histopathology can then be evaluated by the following inflammatory parameters, which are scored between 0 (absent) and 3 (severe): mononuclear and polymorphonuclear cell infiltration; airway epithelial cell hyperplasia and injury; extravasation; perivascular and peribroncheolar cuffing; and percent of the lung involved with inflammation. These parameter scores can then be averaged for a total histology score or used individually to quantify specific aspects of disease progression. Scoring should always be conducted in a double-blind fashion, with reviewers blinded to both genotype and treatment. This scoring system has been previously described [13–17].
11. Evaluate collagen and pre-collagen deposition. Collagen and pre-collagen deposition is often a feature of long-term, chronic models of allergic airway inflammation. To evaluate collagen deposition in the lungs, histology sections can be prepared as described above and stained with Masson's Trichrome. Masson's Trichrome results should be assessed and scored by an experienced reviewer who is blinded to genotype and treatment, as previously described [17]. This technique generates a qualitative or a semiquantitative dataset. However, collagen levels in the lungs can be accurately quantified using biochemical assays, such as the hydroxyproline assay.
12. Evaluate goblet cell hyperplasia. Goblet cell hyperplasia is also a characteristic feature of allergic airway disease and can be assessed in the disease models using AB/PAS staining. Sections of the left lung lobes should be sectioned, as described above, and stained with AB/PAS. For proper evaluation of mucus production and in an effort to avoid bias, the identical area from all lungs should be evaluated. A 2 mm length of airway located midway along the length of the main axial airway should be marked and digitally imaged at 10× and 20× magnification. Using ImageJ software (NIH, National Technical Information Service, Springfield, VA), the length and area of the AB/PAS-stained region in the lung sections can be imaged

and measured (see user guide for software use). The resultant data is expressed as the mean volume density (Vs = nl/mm^2 basal lamina + SEM of AB/PAS-stained material within the epithelium), as previously described [18].

4 Notes

1. Female mice are preferred in these assays due to their more docile nature. There is an increased probability that adult male animals will become aggressive during the course of this type of long-term experiment. If male mice are to be utilized, consider individual housing.
2. We have successfully utilized 6–12-week-old C57Bl/6, 129SvEv, and BALB/c mice in these assays. If strain is not a limiting factor, BALB/c mice are preferred due to their Th2 skewing and robust response. It is possible that some aspects of this protocol may need to be adjusted and further optimized when using mice from different genetic backgrounds.
3. All studies should be conducted in accordance with the local and institutional animal care and use guidelines and in accord with the prevailing national regulations.
4. Mice were exposed i.n. to 0.05 AU/ml of purified 50:50 DerP and DerF whole-body extract. There are a variety of sensitization protocols and dosing parameters reported in the literature for house dust mite exposure. It is also common practice to use either DerP or DerF unmixed. In our experience, all of these procedures appear to work equally well under the conditions described in this protocol.
5. 2,2,2 Tribromoethanol (Avertin) is a common substitute for drop method isoflurane anesthesia in allergic airway inflam mation protocols that require fewer rounds of sensitization (i.e., many ovalbumin models). However, in our experience, the deep plain of anesthesia induced by avertin can actually reduce the effectiveness of the intranasal administrations. Likewise, for the dust mite protocol, the frequency of i.n. administrations (5/week) make i.p. anesthesia impractical and likely to induce significant pain and distress in the animals.
6. We recommend the use of specialized, commercially available tracheal cannulas. However, 16 gage needles can be used as substitutes. In our experience, this alternative works best when the needles are ground down to a blunt end.
7. There are many allergens that could be substituted for DMA using this protocol, including *Aspergillus* sp. and cockroach antigen. However, the sensitization protocols for each allergen should be empirically determined. We have found that the use

of DMA is preferable to ovalbumin in chronic models due to the following: (a) repeated challenges of OVA will eventually result in tolerance; (b) HDM, *Aspergillus* sp., and cockroach antigen are clinically relevant to the human disease; and (c) the robust nature of OVA-induced inflammation typically obscures subtle, yet highly relevant, aspects of disease pathogenesis.

8. Intranasal administration requires extensive practice to achieve proficiency. Improper technique can result in sinus deposition and inefficient sensitization, which result in weak and highly variable inflammatory responses. In our hands, we have found that EBD is an effective training tool. A 1 % solution of EBD in 1× PBS can be generated, filter sterilized, and administered i.n. To quantify the efficiency of the i.n. administration, the lungs can be removed and incubated in formamide for 48 h at room temperature to extract the EBD. The absorption of Evans blue can be measured using a standard plate reader at 620 nm and deposited Evans blue can be calculated against a standard curve to quantify efficiency.
9. Drop method isoflurane induces a low level of anesthesia that is recommended for this procedure. We have found that light anesthesia allows for more effective antigen instillation compared to other techniques, which often suppress breathing volumes and rates. Drop method isoflurane induces anesthesia within 30 s and will lightly anesthetize the mouse for approximately 30 s. Each individual institution will have specific guidelines regarding the use of drop method anesthesia.
10. Note that inhalation anesthetics, such as isoflurane, may result in confounding issues when studying lung physiology. Therefore, ensure that control animals are properly utilized and limit the animal's exposure to the anesthetic as much as possible.
11. We have successfully utilized the described DMA protocols for both short-term (4–6 weeks) and chronic sensitization (12–16 weeks). The short-term models are ideal to evaluate elements associated with inflammation; however, the long-term exposures provide a more physiologically relevant model of the human disease and allow assessments of airway remodeling that is absent in the short-term exposure.
12. All studies should be conducted in accordance with the local and institutional animal care and use guidelines and in accord with the prevailing national regulations.
13. The blood should be harvested by heartstick using the 1 ml syringe with a 27 gage needle attached. There are multiple

approved methods of conducting the heartstick. We have found that it is most effective when performed prior to making any incisions on the animal. Immediately after removal from the CO_2 chamber, ensure proper euthanasia by toe pinch reflex and pin the mouse to a surgical board. Spray the animal with 70 % ethanol and locate the base of the sternum. Insert the needle between the last two ribs slightly to the right of the center. Using a controlled and singular motion, begin withdrawing the blood from the heart. With practice, this procedure can typically recover 500–800 μl of whole blood. Transfer the blood from the syringe to a labeled 1.5 ml microcentrifuge tube. Critical note: Remove the needle from the syringe prior to transferring the blood. Forcing the blood through the needle will induce cell lysis and inhibit serum collection.

14. For optimal results, the lungs must be inflated with O.C.T. As an alternative to utilizing the cannula, the lungs can be inflated through simple injection with O.C.T. using a 27 gage needle. Lung inflation is critical as it allows for observation of the lungs in the most physiologically relevant state.

15. There are many different protocols for red blood cell lysis. The protocol described here is optimized for the subsequent basic morphology assessments by differential staining and total cell counts. However, this procedure results in suboptimal results in higher resolution analyses, such as FACs. Red blood cell lysis via AKT is a viable alternative for procedures requiring less background and higher resolution.

16. Differential staining allows for morphology-based identification of BALF cellularity. To ensure the optimal results, the samples should be cytospun on the same day they were collected and the staining reagents should be prepared fresh prior to each use. DiffQuick-based protocols allow the differentiation of eosinophils (granules stain red) and neutrophils (granules do not stain). Monocytic cells can be easily identified, but are difficult to distinguish. Therefore, these cells should be identified as monocytes, rather than macrophages. Likewise, lymphocytes are also commonly observed in the BALF. However, it is also unlikely that typical researchers can distinguish T-cells from B-cells based on morphology alone. Thus, many investigators have modified these procedures for use with flow cytometry. The only limiting factor is the low number of total cells typically harvested from control animals. Even with flow cytometry, differential staining should be used to confirm the results.

References

1. Busse WW, Lemanske RF Jr (2001) Asthma. N Engl J Med 344:350–362
2. Drazen JM, Silverman EK, Lee TH (2000) Heterogeneity of therapeutic responses in asthma. Br Med Bull 56:1054–1070
3. Wardlaw AJ, Brightling CE, Green R, Woltmann G, Bradding P, Pavord ID (2002) New insights into the relationship between airway inflammation and asthma. Clin Sci (Lond) 103:201–211
4. Downie SR, Salome CM, Verbanck S, Thompson B, Berend N, King GG (2007) Ventilation heterogeneity is a major determinant of airway hyperresponsiveness in asthma, independent of airway inflammation. Thorax 62:684–689
5. Hershenson MB, Brown M, Camoretti-Mercado B, Solway J (2008) Airway smooth muscle in asthma. Annu Rev Pathol 3:523–555
6. Canning BJ (2003) Modeling asthma and COPD in animals: a pointless exercise? Curr Opin Pharmacol 3:244–250
7. Dye JA, McKiernan BC, Rozanski EA, Hoffmann WE, Losonsky JM, Homco LD, Weisiger RM, Kakoma I (1996) Bronchopulmonary disease in the cat: historical, physical, radiographic, clinicopathologic, and pulmonary functional evaluation of 24 affected and 15 healthy cats. J Vet Intern Med 10:385–400
8. Lavoie JP, Maghni K, Desnoyers M, Taha R, Martin JG, Hamid QA (2001) Neutrophilic airway inflammation in horses with heaves is characterized by a Th2-type cytokine profile. Am J Respir Crit Care Med 164:1410–1413
9. Leguillette R (2003) Recurrent airway obstruction–heaves. Vet Clin North Am Equine Pract 19:63–86
10. Taube C, Dakhama A, Gelfand EW (2004) Insights into the pathogenesis of asthma utilizing murine models. Int Arch Allergy Immunol 135:173–186
11. Kumar RK, Foster PS (2002) Modeling allergic asthma in mice: pitfalls and opportunities. Am J Respir Cell Mol Biol 27:267–272
12. Yu M, Tsai M, Tam SY, Jones C, Zehnder J, Galli SJ (2006) Mast cells can promote the development of multiple features of chronic asthma in mice. J Clin Invest 116(6):1633–1641
13. Allen IC, Pace AJ, Jania LA, Ledford JG, Latour AM, Snouwaert JN, Bernier V, Stocco R, Therien AG, Koller BH (2006) Expression and function of NPSR1/GPRA in the lung before and after induction of asthma-like disease. Am J Physiol Lung Cell Mol Physiol 291:L1005–L1017
14. Allen IC, Scull MA, Moore CB, Holl EK, McElvania-TeKippe E, Taxman DJ, Guthrie EH, Pickles RJ, Ting JP (2009) The NLRP3 inflammasome mediates in vivo innate immunity to influenza A virus through recognition of viral RNA. Immunity 30:556–565
15. Willingham SB, Allen IC, Bergstralh DT, Brickey WJ, Huang MT, Taxman DJ, Duncan JA, Ting JP (2009) NLRP3 (NALP3, cryopyrin) facilitates in vivo caspase-1 activation, necrosis, and HMGB1 release via inflammasome-dependent and independent pathways. J Immunol 183:2008–2015
16. Allen IC, Jania CM, Wilson JE, Tekeppe EM, Hua X, Brickey WJ, Kwan M, Koller BH, Tilley SL, Ting JP (2012) Analysis of NLRP3 in the development of allergic airway disease in mice. J Immunol 188(6):2884–2893
17. Allen IC, Lich JD, Arthur JC, Jania CM, Roberts RA, Callaway JB, Tilley SL, Ting JP (2012) Characterization of NLRP12 during the development of allergic airway disease in mice. PLoS One 7(1):e30612
18. Cressman VL, Hicks EM, Funkhouser WK, Backlund DC, Koller BH (1998) The relationship of chronic mucin secretion to airway disease in normal and CFTR-deficient mice. Am J Respir Cell Mol Biol 19(6):853–866

Chapter 14

An Inhalation Model of Allergic Fungal Asthma: *Aspergillus fumigatus*-Induced Inflammation and Remodeling in Allergic Airway Disease

Jane M. Schuh and Scott A. Hoselton

Abstract

The ability to accurately mimic normal processes for sensitization and allergen challenge in an experimental animal model are useful in that they allow researchers to critically manipulate the complex interactions of multiple cell types. In the context of the allergic lung, multiple cell types form complex cellular networks and function to regulate a variety of temporal and spatial changes. Mouse models of allergic airway disease have proven to be highly useful for dissecting these complex interactions, particularly in addressing remodeling of the allergic airway in chronic asthma. Until we can better represent the normal processes that initiate and perpetuate asthma, our understanding of the mechanisms of tissue injury leading to chronic remodeling of the airways and effective therapeutic strategies to treat this disease will remain limited. It was with this goal in mind that we set about devising an inhalational model of *Aspergillus fumigatus*-induced fungal asthma in a murine experimental system.

Key words Asthma, Allergy, Model, Aspergillus, Remodeling, Inhalation, Fungus

1 Introduction

The lung is a fabulously complex organ that employs over 50 cell types to carry out its primary function of gas exchange. From our first breath to our last, its delicate network of air spaces with walls comprising a single cell's thickness is constantly under mechanical stress as the alveoli are stretched and released. Its function and composition dictate that it must routinely rid itself of inhaled and cellular debris. The lung must withstand the regular assault of toxic exposures in the form of chemicals ranging from cigarette smoke to air fresheners. Often the assault is in the form of microorganisms that may be ignored, blocked, or attacked depending upon the level of threat. Not only does the immune response in the lung need to quickly block or eliminate and remove microbial pathogens from infecting the body through this highly vulnerable site of

Irving C. Allen (ed.), *Mouse Models of Allergic Disease: Methods and Protocols*, Methods in Molecular Biology, vol. 1032, DOI 10.1007/978-1-62703-496-8_14, © Springer Science+Business Media, LLC 2013

entry, but it must also retain function through the response and repair process. It is little wonder, then, that sometimes the pulmonary immune response is associated with a host-derived pathology. Whether the immunopathology of allergic asthma is a result of an aberrant response that incorrectly interprets an innocuous antigen as a pathogenic threat or a vestige of an appropriate immune response that has unintended consequences, the resulting response can lead to acute and chronic pulmonary dysfunction.

Asthma is a clinical condition affecting more than 300 million persons worldwide [1]. Its treatment is expensive both in personal expense, which can include medication costs, office and emergency center visits, and hospitalization, and reduced workforce productivity. In the USA alone, the economic burden associated with asthma is $56 billion annually [2] and continues to increase. As a disease that can develop in childhood and persist into senescence, the cost for an individual may be accrued for decades.

Asthma is characterized by acute exacerbations punctuating a persistent disease. The cumulative effects of these exacerbations may lead to permanent damage of the airways, particularly when the individual is sensitized to fungal allergens. Sensitization to fungi in the context of asthma presents a severe clinical scenario that is difficult to treat, accounting for a disproportionately large number of emergency center visits and hospitalizations [3, 4]. The inflammation and airway hyperresponsiveness that accompany an acute asthma attack are well-recognized factors that demand immediate medical intervention. However, while the chronic dysfunction that is associated with the remodeling of the airway wall may be less obvious, it is responsible for considerable morbidity associated with allergic asthma. This immunopathologically mediated transformation of the airway is typified by airway and blood vessel smooth muscle cell hyperplasia, increased mucus production, and peribronchial fibrosis. Airway obstruction in acute asthma is reversible; in contrast, the cumulative dysfunction caused by long-term airway remodeling is not.

The experimental model that is explained here was built upon the foundation of other intratracheal inoculation models of *A. fumigatus*-induced disease [5]. The nose-only inhalation of aerosolized *Aspergillus* conidia by a mouse that has been sensitized to *Aspergillus* antigens elicits an allergic phenotype with many of the immunological signs and physiological parameters that afflict human patients with asthma, including airway wall remodeling and exacerbation following rechallenge [6, 7].

The model entails allergen sensitization through injections of soluble fungal extracts in adjuvant followed by an inhalation challenge with unmanipulated, airborne fungal spores. Directions for assembling a simple apparatus that allows the hydrophobic fungal spores to be blown into a nose-only inoculation chamber are included in the notes section (*see* **Note 1**). At prescribed time points after fungal inhalation, restrained plethysmography is employed to assess airway responses before and after acetyl-β-methacholine injection. Blood, BAL fluid, and lung tissue may then be collected from each animal and stored or prepared for further analyses, which may include morphometric analysis of airway cells, histological visualization of inflammation and airway remodeling, protein and nucleic acid assessment, flow cytometry, and other measurements of the disease process.

2 Materials

2.1 Airborne Fungal Inhalation Apparatus (See Note 1)

1. Apparatus assembly: ¾-in. barbed female thread fitting; 1-in. × ¾-in. female threaded coupler; 1-in. coupler; 1-in. schedule 40 PVC; ¾-in. × 1-in. male threaded adaptor; ¾-in. male threaded to ½-in. barbed fitting; PVC cement; jigsaw with a PVC blade; drill with ⁵⁄₁₆-in. drill bit or a drill press; ½-in. tubing; ¾-in. tubing; two 500-ml vacuum flasks; acidic sporicidal solution.

2.2 Fungal Sensitization and Challenge

1. Animals and husbandry: Specific pathogen-free C57BL/6 or BALB/c mice; Alpha-dri paper bedding.
2. Sensitizing fungal antigen and adjuvant for injections: 100 μg/ml of *Aspergillus fumigatus* antigen (Greer Laboratories, Lenoir, NC, USA) in normal saline (NS) that has been mixed immediately before injection with an equal volume of Imject Alum (Pierce, Rockford, IL, USA); 100 μl is required per injection.
3. Sensitizing fungal antigen for intranasal inoculation: 1 mg/ml of *Aspergillus fumigatus* antigen extract (Greer Laboratories) in NS delivered with a micropipette; 20 μl is required per inoculation.
4. Fungal culture for airborne challenge: *Aspergillus fumigatus, Fresenius* fungal culture stock (strain NIH 5233, American Type Culture Collection (ATCC), Manassas, VA, USA); 1× PBS; 0.4-ml Eppendorf tubes; 4 °C refrigerator; 25-cm^2 cell culture flasks coated on one large surface with 10–12 ml of Sabouraud Dextrose Agar (SDA).
5. Airborne delivery: Assembled apparatus (*see* **Note 1**), set up in a class II biological safety hood; anesthesia cocktail of 75 mg/kg of ketamine and 25 mg/kg of xylazine (*see* **Note 2**) delivered by injection with a tuberculin syringe with 26-gauge needle; warming blankets or heaters for post-anesthesia recovery.

2.3 Airway Plethysmography and Ventilation

1. Anesthesia: 0.01 mg of sodium pentobarbital/g body weight in a volume of <0.5 ml of sterile PBS per mouse (*see* **Note 2**).
2. Airway canulation: Small animal restraint board; 70 % EtOH; surgical scissors; forceps; 19-gauge beveled tracheal tube; surgical sutures.

3. Airway assessment: whole body, restrained plethysmograph for mouse (for example, Buxco, Troy, NY, USA, or flexiVent, SciReq, Montreal, Canada); small animal respirator (Harvard Apparatus, Holliston, MA, USA); 480 μg/kg of acetyl-β-methacholine in a 0.1-ml volume.

2.4 Tissue Collection, Processing, Storage

1. Bronchoalveolar lavage (BAL) cells and fluid: Tuberculin syringe with sterile NS fitted with a blunt 19-G needle; 1.5-ml Eppendorf tubes; ice bucket.
2. Blood collection: Forceps; sterile 1.5-ml Eppendorf tubes; micropipettors; microfuge; –20 °C freezer.
3. Lung tissue collection for protein or nucleic acid, histological, and flow cytometric analyses: Surgical scissors; forceps; 5-ml snap top tubes; liquid nitrogen in a dewar; –80 °C freezer; tuberculin syringes with 26-gauge needles; 10 % neutral buffered formalin; 50-ml tubes; 5-ml snap top tubes with cell culture medium; ice buckets.
4. Tissue preparation for nucleic acid or protein analysis: Tissue homogenizer (Tissue-Tearor, BioSpec Products, Bartlesville, OK); cold DMEM with a protease inhibitor cocktail (Roche Complete Mini or similar, Roche Applied Science, Indianapolis, IN); micropipettors, nucleic acid isolation kits (any); ELISA Abs and kits (R&D Systems, Minneapolis, MN, or others).

3 Methods

3.1 Murine Sensitization and Challenge with Live, Airborne Cultures of A. fumigatus

1. Obtain prior approval for these studies from the appropriate institutional office(s) for the use of animals in research and for the use of biological safety level (BSL) 2 biological organisms.
2. Reconstitute a single lyophilized *A. fumigatus* culture in PBS in a volume recommended by ATCC and store 60-μl aliquots of the suspension in 0.4-ml Eppendorf tubes at 4 °C until use.
3. Purchase animals from a reputable laboratory animal facility and maintain them in a specific pathogen-free facility for the duration of the study. Feed and water animals ad libitum throughout the study on a general mouse chow diet and house them on Alpha-dri paper bedding or a similar low-microbial bedding choice.
4. Divide mice into groups of 5–6 animals (*see* **Note 3**) for each time point. Sensitize mice with a subcutaneous (SC) and an intraperitoneal (IP) injection of 5 μg of soluble *A. fumigatus* antigen dissolved in 0.05 ml of PBS and 0.05 ml of Imject Alum totaling 10 μg between the two injections. Two weeks after the injections, inoculate the mice with a series of 3, weekly 20-μg intranasal (IN) inoculations consisting of soluble *A. fumigatus* antigen dissolved in 20 μl of NS (*see* **Note 4**).

5. One week after the final sensitizing inoculation, prepare the inhalation challenge chamber in a class II biological safety hood by fitting the neck of the culture flask to the input end (*see* **Note 5**). Deliver air through the culture flask at 2 psi to liberate the hydrophobic spores and allow their delivery through the inoculation port. For the initial run, place tape over each of the nose holes in the inoculation apparatus to allow the airborne spores to coat the inside of the apparatus. Turn off the air, remove the tape, and replace the culture flask with a new one for the first group of animals.
6. To expose the animals to live airborne conidia, anesthetize three mice with a ketamine/xylazine anesthesia cocktail and place their noses in one of the three inoculation ports. Adjust the airflow to 2 psi and allow the animals to breathe aerosolized conidia for 10 min. Return the animals to clean cages with heat support and monitor until they recover from anesthesia. Change the *Aspergillus* culture with each set of three mice. After the last group has been treated, decontaminate the apparatus (*see* **Note 6**).

3.2 AHR: Plethysmography and Ventilation by Cannulated Trachea

1. At the appropriate time point after allergen challenge, anesthetize the mice in a group one at a time with an SC injection of sodium pentobarbital. This will be the terminal procedure for each group of mice. Place the animal on a surgical restraint board, and tracheostomize. For tracheostomy, a length of surgical suture taped to the top of the restraint board should be used to catch the animal's front teeth to restrain the head for tracheal surgery. A drop of 70 % EtOH on the trachea helps to wet the fur, making surgery easier. Tracheostomize the mouse by opening the hide with a small snip along the trachea. Put the point of the surgical scissors in the cut and open the blades to extend the opening sagittally. Expose the trachea. Make a small snip in the membrane that covers the trachea. Insert the tip of the surgical scissors in the cut and open the blades to extend the opening sagittally. Using curved, sharp-nosed forceps, make a path behind the trachea and pull a 4-in. length of suture around the back of the trachea. Make a horizontal cut across the front of the trachea anterior to where the surgical suture is positioned, being careful not to cut through the back of the trachea. Insert the 19-gauge bevel tracheal tube and tie it into place securely with surgical suture. Connect the trachea tube to the ventilator. Measure and record the baseline compliance/resistance for airway response (per optimized settings for the plethysmography of choice). Inject 0.1 ml of methacholine (480 μg/kg) by tail vein injection (*see* **Note 7**), and record the postinjection peak airway resistance (Fig. 1).

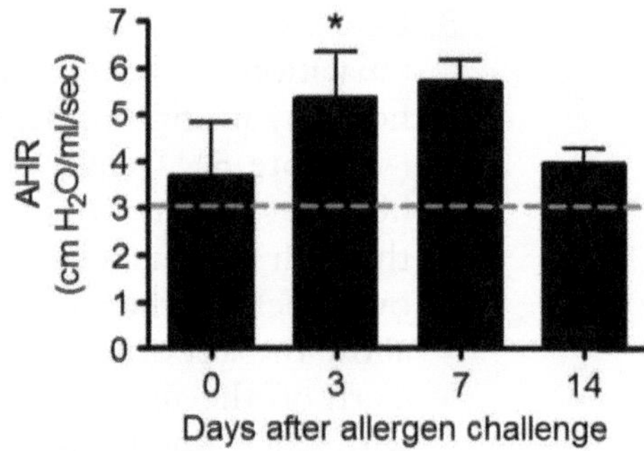

Fig. 1 Airway hyperresponsiveness at days 0, 3, 7, 14, 21, and 35 after conidia challenge in *A. fumigatus*-sensitized BALB/c mice challenged with airborne conidia. The baseline airway resistance in all groups was similar prior to the methacholine provocation (1.52 ± 0.061 cm H_2O/ml/s). Peak increases in airway resistance were stimulated by using an intravenous methacholine injection dose of 480 μg/kg. Naïve values after methacholine are represented with a *dashed line*. Values are expressed as the mean ± SEM; $n = 5$ mice/group (Modified from data originally published in [8] and reproduced with permission from Informa Healthcare)

3.3 Blood Collection per Orbital Bleed Exsanguination

1. Remove the mouse from the ventilator and, under anesthesia, exsanguinate the animal by removing one or both eyeballs. Collect the blood in a 1.5-ml Eppendorf tube. Approximately 500 μl of blood can be collected efficiently by this method. Centrifuge the blood at 15,000 × *g* for 10 min and transfer the serum to a new tube. Store the serum at −20 °C until use. Sera can be used for various protein analyses by standard ELISA methods (Fig. 2a, c, d).

3.4 BAL Fluid Collection via Trachea Tube Cannula, Cell Differential, and Fluid Collection

1. Open the chest cavity, exposing the lungs. Connect a 19-gauge blunt needle fitted to a tuberculin syringe loaded with 1.0 ml of sterile PBS to the tracheal tube and lavage the bronchoalveolar space. Place the lavage fluid in a 1.5-ml Eppendorf tube on ice. After all samples are collected, centrifuge to pellet cells. Remove the supernatant, transfer the BALF to a clean tube, and freeze at −20 °C until use for protein analysis (Fig. 2b). Resuspend the cells in PBS (*see* **Note 8**) and cytospin onto coded glass microscope slides. Dry the slides and perform a standard quick dip differential stain. Differential counts on lymphocytes (B and T cells), monocyte/macrophages, neutrophils, and eosinophils can be recorded by counting at least 300 cells per slide from 1,000× random fields (Fig. 3).

3.5 Lung Dissection for Histology, Nucleic Acid Assessment, or Protein Analysis

1. Dissect whole left lungs from each mouse. Inflate the lung ex vivo by injecting 1 ml of 10 % neutral buffered formalin (NBF) through a single injection into the peripheral lung tissue until the entire left lung is inflated. Place the left lungs from one group in a 50-ml tube containing 10 % NBF and fix overnight for histological processing and staining (Fig. 4, *see* **Note 9**).

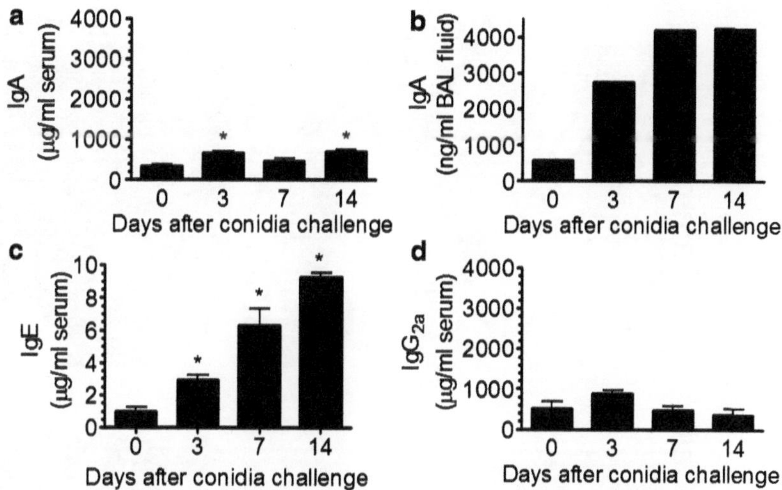

Fig. 2 Antibody levels from serum and BAL fluid after allergen challenge with aerosolized *A. fumigatus* conidia in BALB/c mice. Ab isotypes were quantified by specific ELISA in serum and BAL fluid at days 3, 7, and 14 and compared to sensitized mice that were not challenged with inhaled fungal conidia (day 0). Serum levels were analyzed using an unpaired, student's two-tailed t test with Welch's correction. All values are expressed as the mean ± SEM. $n = 4–5$ mice/group, $^{*}p < 0.05$ was considered statistically significant. BAL samples were pooled, and no statistical analysis was run on them

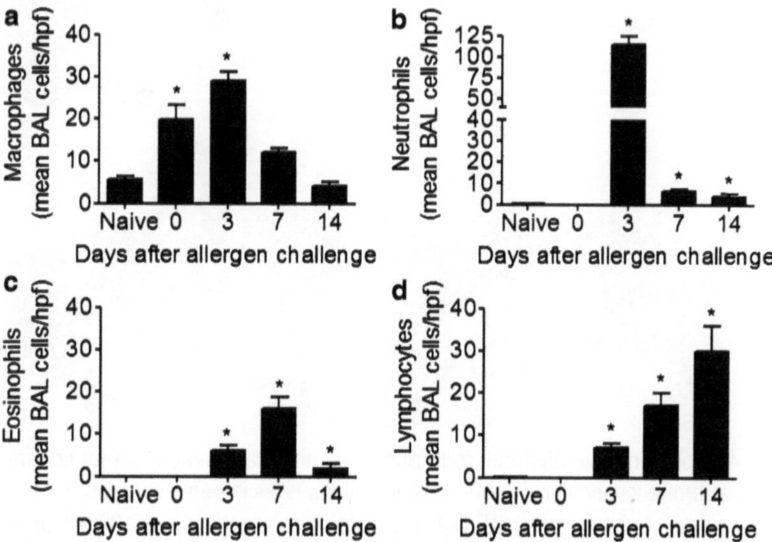

Fig. 3 BAL leukocyte counts in *A. fumigatus*-sensitized BALB/c mice at days 0, 3, 7, 14, and 21 after airborne conidia challenge. Cells washed from the airways at various times after allergen challenge were cytospun onto coded microscope slides and assessed by morphometric characteristics. Data are expressed as the mean number of cells per HPF (1,000×) ± SEM; $n = 5$ mice/group

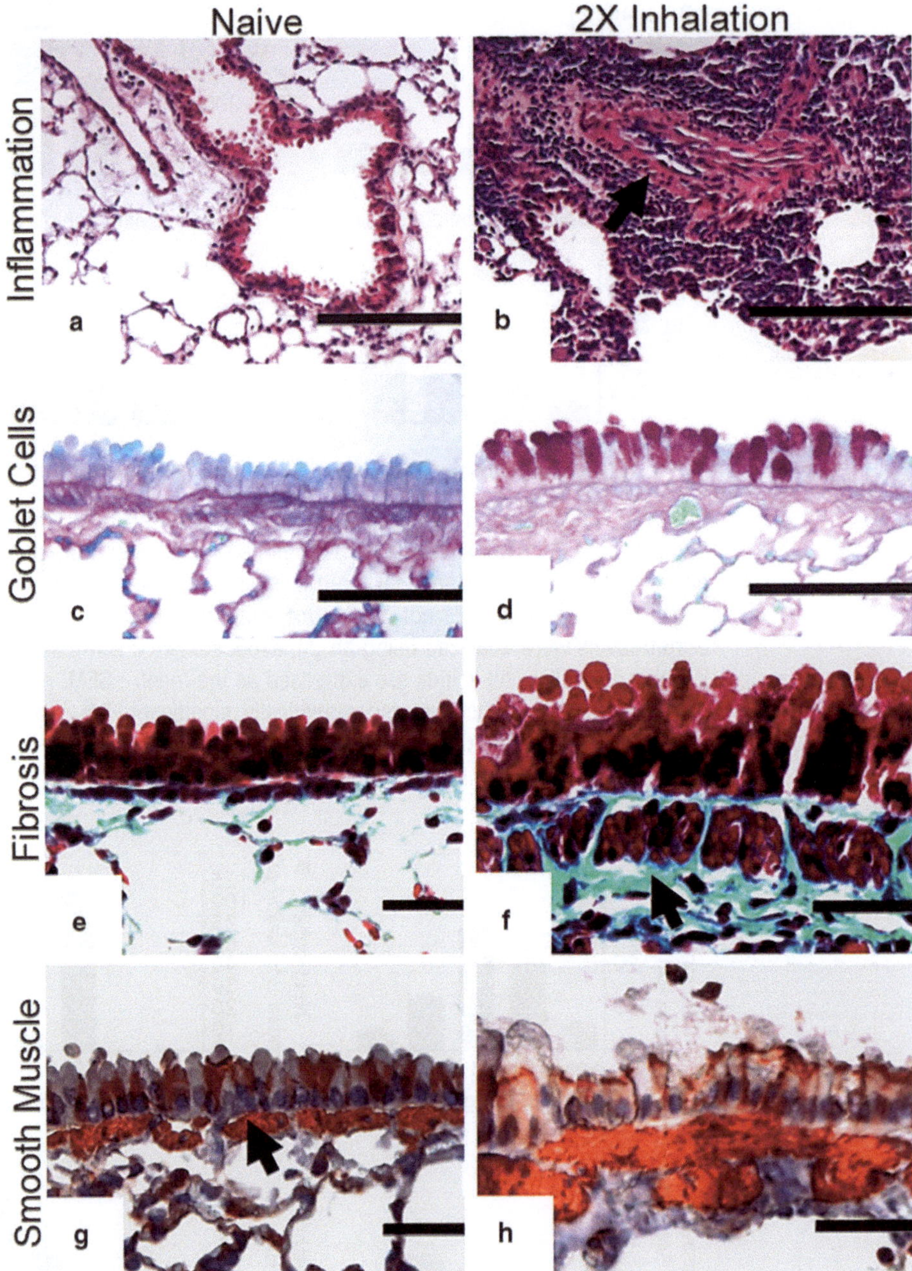

Fig. 4 Representative photomicrographs showing inflammation, goblet cell metaplasia, subepithelial fibrosis, and peribronchovascular smooth muscle cell changes in naïve controls or at day 7 after two inhalational challenges with *A. fumigatus*. H&E-stained histological sections from naive (*left*) and fungus-challenged (*right*) lungs were assessed for inflammation by H&E stain (**a** and **b**, *arrows* indicate perivascular smooth muscle cell increases), goblet cell metaplasia by periodic acid Schiff's stain (**c** and **d**, *magenta* stain), fibrosis by Gomori's trichrome stain (**e** and **f**, *blue* stain), and peribronchial smooth muscle by IHC for α-smooth muscle actin (**g** and **h**, *red* stain). Scale bars for **a**, **b** = 200 μm; for **c**, **d** = 100 μm; for **g**, **h** = 50 μm (Modification of original reproduced from [6] with permission from Elsevier)

Alternatively, each lung can be processed separately for paired analysis with AHR or other measurements.

2. Dissect a small piece of the right lung for nucleic acid analysis and a large piece for protein analysis. Snap freeze in liquid N_2 and store at −80 °C until use. Process the tissues for real-time RT-PCR by isolating total RNA by standard methods. Process the tissues for protein analysis by grinding with a tissue homogenizer in cold DMEM with a protease inhibitor cocktail and analyzing by standard ELISA methods (*see* **Note 10**).

4 Notes

1. Using a jigsaw with a PVC blade, cut the schedule 40 PVC into a 10¾-in. length. Using a 5⁄16-in. drill bit, make nose holes for exposure by first drilling one hole into the middle of the pipe, and then drilling one hole to the left and one to the right of the central hole with approximately 2.5-in. spacing. It is important that the holes are exactly in line. We suggest drilling the holes prior to assembling the apparatus as it may take multiple attempts to achieve this without a drill press.

   Place the ¾-in. × 1-in. male threaded adaptor on the right end of the PVC pipe and the 1-in. PVC coupler on the left end. Insert the 1 × ¾-in. female adaptor into the 1-in. coupler on the left end. Fasten all of these together using PVC cement. Once the cement has dried, place the ¾-in. female adaptor on the right end and the ¾-in. male thread × ½-in. barbed fitting on the opposite end. Attach a short length of ¾-in. tubing to the right side and approximately 2.5-ft of ½-in. tubing to the left side.

   Assemble the inoculation chamber in a class II biological safety hood (Fig. 5). Prepare the 25 cm² cell culture flask containing an 8-day-old culture of *A. fumigatus* by boring a hole into the rear top and back end of the flask (distal from the neck) with a ½-in. cork hole borer heated over a Bunsen burner. The air input tubing is placed into these holes and adjusted to 2 psi. to liberate the spores when the animals are in place. Attach the culture flask neck to the ¾-in. tubing on the right side of the inoculation chamber. The ½-in. tubing on the left end is used to connect the apparatus to two vacuum flasks containing a sporicidal agent. Connect the vacuum flasks in a series so that the incoming air flows into the top of the first flask down through a plastic pipette fitted through a rubber stopper and into the liquid. The air and spores should bubble into the liquid of flask 1 and the exhaust air and any residual spores from that flask will continue out the side port, through another length of ½-in. tubing into the top of a second

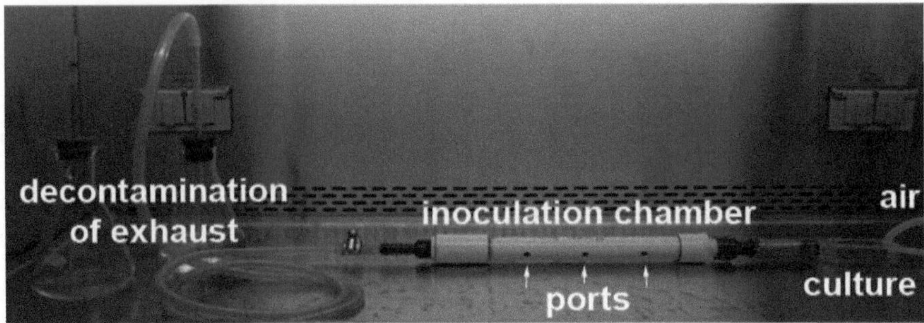

Fig. 5 Airborne inoculation apparatus. From *right* to *left*, the *Aspergillus* inoculation apparatus consists of two air inputs that blow air over a mature, sporulating culture that has been grown on a solid SDA medium in a 25-cm^2 culture flask. Two holes are bored into the plastic immediately before use to provide access for the air hoses. The culture is connected to the inoculation chamber by a short piece of flexible tubing. The inoculation chamber has three, nose-only ports where the anesthetized animals are placed for inoculation. The exhaust air is decontaminated by bubbling through two flasks of sporicidal liquid. The entire apparatus is contained in a class II biological safety hood

flask and down into another volume of sporicidal agent. Finally, the air is allowed to escape from that flask through the side port.

2. Ketamine is a USDEA Schedule III drug, and pentobarbital is a USDEA Schedule II drug. They are controlled substances for which appropriate drug licensure is required for purchase. The University's Attending Veterinarian in charge of animal care may be an appropriate point of contact to procure regulated drugs and to ensure the proper use, storage, documentation, and disposal of the same.
3. Male and/or female mice can be used but should be age and sex matched for each study. In our experience, 5–6 animals per time point provide a reliable assessment of the inflammatory and remodeling aspects of the model. However, a larger sample size may be required for other types of assessments, for example cell sorting for ex vivo experiments. By convention, the day 0 time point represents sensitized animals that have not received the allergen inhalation challenge. These and/or naïve mice are used as controls. In groups that are to receive two or more aerosol challenges, we have found that a 1–2-week interval between inoculations provides robust responses, but does not result in observable physical difficulties for the animals. Likewise, they do not succumb to fungal outgrowth.
4. For intranasal inoculation, pick up the mouse with a hold that immobilizes the head. Draw up the entire 20-μl volume with a micropipettor and deliver half of the volume to each nare allowing the animal to sniff in the inoculum before returning it to the cage.

5. To bore holes through the top and back end of the fungal culture flask, heat a ½-in. metal cork borer over a Bunsen burner and bore holes through the plastic.
6. The interior space of the safety cabinet should be considered contaminated with spores throughout the experiment and until it is thoroughly wetted and wiped down with sporicidal solution. Typically, UV irradiation is insufficient to kill *Aspergillus fumigatus* spores. For decontamination of the apparatus, submerge it in a sporicidal bath in the hood after each use.
7. Warming lights or oil of wintergreen help to vasodilate the tail vein for methacholine injections. The 480 μg/kg dose for tail vein injection has been shown to double the baseline AHR in a naïve mouse, which is then used as the definition of "airway hyperresponsiveness" for the study. Alternatively, a range of increasing injected doses may be used sequentially or inhaled methacholine can be introduced through a nebulization port. If nebulized methacholine is used, care must be taken to prevent the inadvertent exposure of methacholine in the apparatus for the next baseline measurement.
8. To ensure countable BAL cell differentials, we have found that reconstitution in 200 μl of PBS is appropriate for day-0, -7, and -14 samples from a single challenge. Reconstitution in 1 ml of PBS is needed for day-3 samples from a single or a double challenge and for day-7 samples from a double challenge.
9. Columnar epithelial thickness and peribronchial fibrosis can be quantified by measuring the thickness of the cell layer (for epithelial cells) or stained collagen (fibrosis) perpendicularly to the basement membrane. We find that the second (L2) and third (L3) lateral branch of the large airway is an appropriate location to measure continuous lengths of airway to get a representative sampling. Although a skilled technician is still required, L2 and L3 are landmarks that are most easily reproduced when samples are sectioned. At least 50 discrete points for epithelium and at least 100 discrete points for collagen should be measured at intervals of 50 μm, taking care not to include those points that are directly adjacent to a blood vessel as this would artificially increase the measurement.
10. Care should be exercised when interpreting data from ELISAs run on whole-lung homogenates. While serum or BAL fluid results in data that is linear with dilution and reproducible across different manufacturers' platforms, this is not necessarily the case with whole-lung homogenates. Our assessment is that as the protein content of the lung changes dramatically over the course of the model, it may adversely impact the signal-to-noise ratio of antibody-based ELISAs.

Acknowledgments

This work was supported by NIH grant 1R15AI69061 to J.M.S. and an NIH Center grant 2P20RR015566 to Sibi. Core Biology Facilities and microscopy through the Advanced Imaging and Microscopy laboratory at NDSU were funded through grants 2P20RR015566 to Sibi and NSF MRI-R2 DBI-0959512 to Grazul-Bilska, respectively. The authors would also like to acknowledge the outstanding undergraduate, graduate, and postdoctoral trainees who have contributed their effort, intellect, and enthusiasm to this project.

References

1. WHO (2007) Global surveillance, prevention and control of chronic respiratory diseases: a comprehensive approach, 2007. World Health Organization, Geneva
2. Centers for Disease Control and Prevention (CDC) (2011) Vital signs: asthma prevalence, disease characteristics, and self-management education: United States, 2001–2009. MMWR Morb Mortal Wkly Rep 60:547–552
3. Schwartz HJ, Greenberger PA (1991) The prevalence of allergic bronchopulmonary aspergillosis in patients with asthma, determined by serologic and radiologic criteria in patients at risk. J Lab Clin Med 117:138–142
4. Mari A, Schneider P, Wally V, Breitenbach M, Simon-Nobbe B (2003) Sensitization to fungi: epidemiology, comparative skin tests, and IgE reactivity of fungal extracts. Clin Exp Allergy 33:1429–1438
5. Hogaboam CM, Blease K, Mehrad B, Steinhauser ML, Standiford TJ, Kunkel SL, Lukacs NW (2000) Chronic airway hyperreactivity, goblet cell hyperplasia, and peribronchial fibrosis during allergic airway disease induced by *Aspergillus fumigatus*. Am J Pathol 156:723–732
6. Samarasinghe AE, Hoselton SA, Schuh JM (2011) A comparison between intratracheal and inhalation delivery of Aspergillus fumigatus conidia in the development of fungal allergic asthma in C57BL/6 mice. Fungal Biol 115:21–29
7. Ghosh S, Hoselton SA, Schuh JM (2012) mu-chain-deficient mice possess B-1 cells and produce IgG and IgE, but not IgA, following systemic sensitization and inhalational challenge in a fungal asthma model. J Immunol 189:1322–1329
8. Hoselton SA, Samarasinghe AE, Seydel JM, Schuh JM (2010) An inhalation model of airway allergic response to inhalation of environmental Aspergillus fumigatus conidia in sensitized BALB/c mice. Med Mycol 48: 1056–1065

Chapter 15

PAMPs and DAMPs in Allergy Exacerbation Models

Monique A.M. Willart, Philippe Poulliot, Bart N. Lambrecht, and Mirjam Kool

Abstract

Sensitization of mice to real-life allergens or harmless antigen with the use of adjuvants will lead to the induction of DAMPs in the immune system. We have shown that the Th2-inducing adjuvant aluminum hydroxide or exposure of the airways to house dust mite leads to the release of DAMPs: uric acid, ATP, and IL-1. Exposure to DAMPs or PAMPs present in allergens or added to harmless allergens, such as the experimental allergen ovalbumin, induces several immune responses, including cellular influx and activation. Cellular influx can be analyzed by flow cytometry. Likewise, cellular activation can be assessed by measuring increased expression and release of chemokines and cytokines. These inflammatory mediators can be analyzed by ELISA or confocal microscopy. Here, we describe the protocols for these assessments and a protocol that takes advantage of bone marrow chimeric mice to further elucidate mechanism.

Key words Damage-associated molecular pattern, Pathogen-associated molecular pattern, Lung, Dendritic cell, Lung epithelium, Allergy, Asthma, Adjuvant

1 Introduction

In addition to the necessary O_2/CO_2, one breath contains many allergens and pollutions, like diesel and ozone. Individuals that are susceptible to these agents mount Th2 responses to the respective allergens. Common allergens include house dust mite antigen, various molds, and many types of pollen [1]. Allergic inflammation is characterized by an influx of eosinophils, goblet cell metaplasia, Th2 T cell responses, increased serum IgE levels, and, in the case of asthma, increased airway hyper-responsiveness. The development of Th2 responses is dependent on the innate arm of the immune system, which includes the release of both cytokines and chemokines by stromal cells and hematopoietic cells. These proinflammatory mediators can also be released by recruited cells, like neutrophils, monocytes, and dendritic cells (DCs). DCs are at the gateway between innate and adaptive immunity. DCs can phagocytose antigens and process them for presentation to antigen-specific T cells, which initiates a proper

Irving C. Allen (ed.), *Mouse Models of Allergic Disease: Methods and Protocols*, Methods in Molecular Biology, vol. 1032, DOI 10.1007/978-1-62703-496-8_15, © Springer Science+Business Media, LLC 2013

immune response [1, 2]. However, in the airway, the interaction between DCs and lung epithelial cells is crucial [3]. Lung epithelial cells release several chemokines and cytokines shortly after exposure to allergens or pollutions that recruit and mature DCs to induce a immune responses [4]. Allergens can be accompanied by pathogen-associated molecular patterns (PAMPs) and damage-associated molecular patterns (DAMPs) can be induced and produced by host cells. PAMPs and DAMPs can both act as adjuvants to further strengthen the immune response. DCs, macrophages, and epithelial cells in the lung can sense PAMPs and DAMPs by the use of several pattern recognition receptors (PRRs) on their surface, such as Toll-like receptors (TLRs), Nod-like receptors (NLRs), and purinergic receptors (P2X- and P2Y-receptors).

As an example of PAMPs, lipopolysaccharide (LPS) is a commonly used stimulus in experiments to induce maturation on DCs via TLR4 signaling. It even has been shown to induce Th2 sensitization to a harmless antigen, whereof the amount of LPS is able to shift the balance to Th1 or Th2 [5, 6]. Another well-known DAMP, adenosine triphosphate (ATP), is able to signal on DCs via the P2X7 receptor [7, 8]. TLR4 signaling on DCs will lead to NF-κB activation, which subsequently leads to the secretion of inflammatory cytokines, such as pro-IL-1β and pro-IL-18. A second signal, like ATP binding, activates potassium efflux via the P2X7R and, when combined with pannexin-1, leads to the activation of the NLRP3 inflammasome. NLRP3 inflammasome activation results in the activation of caspase-1. This enzyme cleaves pro-IL-1β and pro-IL-18 into their bioactive forms and these cytokines will be secreted [9].

Aluminum-containing adjuvants, which are used in many vaccines, stimulate the release of uric acid (UA). UA crystals are another proinflammatory DAMP that can directly activate the NLRP3 inflammasome [10, 11]. However, recently we have shown that UA does not need the NLRP3 inflammasome or IL-1 axis to induce Th2 immunity. Instead, UA activation of the immune system for Th2 induction is dependent on spleen tyrosine kinase (Syk) and PI3-kinase delta signaling [12, 13].

Sensitization of mice to real-life allergens or harmless antigens with the use of adjuvants will lead to the induction of DAMPs by the immune system. We have shown that the Th2-inducing adjuvant aluminum hydroxide or exposure of the airways to house dust mite leads to the release of the DAMPs: uric acid, ATP, and IL-1. This release is measured in either the peritoneal lavage (PL), in the case of an intraperitoneal antigen injection combined with adjuvant, or the broncho-alveolar lavage (BAL), in the case of airway sensitization. Here, we describe a set of protocols to induce and analyze the release of different DAMPs and PAMPs with particular emphasis on ATP, IL-1, and UA.

Table 1
Mouse strains available to study the role of TLRs and signaling pathways

Knockout strain	Reference
IRAK1-/-	Thomas J.A., et al.; J Immunol 1999
IRAK2-/-	Wang Y., et al; J Biol Chem 2009
IRAK4-/-	Suzuki N., et al; Nature 2002
IRF3-/-	T. Taniguichi (Tokyo, Japan)
IRF7-/-	Riken BioResource Center (Tsukuba, Japan)
MyD88-/-	Adachi O., et al.; Immunity 1998
TBK-/-	Sato S., et al.; J Immunol 2003
TLR1-/-	Alexopoulou L., et al.; Nat Med 2002
TLR2-/-	Wooten R.M., et al; J Immunol 2002
TLR3-/-	Alexopoulou L., et al.; Nature 2001
TLR4-/-	Poltorak A., et al.; Science 1998
TLR5-/-	Vijay-Kumar M., et al.; J Clin Invest 2007
TLR6-/-	Sugawara I., et al.; Microbiol Immunol 2003
TLR7-/-	Hemmi H., et al.; Nat Imm 2002
TLR8-/-	Demaria O., et al.; J Clin Invest 2010
TLR9-/-	Hemmi H., et al.; Nature 2000
TLR11-/-	Zhang D., et al.; Science 2004
TLR13-/-	Shi Z., et al.; J Biol Chem 2010
TRAF6-/-	Lomaga M.A., et al.; Genes Dev 1999
TRIF-/-	Hoebe K., et al.; Nature 2003

The TLRs play an important role in the recognition of PAMPs. The TLR family in mice consists of 12 family members. TLR1, TLR2, TLR4, TLR5, and TLR6 are localized on the cell surface mainly recognizing microbial membrane components, such as LPS and flagellin, whereas TLR3, TLR7, TLR8, and TLR9 are expressed within intracellular vesicles and recognize dsRNA, ssRNA, CPG, and DNA [14]. Downstream of TLR signaling, adaptor molecules like MyD88, BTK, IRAK4, IRAK1, and IRAK2 eventually lead to TRAF6 ubiquitination and NF-κB activation. Another activation pathway via TRAM/TRIF forms complexes with TBK1 and subsequently activates IRF3. Activation of IRF3 leads to type I IFN production [14, 15].

To study the role of these TLRs and their signaling molecules in allergic asthma models, various knockout strains are available as summarized in Table .1.

Table 2
Mouse strains available to study the role of DAMPs and signaling pathways

Knockout strain	Reference
ASC−/−	Mariathasan S., et al.; Nature 2004
Caspase1−/−	Kayagaki N.; Nature 2011
IL-1RI−/−	Labow M., et al.; J Immunol 1997
Ipaf−/−	Franchi L., et al.; Nat Imm 2006
NLRP3−/−	Kanneganti T.D., et al.; Nature 2006
NLRP6−/−	Chen G.Y., et al.; J Immunol 2011
P2X1R−/−	Mulryan K., et al.; Nature 2000
P2X2R−/−	Cockayne D.A., et al.; J Physiol 2005
P2X3R−/−	Cockayne D.A., et al.; Nature 2000 and Zhong Y., et al.; Eur J Neurosci 2001
P2X7R−/−	Pelegrin P. and Suprenant A.; EMBO 2006
Pannexin-1−/−	Qu Y., et al.; J Immunol 2011
RAGE−/−	Lexicon Genetics Incorporated, Woodlands, TX, USA
Uricase−/−	Wu X., et al.; Proc Natl Acad Sci U S A 1994
Uricase-Tg	Kono H., et al.; J Clin Invest 2010

Multiple mouse strains are also available to study the role of DAMPs in allergic asthma (Table 2). Some well-known DAMPs that have been shown to have adjuvant activity are IL-1α, high-mobility-group protein 1 (HMGB1) and ATP [16–18]. For these, the danger signals are also defined receptors like IL-1RI, RAGE, and the P2X receptors. However, the receptors for many DAMPs are not known. For example, uric acid is a potent inducer of Th2 immunity [12, 19]; however, the receptor that senses uric acid has not been identified. Therefore, to study the role of uric acid, uricase-deficient mouse strains can be used.

Some DAMPs activate the intracellular NALP/IPAF-inflammasomes [20]. For example, NLRP3 can be activated by uric acid crystals, alum adjuvant, and potassium efflux via pannexin-1 hemichannels. Inflammasome activation leads to recruitment of the adaptor molecule ASC and the subsequent activation of caspase-1, which is needed to cleave an assortment of pro-cytokines into their bioactive forms [21]. Knockout mouse lines have proven to be vital for these studies.

Here, we describe methods used to evaluate DAMPs, with special emphasis on uric acid, during the induction of allergic airway inflammation. We also describe methods to use DAMPs and PAMPs as adjuvants and protocols to evaluate cytokine and chemokine production. Finally, we detail the process of generating bone marrow chimera mice and steps to evaluate dendritic cell migration.

2 Materials

2.1 Peritoneal Lavage and Broncho-Alveolar Lavage

1. C57BL/6 or BALB/c mice can be obtained from certified providers such as Harlan or Jackson Labs (*see* **Note 1**).
2. Pipet for 50 μl administration (required for intratracheal/intranasal administration).
3. Inhalation anesthesia administration station (preferentially for isoflurane).
4. Allergen—House Dust Mite Antigen (Greer Laboratories).
5. Allergen—Ovalbumin (OVA).
6. Adjuvant (Imject alum, Pierce).
7. Trachea catheter for BAL (23 G needle with a piece of PE50 tubing).
8. Suture: 3-0 silk thread.
9. 23 G needle with a 2.5 ml syringe for PL.
10. 0.5 mM EDTA/PBS.
11. Ice.

2.2 ATP Measurement in BAL and PL

1. ATPlite™ Luminescence Assay System (Perkin Elmer).
2. Plate reader to detect luminescence.

2.3 Uric Acid Measurement in BAL and PL

1. Amplex® Red Uric Acid/Uricase Assay Kit (Invitrogen).
2. Plate reader to detect luminescence.

2.4 Uric Acid Detection on Cryosections

1. Tissue-Tek (Sakura)/PBS solution, ratio 1:1 (*see* **Note 2**).
2. Liquid nitrogen.
3. Cryostat.
4. Adhesive microscope slides and coverslips.
5. 4 % Paraformaldehyde (PFA) in PBS.
6. Block buffer: 1 % Blocking reagent (Roche) in PBS.
7. Anti-uric acid antibody (Abcam).
8. Goat-anti-rabbit Ig-Cy3 (Jackson Immunoresearch).
9. 4′,6-Diamidino-2-Phenylindole dihydrochloride (DAPI).
10. Polyvinyl alcohol mounting medium with DABCO®, anti-fading.

2.5 Lung Homogenates

1. C57BL/6 or BALB/c mice can be obtained from certified providers such as Harlan or Jackson Labs.
2. Allergens, DAMPs, and PAMPs of interest.
3. Trachea catheter: 23 G needle with piece of PE50 tubing.
4. Suture: 3-0 silk thread.
5. 0.5 mM EDTA/PBS.
6. Liquid nitrogen.
7. Tissue homogenizer: IKA T10 rotor-stator homogenizer, with a 5 or a 7 mm generator.
8. 2 ml safe-lock tubes.
9. Cold lysis buffer: 20 mM Tris–HCl (pH 8.0), 0.14 M NaCl, 10 % glycerol (v/v), 1 mM PMSF, 1 mM sodium orthovanadate (Na_3VO_4), 1 μM NaF, 40 mg/ml aprotinin, and 20 mg/ml of leupeptin. Protease inhibitors should be prepared fresh on the day of use (*see* **Notes 3** and **4**).
10. Igepal (US Biological).
11. NanoOrange protein quantitation assay (Invitrogen).
12. Plate reader to detect fluorescence.
13. Eppendorf centrifuge.
14. Mini-labroller.

2.6 ELISA

1. Half area plate Microlon 600 (Greiner) or 96 well plate Maxisorp (NUNC). In the Greiner plate, 50 μl samples are required per well. If NUNC plates are used, 100 μl samples are required per well.
2. Coating buffer: The choice of coating buffer depends on the antibody used. Typical coating buffers are either 0.1 M sodium carbonate, pH 9.5 or 0.2 M sodium phosphate, pH 6.5.
3. Wash buffer: 0.05 % Tween-20 in 1× PBS.
4. 10 % Fetal calf serum (FCS) in 1× PBS.
5. Purified antibody (coating), biotinylated antibody (detection), and streptavidin–HRP for the specific protein being assayed.
6. TMB substrate solution.
7. Stop solution: 2.5 N H_2SO_4.
8. Plate reader.

2.7 MCP-1 Staining on Lung Sections

1. Cryostat.
2. Tissue-Tek (Sakura)/PBS solution, ratio 1:1.
3. Liquid nitrogen.
4. Adhesive microscope slides and coverslips.
5. PBS, pH 7.4–7.8.

6. 4 % PFA at 4 °C (1:10 dilution of 37 % PFA in PBS).
7. 1 % Blocking reagent (Roche Applied Science) in PBS.
8. Normal donkey serum.
9. Normal goat serum and normal mouse serum.
10. Rat anti-MCP-1 (Abcam).
11. Donkey anti-rat conjugated with Cy3 (Jackson Immunoresearch).
12. 1 mg/ml of DAPI, stock.
13. Polyvinyl alcohol mounting medium with DABCO.
14. Confocal microscope.

2.8 Bone Marrow Chimeric Mice

1. Bone marrow donor mice of WT and KO origin.
2. Bone marrow acceptor mice of WT and KO origin, which will be irradiated.
3. Irradiation device (X-Rad 320, RPS).
4. Enrofloxacin (antibiotic).
5. Heating lamp.
6. Inverted microscope.
7. Sterilized pestle and mortar.
8. Red blood cell (RBC)-lysis buffer: 0.15 M NH_4Cl, 1 mM $KHCO_3$, 0.1 mM Na_2EDTA. Filter-sterilize before use.
9. 1× HBSS and D-PBS.
10. 100 μm cell strainer.
11. 0.4 % Trypan blue solution, diluted 1:10 in 1× PBS.
12. Tubes, pipets, pipet tips, syringes, needles.

2.9 Innate Cellular Influx and DC Migration

1. FACS buffer: 1× PBS, 0.25 % BSA, 0.5 mM EDTA, 0.05 % NaN_3.
2. Low-binding flexiplates.
3. OVA-Alexa Fluor 647.
4. DAPI.
5. Fixable live/dead Aqua.
6. FACS tubes.
7. 1× HBSS.
8. Multi-well plates and 15 ml tubes.
9. Tweezer and curved iris scissor.
10. 35 mm petri dishes.
11. 100 μm cell strainers.
12. Pasteur pipets.

13. Digestion medium: Liberase™ (Roche) and DNase I in RPMI generated as directed by manufacturer.
14. 14. RBC-lysis buffer: 0.15 M NH_4Cl, 1 mM $KHCO_3$, 0.1 mM Na_2EDTA. Filter-sterilize before use.
15. Water bath at 37 °C.
16. 96-Well filter plate or cell strainer-capped tubes.
17. Flow cytometer (equipped with a 405, 488, and 633 nm laser).

3 Methods

3.1 Intratracheal Injection of Allergens

1. Anesthetize mice according to local guidelines.
2. Suspend the anesthetized mouse by the upper front teeth. This puts the mouse in a position where the head is vertical, and the body is suspended on the apparatus. It is an optimal position for the trachea to be vertical, which allows the liquid to effectively reach the airways.
3. Pull the tongue out of the mouth of the animal using blunt forceps. Hold the tongue on one side of the mouth while maintaining it in an extended position. This is extremely important, as it ensures that the mouse is not able to swallow and allows the allergen to reach the trachea.
4. Inject liquid just above the vocal cords in the mouth of the mouse. The mouse will gradually inhale the liquid.
5. Once the liquid is inhaled and the breathing rate has returned to normal, release the tongue.
6. If an injectable anesthesia is utilized, place the mouse on a heating mat to recover.
7. At the desired time point, euthanize mice and expose the trachea.
8. Insert the suture thread between the esophagus and the trachea.
9. With scissors, make a small incision into the trachea between the cartilage rings. The incision should be large enough to insert the catheter. Care should be taken to avoid cutting the trachea completely.
10. Insert the catheter into the trachea towards the lungs. Secure the catheter in place with the ligature.
11. Using EDTA/PBS at RT, wash the lung three times through the catheter with the same 1 ml. Place the retrieved BAL-fluid in a 15-ml tube. The whole 1 ml must be injected and slowly retrieved (*see* **Note 5**).
12. Keep the BAL fluid on ice during the procedure.
13. Centrifuge BAL samples at 400 ×*g* at 4 °C for 7 min and transfer the supernatant into a new tube (*see* **Note 6**). It is very important

that samples be kept cold. Samples should be used immediately for the measurement of ATP. For uric acid and IL-1 measurements, the supernatant can be stored at −20 °C until further analysis.

14. The measurement of ATP and uric acid in the supernatant is done according to the manufacturer's protocol.

3.2 Intraperitoneal Injection of Allergens Combined with Adjuvant

1. Inject 10 μg of allergen, such as OVA, combined with 1 mg of alum in 500 μl of saline intraperitoneally (i.p.).
2. Sacrifice the mouse after 2 h by CO_2 inhalation (*see* **Note 7**).
3. Gently cut the skin of the abdomen. Incisions should begin as close as possible to the leg area and care should be taken to avoid cutting the muscles of the abdomen.
4. Cut from the lowest part of the abdomen to the thorax and gently remove the skin from the muscles.
5. Inject 3 ml of warm EDTA/PBS i.p.
6. Gently massage/shake the mouse and recollect the EDTA/PBS back into the syringe. Usually, 2–2.5 ml is collected.
7. Store on ice immediately.
8. Centrifuge PL samples at 400 × *g* at 4 °C for 7 min and transfer the supernatant into a new tube (*see* **Note 6**). It is very important that samples be kept cold. Samples should be used immediately for the measurement of ATP. For uric acid and IL-1 measurement, the supernatants can be stored at −20 °C until further analysis.
9. The measurement of ATP and uric acid in the supernatant is done according to the manufacturer's protocol.

3.3 Uric Acid Measurement on Cryosections

1. Inflate the mouse lung via the trachea with 1 ml of Tissue-Tek/PBS solution via the trachea-catheter used to collect the BAL.
2. Lungs should be snap frozen in liquid nitrogen and kept at −80 °C until further use.
3. Make 6-μm-thick cryosections.
4. Dry sections before storage at −80 °C or before staining.
5. Fix the slides in 4 % PFA for 10 min at room temperature (*see* **Note 8**).
6. Wash the slides two times with PBS for 5 min per wash.
7. Block the slides with 10 % normal goat serum in block buffer for 10 min.
8. Wash the slides two times with PBS for 5 min per wash.
9. Incubate the sections for 1 h with anti-uric acid antibody (rabbit Ig) in block buffer (*see* **Note 9**).

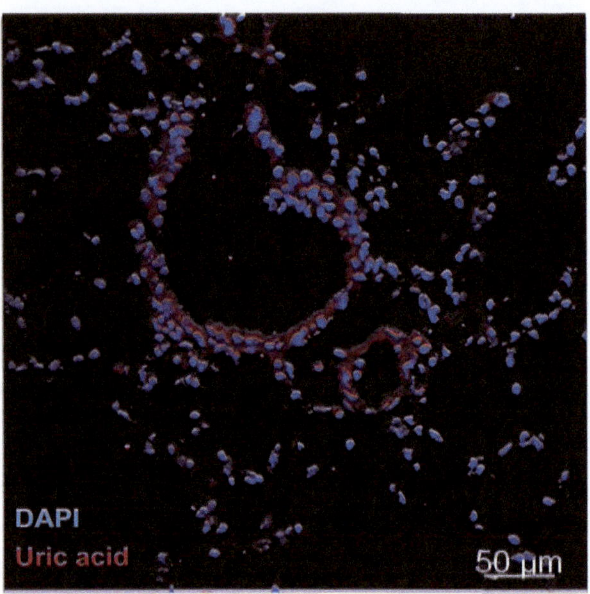

Fig. 1 Picture of a lung section stained for uric acid and DAPI. Bronchial epithelial and endothelial cells stain positive for uric acid

10. Wash the slides two times with PBS for 5 min per wash.
11. Incubate the sections for 30 min with goat anti-rabbit Ig-Cy3 in block buffer.
12. Wash the slides two times with PBS for 5 min per wash.
13. If other markers are to be evaluated, additional antibodies can be utilized to stain the sections.
14. Stain nuclei using DAPI (1 μg/ml in PBS) for 5 min.
15. Wash the slides two times with PBS for 5 min per wash.
16. Wash the slides with H_2O for 5 min.
17. Mount slides with polyvinylethanol.
18. Analyze slides with a confocal microscope (Fig. 1).

3.4 Preparation of Lung Homogenates

1. Inject the allergens intratracheally and perform BAL as described in Subheading 3.1.
2. To analyze lung cellular influx and cytokine/chemokine responses to allergens, DAMPs or PAMPs, harvest the BAL and lung tissue at several time points after exposure. Samples should be collected at time points between 2 and 48 h.
3. BAL supernatant can be used for ELISA to determine the levels of cytokines and chemokines. The cells in the BAL can be analyzed for cellular influx by FACS-analysis (described in Subheading 3.9).
4. Open the chest of the mouse, dissect the left lobe of the lung, and collect it in the 2 ml tube. Snap-freeze the lung lobe in

liquid nitrogen and store at −80 °C until homogenates are made. The right lobes can be dissected and maintained in HBSS on ice for the generation of cell suspensions for FACS-analysis.

5. Homogenize the lung. Add 400 μl of cold lysis buffer to the frozen lung samples and immediately homogenize them using a rotor-stator homogenizer equipped with a 5 or a 7 mm generator for 1.5 or 2 ml Eppendorf tubes. Tube sizes may extend up to 5 ml tubes, depending on lab availability. The speed of the homogenizer should be adjusted to avoid foaming. Foaming could alter the quality of the proteins and reduce the practical volume recovered. The homogenization is complete when no macroscopic pieces of lung are visible in the solution. Place the samples on ice until all of the samples are homogenized.
6. Add 1 % v/v Igepal to each sample, vortex for 5 s, and place the sample back on ice (*see* **Note 10**).
7. Place all of the samples in a mini-labroller for 20 min at 4 °C. Alternatively, samples can be left on ice for 45 min with vortexing occurring every 5 min.
8. Centrifuge the samples at 16,000 × *g* at 4 °C for 15 min and transfer the supernatant into a new tube. Collect 10 μl of each sample for NanoOrange protein content measurements.
9. Store supernatant at −80 °C until ELISA is performed. Use the NanoOrange kit to measure and normalize the protein content.

3.5 Cytokine Measurement by ELISA

1. Coat the ELISA plates with purified antibody in an appropriate coating buffer overnight at 4 °C. For half-area plates, use 50 μl/well; otherwise double all volumes described below.
2. Wash the wells three times with 150 μl/well of wash buffer and empty wells by blotting the plate on an absorbent towel.
3. Block the uncoated spots in wells with 150 μl/well of 10 % FCS/PBS and incubate the plate for 1 h at room temperature.
4. Wash the wells once with 150 μl/well of wash buffer and empty the wells by blotting the plate on an absorbent towel.
5. Add 50 μl/well of samples, standards, and blank (in either duplicate or triplicate) and incubate the plate for 2–2.5 h at room temperature.
6. Wash the wells five times with 150 μl/well of wash buffer and empty the wells by blotting the plate on an absorbent towel.
7. Add 50 μl/well of detection antibody diluted in 10 % FCS/PBS. Incubate the plate for 1–2 h at room temperature.
8. Wash the wells five times with 150 μl/well of wash buffer and empty the wells by blotting the plate on an absorbent towel.

9. Add 50 μl/well of streptavidin diluted in 10 % FCS/PBS. Incubate the plate for 30 min at room temperature.
10. Wash wells five times with 150 μl/well of wash buffer and empty the wells by blotting the plate on an absorbent towel.
11. Add 50 μl/well of TMB substrate solution into each well and incubate the plate for 10–30 min in the dark at room temperature.
12. Stop the reaction by adding 25 μl/well of stop solution and measure the wavelength using a plate reader set at 405 nm and reference at 650 nm.

3.6 Chemokine Measurement by Confocal Microscopy

1. Inflate the mouse lung via the tracheal catheter with 1 ml of Tissue-Tek/PBS solution.
2. The lungs should be snap frozen in liquid nitrogen and stored at –80 °C until further use.
3. Make 6-μm cryosections using a cryostat and store these sections at –80 °C. However, if the staining is to be performed on the same day, air-dry the sections for 1 h prior to staining.
4. Fix the slides for 10 min in 4 % PFA at 4 °C.
5. Incubate the sections with 10 % normal donkey serum in 1 % blocking reagent (*see* **Note 8**) for 10 min at room temperature.
6. Rinse slides with PBS for 2 min.
7. Add anti-MCP1 antibody diluted in 1 % blocking reagent to each slide and incubate for 1 h at room temperature (*see* **Note 9**). The antibody dilutions should be optimized prior to use and can vary per lab.
8. Rinse slides with PBS for 2 min.
9. Add donkey anti-rat antibody diluted 1:50 in 1 % blocking reagent and incubate for 30 min at room temperature in the dark.
10. Rinse slides with PBS for 2 min.
11. Add DAPI diluted 1:1,000 in PBS and incubate for 5 min.
12. Rinse slides with PBS for 2 min and ddH_2O for 2 min.
13. Mount slides with mounting medium and a coverslip and leave them overnight at room temperature to allow the mounting medium to polymerize. Analyze the slides under a confocal microscope (Fig. 2).

3.7 Bone Marrow Chimeric Mice

1. 8–10-week-old mice (WT and KO) are sublethally irradiated with 8–10 Gy (X-Rad 320, RPS) (*see* **Notes 11** and **12**). The mice are subsequently placed back into their home cages for at least 4 h.

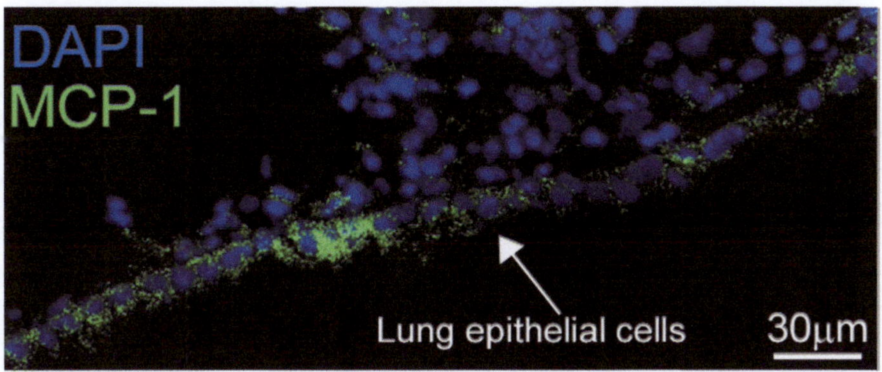

Fig. 2 Picture of a lung section after exposure to LPS and stained for MCP-1 and DAPI. Bronchial epithelial cells stain positive for MCP-1

2. Isolate femurs and tibias from bone marrow donor mice and collect the bones in cold HBSS.
3. Incubate bones for 2 min with 70 % ethanol and wash twice with cold HBSS.
4. Transfer bones in a sterilized mortar and smash the bones in a small volume of HBSS with a pestle.
5. Rinse the pestle and the mortar with a larger volume of 1× HBSS and transfer the cell suspension through a 100 μm cell strainer, placed in a 50 ml tube.
6. Centrifuge the cells at $400 \times g$ for 7 min at 4 °C.
7. Suspend the cell pellet in RBC lysis buffer (1 ml/# of mice).
8. Incubate the cells for 4 min on ice and shake occasionally.
9. Add an excess amount of cold D-PBS to stop the lysis and centrifuge the cell suspension at $400 \times g$ for 7 min at 4 °C.
10. Suspend the cell pellet in D-PBS.
11. Remove an aliquot of each sample and combine with Trypan blue solution in a 1:1 ratio. Count the live cells/ml (dead cells stain blue) using a hemacytometer.
12. Centrifuge the remaining cells at $400 \times g$ for 7 min at 4 °C and suspend the pellet in D-PBS. The final concentration of cells should be 10×10^6 cells/ml.
13. At least 4 h after irradiation the bone marrow cells can be injected intravenously. Warm the irradiated mice under the heating lamp and inject each animal with 200 μl of the bone marrow cells. Each mouse should receive 2×10^6 cells. Return the mice to their original cages and add enrofloxacin to the drinking water for 10 days. After 6–8 weeks, collect blood samples via tail nick to analyze the hematopoietic cell

Table 3
Monoclonal antibodies to analyze innate cellular influx

Marker	Fluorochrome	Clone	Supplier
Ly6C	FITC	AL-21	BD Biosciences
Ly6G	PE	1A8	BD Biosciences
CD11c	PE-Texas Red	N418	Invitrogen
CD8a	PerCP-Cy5.5	53-6.7	BD Biosciences
CD86	PE-Cy7	GL1	BD Biosciences
ratIgG2a	PE-Cy7	eBR2a	eBioscience
OVA	Alexa Fluor 647		Invitrogen
MHC II	Alexa Fluor 700	M5/114.15.2	eBioscience
F4/80	APC-eFluor780	BM8	eBioscience
CD11b	eFluor450	M1/70	eBioscience
FcgRII/III		2.4G2	In house

chimerism of the mice. If the donor is carrying a GFP expression marker or unique cell surface markers, such as CD45.1 or CD45.2, then the extent of chimerism can be analyzed by flow cytometry.

14. Allergic asthma experiments can be initiated 10–12 weeks after irradiation. This will allow the long-lived alveolar macrophages in the lung to be replenished by the newly derived bone marrow.

3.8 DAMP and PAMPs as Adjuvants

1. Resuspend the PL or BAL cell pellet in 200–500 μl of FACS buffer.
2. Count an aliquot of the samples using Trypan blue and a hemacytometer.
3. Transfer 1×10^6 cells to a FACS flexiplate (max 200 μl).
4. Centrifuge the plate for 3 min at 400 × *g* and 4 °C.
5. Remove the supernatant and add 40–50 μl of staining mix, which has been prepared with the monoclonal antibodies described in Table 3 in FACS buffer.
6. Incubate the supernatant for 30 min at 4 °C or 15 min at room temperature.
7. Add 150 μl of FACS buffer.
8. Centrifuge the plate for 3 min at 400 × *g* and 4 °C.

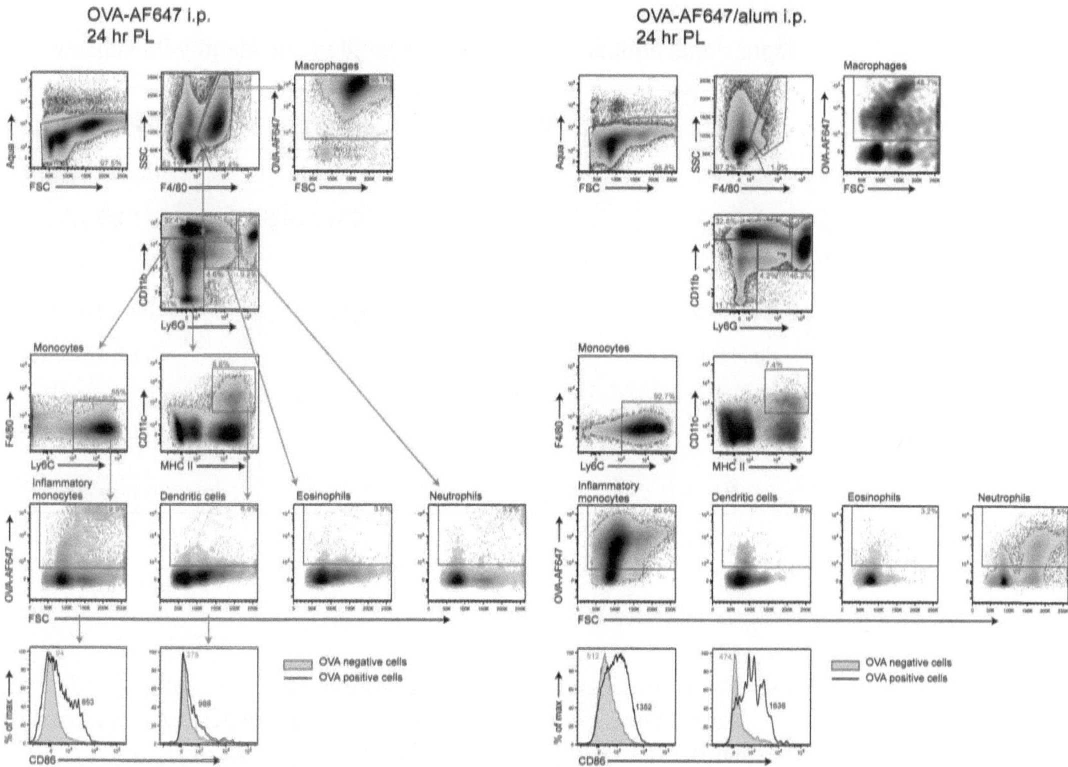

Fig. 3 Gating strategy with and without adjuvant in PL

9. Remove the supernatant and suspend the cell pellet in 200 μl of FACS buffer. This step is to wash all of the free monoclonal antibodies from the pellet.
10. Centrifuge the plate for 3 min at 400 ×*g* and 4 °C.
11. Remove the supernatant and suspend the pellet in 200 μl of FACS buffer. Transfer the cells to FACS tubes and evaluate using a flow cytometer.
12. Data analysis is done according to Fig. 3 (*see* **Note 13**).

3.9 Dendritic Cell Migration

1. Dissect the lung and LNs and keep them in HBSS on ice.
2. Cut the tissue into small pieces in a 35 mm petri dish using the iris scissors.
3. Transfer the pieces into a 15 ml tube and rinse the petri dish with digestion medium. For each lung half, use 500 μl of medium and for LNs use 200 μl per organ. Keep on ice until all of the samples are processed.

Table 4
Monoclonal antibodies to track DC migration and identify DC subsets

Marker	Fluorochrome	Clone	Supplier
BST-2	FITC	120G8	Made in house
MHC II	PE	M5/114.15.2	BD Biosciences
CD11c	PE-Texas Red	N418	Invitrogen
CD11b	PerCP-Cy5.5	M1/70	eBioscience
CD103	Biotin	2E7	BD Biosciences
Streptavidin	PE-Cy7		eBioscience
OVA	Alexa Fluor 647		Invitrogen
FcgRII/III		2.4G2	In house

4. Place the tubes in the warm water bath two times for 15 min each. After each 15-min incubation, resuspend the suspension vigorously using a Pasteur pipet.
5. Filter the cell suspension over a 100 μm cell strainer and transfer the samples into new 15 ml tubes.
6. Centrifuge all samples at 4 °C at 400 × *g* for 7 min.
7. Resuspend the cell pellet in RBC-lysis buffer. Each LN should be resuspended in 200 μl and each lung half should be resuspended in 1 ml. Leave the cell suspensions on ice for 4 min and shake occasionally.
8. Add excess volumes of FACS-buffer and centrifuge all of the samples at 4 °C at 400 × *g* for 7 min.
9. Resupend the cell pellet in FACS-buffer and count the number of cells in each sample using Trypan blue and a hemacytometer.
10. Proceed with FACS-staining as described in Subheading 3.8 using antibodies described in Table 4.
11. Before acquiring on the flow cytometer, samples should be filtered using a filter plate of tubes with a filter cap to prevent clogs during acquisition.
12. Data analysis is done according to Fig. 4 (*see* **Note 13**).

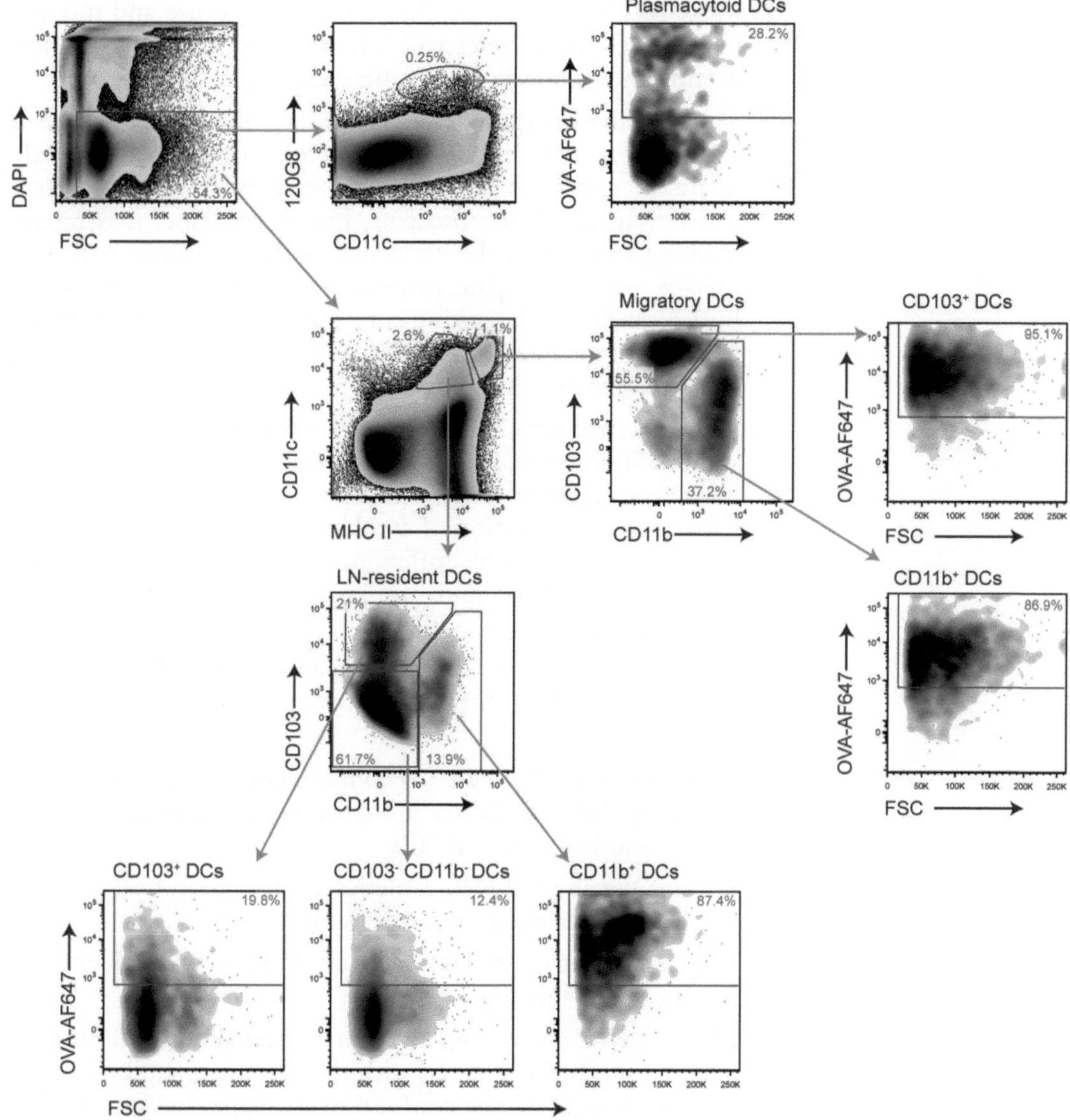

Fig. 4 Gating strategy for DC migration in mediastinal LNs

4 Notes

1. We would like to stress the importance of monitoring the health status of your animal facility. It is known that certain pathogens (containing PAMPs) will greatly influence the outcome of the measurements described throughout this protocol. As far as possible within your facility, housing specific pathogen-free (SPF) mice in individually ventilated cages (IVC) would be optimal.

2. Make solutions no more than 24 h prior to use and mix well before use. Air bubbles will interfere with cutting and interpreting the morphology of lung sections.
3. The cold lysis buffer described here is for the extraction of extracellular and intracellular proteins and is therefore adequate for cytokines and other messengers. It will also extract many transmembrane proteins, but in this case, it is recommended to confirm the efficiency of the technique with your specific transmembrane protein. If ineffective, another lysis buffer can be used, making sure not to include any detergent in the homogenization phase. Omitting the detergent will avoid foaming of the solution.
4. The described lysis buffer contains sodium orthovanadate and sodium fluoride (NaF): these are phosphatase inhibitors. If you have no interest in protein phosphorylation (e.g., STAT proteins to assess activation of cytokine receptors), these reagents are dispensable in the buffer. Aprotinine and leupeptine are protease inhibitors and are necessary to avoid protein degradation.
5. If you do not want to analyze cytokines in the BAL, it is better to take the BAL with three times 1 ml of PBS/EDTA (for a total of 3 ml).
6. Make sure that there are no contaminating cells in the supernatant as this will greatly influence your measurement. Cells are the source of the DAMPs.
7. Do not use injectable anesthetics via the peritoneal route, as they can negatively impact cell viability.
8. Make sure that the slides never run dry; this will influence the result of your staining.
9. Make sure to always take an extra section alone without a primary antibody, but stained with the secondary antibody to set the background on the confocal microscope. Lungs are full of autofluorescent cells.
10. Depending on the techniques applied to the homogenate, some components of the lysis buffer (e.g., Igepal as a detergent) might interfere with the assay. The first attempt should be to dilute the lysate, which should reduce the impact of the lysis buffer components. If this cannot be achieved, modifications of the lysis buffer can be envisaged for the specific protocol. However, for the procedures described here, using recommended dilutions, no interference is expected.
11. The dose of irradiation should be confirmed in each lab. This dose is general enough to deplete all bone marrow cells in C57Bl/6 mice. However, mice on a BALB/c background are more sensitive to irradiation. Thus, it might be necessary to

irradiate the mice twice with 4 Gy at a 4-h interval. The mice are then injected early the next morning with the new bone marrow.

12. Make sure that you have enough mice to make four groups with the following controls: WT into WT; KO into WT; WT into KO; and KO into KO. Irradiation induces changes to the immunological response of mice, which must be controlled for in the experiment. Take cells for compensation. This means that all fluorochromes used in the mix are prepared as a single stain.
13. Take cells for fluorescence minus one (FMO) control staining to optimize your gating strategy [22]. FMO samples contain all fluorochromes except one. When placing your gate on the staining of the fluorochrome missing in the FMO, the background fluorescence is observed. By using FMO samples, you ensure that your gates are placed on positive cells and not on background fluorescence induced by other fluorochromes.

References

1. Lambrecht BN, Hammad H (2010) The role of dendritic and epithelial cells as master regulators of allergic airway inflammation. Lancet 376(9743):835–843
2. Banchereau J, Steinman RM (1998) Dendritic cells and the control of immunity. Nature 392:245–252
3. Hammad H, Lambrecht BN (2011) Dendritic cells and airway epithelial cells at the interface between innate and adaptive immune responses. Allergy 66(5):579–587
4. Willart M, Hammad H (2011) Lung dendritic cell-epithelial cell crosstalk in Th2 responses to allergens. Curr Opin Immunol 23(6):772–777
5. Eisenbarth SC, Piggott DA, Huleatt JW, Visintin I, Herrick CA, Bottomly K (2002) Lipopolysaccharide-enhanced, toll-like receptor 4-dependent T helper cell type 2 responses to inhaled antigen. J Exp Med 196(12): 1645–1651
6. Tan AM, Chen HC, Pochard P, Eisenbarth SC, Herrick CA, Bottomly HK (2010) TLR4 signaling in stromal cells is critical for the initiation of allergic Th2 responses to inhaled antigen. J Immunol 184(7):3535–3544
7. Qu Y, Micaghi S, Newton K, Gilmour LL, Louie S, Cupp JE, Dubyak GR, Hackos D, Dixit VM (2011) Pannexin-1 is required for ATP release during apoptosis but not for inflammasome activation. J Immunol 186(11): 6553–6561
8. McDermott MF, Tschopp J (2007) From inflammasomes to fevers, crystals and hypertension: how basic research explains inflammatory diseases. Trends Mol Med 13(9): 381–388
9. Dinarello CA (2011) Interleukin-1 in the pathogenesis and treatment of inflammatory diseases. Blood 117(14):3720–3732
10. Hornung V, Bauernfeind F, Halle A, Samstad EO, Kono H, Rock KL, Fitzgerald KA, Latz E (2008) Silica crystals and aluminum salts activate the NALP3 inflammasome through phagosomal destabilization. Nat Immunol 9(8): 847–856
11. Martinon F, Petrilli V, Mayor A, Tardivel A, Tschopp J (2006) Gout-associated uric acid crystals activate the NALP3 inflammasome. Nature 440(7081):237–241
12. Kool M, Willart MA, van Nimwegen M, Bergen I, Pouliot P, Virchow JC, Rogers N, Osorio F, Reis E, Sousa C, Hammad H, Lambrecht BN (2011) An unexpected role for uric acid as an inducer of T helper 2 cell immunity to inhaled antigens and inflammatory mediator of allergic asthma. Immunity 34(4):527–540
13. Lambrecht BN, Kool M, Willart MA, Hammad H (2009) Mechanism of action of clinically approved adjuvants. Curr Opin Immunol 21(1): 23–29
14. Kawai T, Akira S (2011) Toll-like receptors and their crosstalk with other innate receptors in infection and immunity. Immunity 34(5): 637–650
15. Barton GM, Kagan JC (2009) A cell biological view of Toll-like receptor function: regulation through compartmentalization. Nat Rev Immunol 9(8):535–542

16. Kono H, Karmarker D, Iwakura Y, Rock KL (2010) Identification of the cellular sensor that stimulates the inflammatory response to sterile cell death. J Immunol 184(8): 4470–4478
17. Scaffidi P, Misteli T, Bianchi ME (2002) Release of chromatin protein HMGB1 by necrotic cells triggers inflammation. Nature 418(6894):191–195
18. Idzko M, Hammad H, van Nimwegen M, Kool M, Willart MA, Muskens F, Hoogsteden HC, Luttmann W, Ferrari D, Di Virgilio F, Virchow JC Jr, Lambrecht BN (2007) Extracellular ATP triggers and maintains asthmatic airway inflammation by activating dendritic cells. Nat Med 13(8): 913–919
19. Kool M, Soullie T, van Nimwegen M, Willart MA, Muskens F, Jung S, Hoogsteden HC, Hammad H (2008) Alum adjuvant boosts adaptive immunity by inducing uric acid and activating inflammatory dendritic cells. J Exp Med 205(4):869–882
20. Martinon F (2008) Detection of immune danger signals by NALP3. J Leukoc Biol 83(3):507–511
21. Petrilli V, Dostert C, Muruve DA, Tschopp J (2007) The inflammasome: a danger sensing complex triggering innate immunity. Curr Opin Immunol 19(6):615–622
22. Roederer M (2002) Compensation in flow cytometry. Curr Prot Cytometry/editorial board, J. Paul Robinson, managing editor. Chapter 1: Unit 1 14

Chapter 16

Assessment of Airway Hyperresponsiveness in Mouse Models of Allergic Lung Disease Using Detailed Measurements of Respiratory Mechanics

John M. Hartney and Annette Robichaud

Abstract

This chapter provides an outline of the procedures necessary to measure airway hyperresponsiveness to inhaled methacholine in mouse models of allergic lung disease. We present a method for acquiring detailed measurements of respiratory mechanics using broadband low-frequency oscillatory waveforms applied at the subject's airway opening and analyzed using the constant phase model of the lung. We acknowledge that there are other methods of measuring airway responsiveness in allergic rodent models. However, a discussion of the merits and or detriments of these various methods have been vigorously debated in the primary literature and are beyond the scope of this chapter. The goal of this chapter is to provide a guide in how to begin these types of assays in laboratories which have little to no experience with these particular types of assessments.

Key words Airway hyperresponsiveness, Respiratory mechanics, Allergic airway disease, Asthma, Forced oscillation technique

1 Introduction

One of the cardinal characteristics of asthma is airway hyperresponsiveness (AHR) [1]. It is defined as an exaggerated bronchoconstrictor response to a given stimuli [1]. Initially, direct measurement of lung responsiveness in mice was performed by a handful of labs that had developed custom equipment which was sensitive enough to detect changes in the mouse lung [2, 3]. More recently, commercial systems have become available allowing a wide range of researchers to measure changes in the mechanics of the respiratory system. This chapter attempts to provide an outline of how to assess responsiveness to inhaled methacholine in the mouse lung for laboratories with little or no experience in invasive measurements using forced oscillations, a technique allowing partitioning of the respiratory response into airway and parenchymal

Irving C. Allen (ed.), *Mouse Models of Allergic Disease: Methods and Protocols*, Methods in Molecular Biology, vol. 1032,
DOI 10.1007/978-1-62703-496-8_16, © Springer Science+Business Media, LLC 2013

Table 1
Constant phase model parameters [4, 8, 9]

Parameters	Name	Layman's term definition
R_N	Newtonian resistance	Term reflecting the opposition of the airways to a flow of air. It is inversely related to the caliber of the large conducting airways.
I	Inertance	Term related to the amount of air in the airways. It has a negligible value in mice below 20 Hz and is not reported.
G	Tissue damping	Term describing the loss of energy to heat in the lung tissue during a forced oscillation maneuver. It is closely related to tissue resistance and will increase with contraction of the airway smooth muscle.
H	Tissue elastance	Term describing the storage of energy in the lung tissue during a forced oscillation maneuver. It reflects the elastic recoil of the lung (or tissue stiffness) that permits its return towards an initial form after a deformation.
η (eta)	Hysteresivity	It is the ratio of G/H. A comparative change in both parameters was described as reflecting airway closure or collapse while a larger change in G relative to H was associated to heterogeneity in ventilation [8].

lung tissue mechanics through the use of advanced mathematical models. The results presented in this chapter were generated using broadband low-frequency forced oscillations (1–20 Hz) delivered at the subject's airways by a piston-ventilator. The resulting respiratory input impedance was then fit to the constant phase model [4] of the lung by the operating software in order to extract physiological significance (Table 1).

2 Materials

2.1 Equipment for Aerosol Generation and Measurement of Respiratory Mechanics

The authors will describe procedures that are specific to the *flexiVent* (SCIREQ Inc, Montreal, QC, Canada) system, the only commercial system currently employing the forced oscillation technique in small rodents. To generate the results presented here, the system was equipped with a standard particle size (4–6 μm MMAD) Aeroneb Lab nebulizer (Aerogen Ltd, Ireland) for aerosol generation. The surgical procedures and pharmacological principles described apply to any type of invasive measurement of airway responsiveness.

2.2 Surgical Equipment

1. Two sets of small curved forceps.
2. Blunt lexer-baby scissors.
3. Fine scissors, sharply angled.

4. Non-sterile size three braided silk suture thread.
5. Stainless steel tracheal cannula with Luer-adapter (20 mm long). Experiments were done using three different sizes of outer diameter (1.0, 1.2, or 1.3 mm) for different strains or ages of mice.
6. Homeothermic heating pad and rectal temperature probe.
7. Scale to weigh live mice.

2.3 Reagents

1. Anesthetic agents (e.g., sodium pentobarbital:nembutal sodium solution 50 mg/ml).
2. Muscle relaxant (e.g., pancuronium bromide: 1 mg/ml).
3. Acetyl-β-methyl choline chloride (methacholine).
4. Phosphate-buffered saline, 1×.
5. 70 % Ethanol.

3 Methods

3.1 Preparation

1. Prepare the anesthetic agent. Results presented in this protocol were generated under sodium pentobarbital-induced anesthesia. Thus, procedures described here are specific to that regimen. Dilute the stock solution based on the desired dose and the injection volume (*see* **Notes 1**, **4**, and **5** and Table 2).
2. Prepare the muscle relaxant. Pancuronium bromide is typically used in this assay. Prepare a dilution based on the desired dose and the injection volume (*see* **Notes 1**, **5**, **8**, and **9** and Table 2).
3. Prepare the methacholine. Typically a stock solution of 50 mg/ml is made in PBS and serial dilutions are performed to generate concentrations of 25, 12.5, 6.25, and 3.125 mg/ml or less, if needed (*see* **Notes 5**, **9–11**).

Table 2
Preparation of surgical reagents

Agent	Desired dose (mg/kg ip)	Injection volume (ml/kg)	Dilute to	Administer
Sodium pentobarbital (stock solution at 50 mg/ml)	70	10	7 mg/ml (i.e., for 5 ml: 0.7 ml of stock + 4.3 ml of saline)	0.2 ml for 20 g mice
Pancuronium bromide (stock solution at 1 mg/ml)	0.8	10	0.08 mg/ml (i.e., for 5 ml: 0.4 ml of stock + 4.6 ml of saline)	0.2 ml for 20 g mice

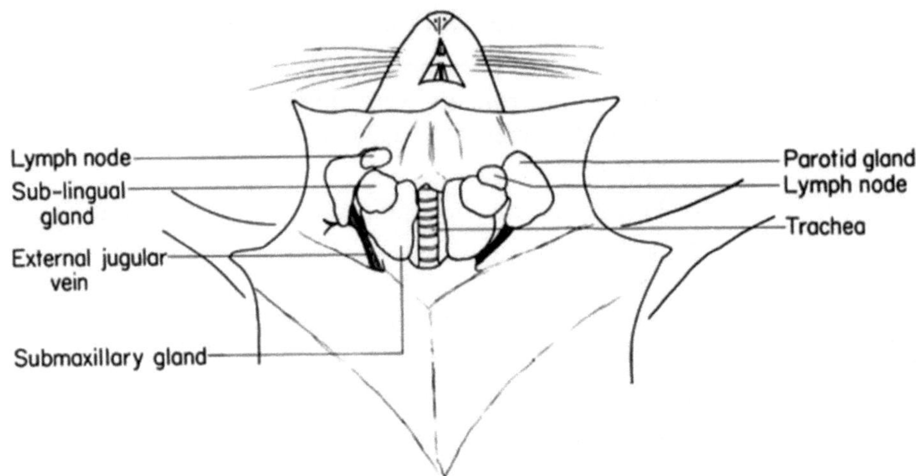

Fig. 1 Drawing of ventral dissection of neck region in mouse. Reproduced from Cook [11]. Copyright holder, Elsevier. Reproduced with permission

4. Calibrate the *flexiVent* system. Weigh the animal, enter its weight and an identifier in the *flexiVent* operating software, and proceed with the calibration of the system using the appropriate endotracheal cannula (*see* **Note 2**).
5. Anesthetize the mouse. Inject the anesthetic agent intraperitoneally based on the animal's weight and the desired volume of injection (*see* Table 2). Place the animal back in its cage and allow a period of 5–10 min for the drug to reach effect. The animal should become sedated and then lose righting reflex.
6. Verify that a surgical plane of anesthesia has been reached. This can be done by evaluating the animal's toe pinch reflex. A lack of any observable response indicates that a surgical plane of anesthesia has been reached. Prior to advancing to additional steps, verify that the animal's breathing is regular and relaxed.

3.2 Tracheostomy and Cannulation

1. After having established that a suitable plane of anesthesia was reached, place the mouse in supine position typically on a heating pad secured to a moveable board. At this point, the means of measuring and regulating animal's body temperature should also be established (*see* **Note 6**).
2. Wipe down the fur on the neck area with 70 % ethanol. Using blunt-tipped scissors make a centrally located vertical incision starting between the forelimbs and proceeding almost to the chin (Fig. 1). The submaxillary gland should now be visible.
3. Gently tease apart the two lobes of the submaxillary gland. The trachea will now become visible. A sheath of muscular tissue which surrounds the trachea should now be exposed.

4. Dissect a small piece (1 cm) of the ventral portion of this muscular tissue to directly expose the trachea at which point the trachea rings should be clearly visible.
5. Guide a piece of surgical thread underneath the trachea and between the trachea and muscular tissue. Placing a pair of slightly open (0.5 cm) forceps against the trachea will allow the investigator to push a closed pair of forceps, which are holding the end of a 10 cm piece of surgical thread, underneath the trachea and through to the other side.
6. Once the thread is properly positioned, make a small horizontal incision directly in the trachea between the cartilaginous rings. The higher on the trachea the initial incision is made the more space available to repeat this process if a problem occurs.
7. Insert a tracheal cannula into the incision. Slide the cannula down past the incision until there is an adequate length of cannula inside the trachea so that the thread can be tied around the trachea in order to form an airtight seal with the cannula.

3.3 Mechanical Ventilation and Administration of Muscle Relaxant

1. Maneuver the mouse board so that the cannula can be attached to the ventilator system in a manner that allows the cannula to be directly aligned with the natural direction of the trachea.
2. Start the ventilator and attach the cannula to it (*see* **Note** 7).
3. Administer the muscle relaxant via intraperitoneal injection and allow a period of 3–5 min for the agent to become effective (*see* **Notes 5**, **8**, and **9** and Table 2).

3.4 Measurement of Airway Responsiveness

1. Select a predefined script or create one. Results presented in Figs. 2 and 3 were generated using a predefined script for inhaled methacholine in mice (*see* **Notes 2** and **3**).
2. Initiate automated measurement sequences by activating the script. The operator is guided by the software through all the steps necessary for AHR assessment (*see* **Notes 1** and **14**).
3. When required during the course of the experiment, load increasing concentrations of methacholine in the nebulizer. A typical methacholine challenge includes aerosol challenges at 3, 6, 12, 25, and 50 mg/ml concentrations (Fig. 2).

3.5 Post-methacholine Challenge

1. Upon completion of the last methacholine challenge, stop the ventilator and detach the subject.
2. Remove any leftover solution of methacholine in the nebulizer. Detach the nebulizer from its mount, rinse it with water, and blot dry it.
3. Disconnect the Y tubing, rinse it with water, and dry it using compressed air before reassembling the system.

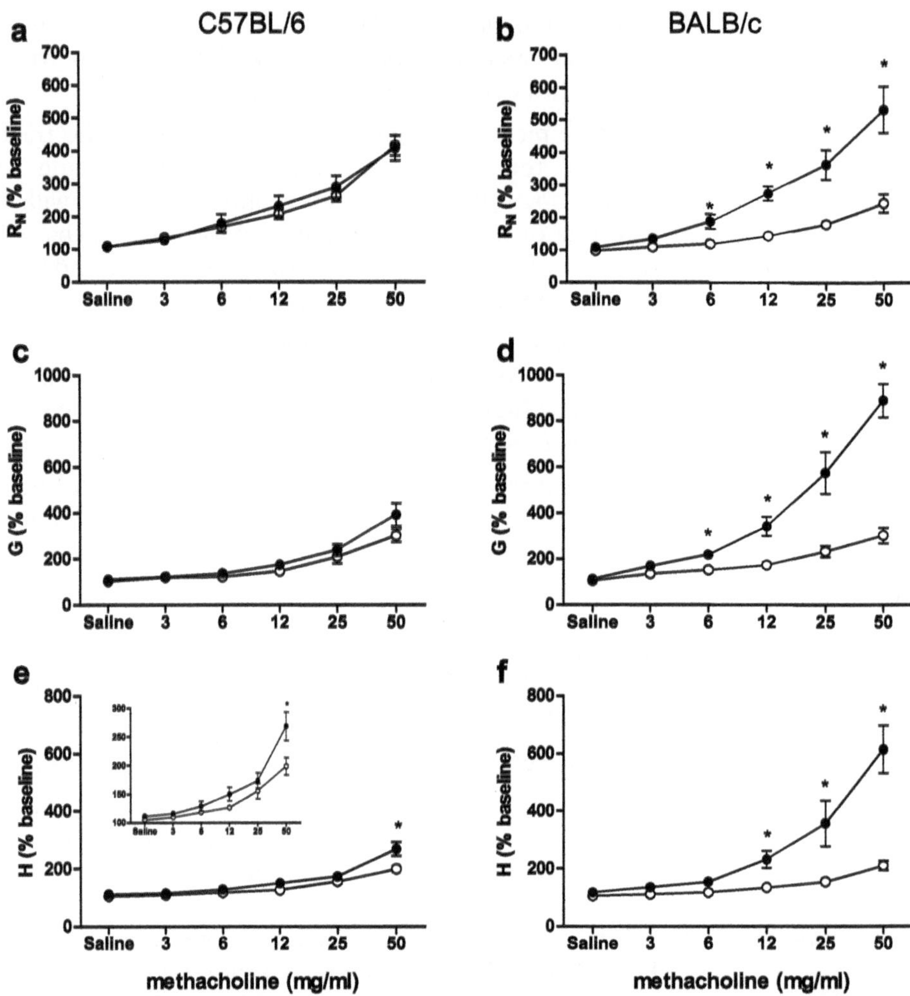

Fig. 2 Assessment of airway hyperresponsiveness in C57BL/6 and BALB/c mice. Allergic pulmonary inflammation was induced using two ovalbumin (OVA) sensitization injections (ip) with alum and three aerosol OVA challenges. Respiratory mechanics were measured using a Prime-4 perturbation with fitting of the respiratory input impedance to the constant phase model of the lung. Individual animal's parameters (R_N, G, and H) were then normalized to percentage of the average baseline measurement for that animal. The average of the group was calculated and all measurements taken were plotted in order to identify the group peak response for each parameter and methacholine concentration. Individual values for each animal at that set time point (i.e., group peak) were then used to generate a dose–response [10]. (**a**, **c**, **e**) Changes in respiratory mechanics as measured by percentage of baseline in wild-type C57BL/6 female mice between 3 and 4 months of age. *Open symbols* represent animals challenged with OVA ($n = 32$); *solid symbols* represent animals sensitized and challenged with OVA ($n = 32$). (**b**, **d**, **f**) Changes in respiratory mechanics as measured in percentage of baseline in wild-type BALB/c female mice between 3 and 4 months of age. *Open symbols* represent animals challenged with OVA ($n = 11$); *solid symbols* represent animals sensitized and challenged with OVA ($n = 12$). Differences between groups were analyzed by analysis of variance (ANOVA) for repeated measures using the logarithm (Log_{10}) of individual responses to ensure homogeneity of variances. This was followed by Bonferroni multiple comparison tests for differences between means. *$p < 0.05$ was considered statistically significant

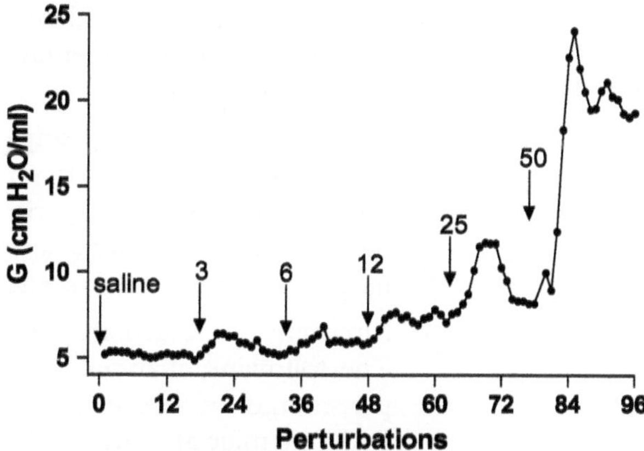

Fig. 3 Plot of automated closely spaced measurements of *G*. Measurements were recorded following increasing methacholine challenges in sensitized and challenged C57BL/6 female mice ($n=32$) [10]. *Arrows* denote time point of saline or methacholine challenge (in mg/ml). Prime-4 perturbations were executed every 10 s following aerosol challenge with a total of 16 measurements for each concentration assessed

4. Run the nebulizer briefly with PBS while holding it in your hand to visualize aerosol production (*see* **Note 12**).
5. Remove any condensation that may have formed at the bottom of the nebulizer or that could have accumulated inside the mount before starting with a new subject.
6. If running a multi-subject experiment, replace the subject with a new one in the *flexiVent* operating software and proceed with the calibration of the system as directed by the software.
7. Repeat all the necessary procedures described above with the following animal.
8. Upon completion of an experimentation session, clean nebulizer and Y tubing as previously described and empty the water PEEP trap (if used). Follow the manufacturer's instructions on module maintenance and expiratory valve cleaning in order to maintain the performance of your system.

3.6 Analysis

1. Export included parameters associated with each perturbation used directly into a spreadsheet (Microsoft® Excel®) (*see* **Note 13**).
2. Look at results in their raw form. Compile the responses for each experimental group and plot group averages for each parameter and condition. This should generate graphs similar to what is shown in Fig. 3. You may then consider the alternatives listed below to further analyze an experiment.
3. Alternative 1: Perform a detailed analysis of the time course curves to gather information relative to the general profile of the curves, the time to reach peak, or the area under the curve.

4. Alternative 2: Normalize individual animal's parameters (R_N, G, and H) to percentage of the average baseline measurement for that animal.
5. Alternative 3: Generate, using either form of data expression mentioned above (raw form or normalized), dose–response curves for each parameter and experimental groups by looking at the response of each animal at a set point (e.g., peak value for individual parameters) or set time after methacholine challenge (Fig. 2).
6. Alternative 4: Calculate the amount of change from baseline. The following changes in airway resistance (R_N; expressed as percentage of baseline; Fig. 2b) were observed in naïve BALB/c mice after methacholine challenge: 3 mg/ml = 110 %, 6 mg/ml = 120 %, 12.5 mg/ml = 145 %, 25 mg/ml = 180 %, and 50 mg/ml = 245 %.
7. Alternative 5: Calculate, from the individual dose–response curves, the concentration (or dose) of methacholine required to induce a doubling of baseline (PC_{200} or PD_{200}) and report an average value for each parameter and experimental condition.

4 Notes

1. Because procedures are performed in living animals, the investigator needs to obtain the appropriate approvals by the Institutional Animal Care and Use Committee (IACUC) prior to conducting any experiments.
2. Familiarize yourself with the *flexiVent* system and its operating software prior to doing any animal experiments. Learn to start an experiment and to calibrate the system. Best practice recommends that the system be calibrated each day before use. The operator is guided through all the steps necessary for calibration by the software at the opening of an experimentation session and also when required during the course of an experiment (e.g., following a change of subject). The operator can also refer to the owner's manual for additional details.
3. Learn to operate the system using automated tasks (referred to as scripts) in order to standardize procedures during aerosol delivery and measurements following methacholine challenge. This step, which can be done using test loads, will help the investigator plan how much time is necessary each day for equipment preparation as well as for animal assessment. It will also provide an opportunity to make adjustments to the script, if needed. A selection of predefined scripts is provided with each *flexiVent* system. Operators can also create or modify scripts. When creating or modifying a script for automated airway responsiveness assessment, care should be taken to include in the specified order the key steps described in Table 3.

Table 3
Key steps to include in a script for automated assessment in mice of airway responsiveness to inhaled methacholine using broadband low-frequency forced oscillation measurements

Steps	Description	Parameters
1. Normalization of lung volume and opening of closed areas	This is done by initiating a large amplitude perturbation, e.g.: • Deep inflation (or TLC in earlier software versions) • PVs-P or PVs-V (stepwise, pressure- or volume-driven pressure–volume curves)	• Deep inflation: IC: Inspiratory capacity • PVs-P or PVs-V: *A*: Salazar–Knowles equation parameter; provides an estimate of inspiratory capacity *K*: Salazar–Knowles equation parameter; assesses the curvature of the upper portion of expiratory limb of the pressure–volume curve. C_{st}: Quasi-static compliance Area: Area between inspiratory and expiratory branches of pressure–volume curve
2. Baseline measurements	Several broadband low-frequency forced oscillation measurements are taken using perturbation(s) of the Primewave family, e.g.: • Quick Prime-3 • Prime-4[a] • Prime-8	Constant phase model parameters (Table 1)
3. Administration of aerosol	Automated activation of the nebulizer is done by adding a command in the script: Output name = "Aeroneb" state = on	
4. Closely spaced measurements	Measurements every 10–15 s for at least 3 min using perturbations of short duration, e.g.: • Quick Prime-3 • Prime-4[a]	Constant phase model parameters (Table 1)

[a]The Prime-4 perturbation was available in earlier *flexiVent* operating software versions. It is mentioned here since results presented in this chapter were generated with it

4. Establish an anesthetic regimen. Sodium pentobarbital is frequently used in this type of experiment. It is administered either alone (by intraperitoneal injections of approximately 70–100 mg/kg body weight) or following preanesthetic medication with agents such as xylazine [5] or a combination of drugs such as ketamine/diazepam [6]. Variations in time to reach a surgical plane of anesthesia can be seen between animals or mouse strains. The addition of a preanesthetic medication can be helpful to standardize this step, minimize any excitation phase associated with anesthesia induction, and reduce the administered

dose of sodium pentobarbital. Under the present protocol of AHR assessment with a graduated methacholine challenge, a typical experiment lasts between 30 and 50 min. Therefore, it would be advisable to establish a regimen providing adequate coverage for this length of time in a few naïve animals that would be mechanically ventilated, but would not undergo AHR assessment. Documenting if and when these animals begin to recover from a surgical level of anesthesia and verifying at the end of that time period that the subjects are still alive would be of particular importance. This step would also allow new operators to familiarize themselves with animal handling, injections, and surgical procedures in a small rodent.

5. Some formulations of sodium pentobarbital can precipitate with time. Prepare a working solution fresh each day. Pancuronium bromide is sensitive to light and oxygen but stable at room temperature. The stock solution should be stored at 4 °C to prolong its shelf life. Methacholine should be stored at −20 °C with desiccant as it is highly hygroscopic.
6. During the surgical preparation, it is helpful to place a loop of thread between the teeth in order to pull the animal's head slightly over the end of the board to fully expose the neck area for the tracheostomy as well as to provide as straight as possible flow of air from the ventilator into the lungs. Ideally the animal should be positioned so as to minimize changes in the direction of the ventilation tubing and tracheal cannula when it is connected to the ventilator. The mouse can be immobilized by taping or restraining the limbs. When using a rectal probe to monitor body temperature, strive to maintain a temperature on the lower end of the acceptable range (35–37 °C) throughout the duration of the assessment. A body temperature over 38 °C can rapidly cause the animal to expire. If necessary, body temperature can be reduced by wiping down part of the animals fur with 70 % ethanol. If during the surgical process any movement is noted, a supplemental dose of sodium pentobarbital should be administered (¼–½ dose).
7. When ready to proceed with mechanical ventilation, start the ventilator before attaching the cannula to assure no interruption in the flow of air into the lungs. If working with an external water trap to establish a positive end-expiratory pressure (PEEP), it would be important to adjust the desired pressure before the start of mechanical ventilation. Typically, ventilation in rodents is performed against a 3 cmH_2O PEEP. It is useful to confirm at the start of mechanical ventilation that the animal is still alive (e.g., using vital sign transducers) and that there is no leak around the cannula. This latter step can be done by initiating a "Deep Inflation" perturbation (also known as "TLC" in earlier *flexiVent* software versions; Table 3). In the absence of

leaks, the system should be able to maintain the set pressure (30 cmH_2O) over a period of 3 s without any significant increase in the volume of air displaced by the piston of the ventilator. Running a "Deep Inflation" perturbation will also standardize lung volume, which contributes to decreasing variability between animals.

8. Under the present protocol, a muscle relaxant was administered in addition to the surgical anesthesia during AHR assessment. The purpose of the muscle relaxant is to prevent any breathing efforts during measurements (perturbations) as these efforts would contaminate the oscillatory airflow signal sent by the system and invalidate measurement outcomes. It is important to remember that once the muscle relaxant has been administered, it will be impossible to ascertain the level of anesthesia by skin or paw pinch. If required, vital sign transducers (e.g., heart rate, blood pressure, body temperature) can be integrated into the *flexiVent* system for online monitoring of the subjects [7].
9. Confirmation of adequate muscle relaxation can be achieved by running a perturbation (e.g., PVs-P; Table 3) and ensuring that the recorded pressure signal traces show no downward drops at each plateau. The absence of spontaneous breathing efforts is critical in order to generate valid data sets.
10. Establish a protocol in which inhalation of aerosolized methacholine produces measurable changes in respiratory mechanics with your specific strain of mice using naïve animals. It is critical that the investigator validates that operators can consistently and reliably measure respiratory mechanics with their particular system before investing effort and resources in generating mice with pulmonary allergic inflammation. It is suggested that new operators perform AHR assessment on at least 6–8 naïve mice on two different occasions. Once a consistent data set of naïve animals has been generated, the investigator should confirm that the protocol produces baseline values in relation to previously published results for that mouse strain (Table 4) and that changes in respiratory mechanics reproduced those presented in Figs. 2 and 3. Following success in naïve animals, proceed to establish cohorts of mice with allergic lung disease to assess AHR.
11. C57BL/6 and BALB/c mice are the mouse strains most commonly used in these types of experiments. BALB/c mice have been shown by multiple investigators to have a robust increase in airway responsiveness to inhaled methacholine when pulmonary allergic inflammation is present. However the majority of gene-targeted mice are available on the C57BL/6 background. The C57BL/6 strain, under most protocols for allergic sensitization, produces much lower levels of AHR than the BALB/c strain. The protocol, as outlined below, produces

Table 4
Baseline values in C57BL/6 and BALB/c mice

Strains	Parameters	Average	Standard deviation	Minimal value	Maximal value	Coefficient of variation	Count
C57BL/6	R_N (cmH$_2$O s/ml)	0.29	0.05	0.22	0.38	0.17	12
	G (cmH$_2$O/ml)	5.22	0.45	4.61	6.08	0.09	12
	H (cmH$_2$O/ml)	23.10	1.45	20.21	25.29	0.06	12
BALB/c	R_N (cmH$_2$O s/ml)	0.37	0.08	0.26	0.50	0.23	12
	G (cmH$_2$O/ml)	4.02	0.26	3.64	4.37	0.07	12
	H (cmH$_2$O/ml)	17.93	0.92	16.66	19.63	0.05	12

significant changes in response to methacholine in sensitized and challenged BALB/c mice in all three constant phase model parameters (Table 1), namely, R_N (airway resistance), G (tissue damping, which is closely related to tissue resistance), and H (tissue elastance) (Fig. 2). The same protocol, when applied to the C57BL/6 animals, produces a much more modest change which reaches statistical significance only at the highest concentration of methacholine and in one parameter (tissue elastance or H) (Fig. 2).

12. Aeroneb nebulizers have a limited life span (between 3 and 24 months). The frequency at which a given unit needs to be replaced depends on the operating conditions (e.g., usage, substance nebulized, or cleaning care). We recommend for facilities with multiple investigators using a single system that each investigator purchases its own unit. The volume of aerosol produced by a nebulizer can be determined gravimetrically and different units or types of nebulizers can produce different volumes of aerosol. Monitoring nebulizer performance on a regular basis, keeping accurate records, and modifying, if needed, the nebulization settings to adjust aerosol output rates should ensure reproducibility of results during and between studies.
13. For each data set, a coefficient of determination (COD) indicates how well the mathematical model fits the data. Typically, parameters of any given perturbation will be included provided that the COD is greater or equal to 0.9. Rejected data sets appear as an open symbol in the software "Trend" view.
14. Despite special attention to key steps (system calibration, positioning of animal, leaks, or breathing efforts), it is possible to see data sets being rejected. If baseline perturbations are being excluded, review each of these key steps. Temporary buildup of aerosolized liquid in the subject's airways can account for perturbations being excluded immediately following methacholine challenge. High levels of bronchoconstriction can also

result in data set exclusion around peak response. In either case, reviewing the nebulization part of the protocol including the concentrations of methacholine at which airway reactivity is assessed should improve the situation. Finally, working with a high-resistance cannula relative to the animal's airway resistance can have a negative impact on the signal-to-noise ratio or even lead to negative R_N values. The resistance of the cannula (R_t) is measured during the open dynamic calibration step and can be monitored. Increasing the diameter of the cannula or shortening its length will result in a reduction of the R_t value.

References

1. Expert Panel Report 3 (2007) Guidelines for the diagnosis and management of asthma – summary report. J Allergy Clin Immunol 120(5 Suppl):S94–S138
2. Martin TR, Gerard NP, Galli SJ, Drazen JM (1988) Pulmonary responses to bronchoconstrictor agonist in the mouse. J Appl Physiol 64(6):2318–2323
3. Takeda K, Hamelmann E, Joetham A, Shultz LD, Larsen LD, Irvin CG, Gelfand EW (1997) Development of eosinophilic airway inflammation and airway hyperresponsiveness in mast cell-deficient mice. J Exp Med 186(3): 449–454
4. Hantos Z, Daroczy B, Suki B, Nagy S, Fredberg JJ (1992) Input impedance and peripheral inhomogeneity of dog lungs. J Appl Physiol 72(1):168–178
5. Takubo Y, Guerassimov A, Ghezzo H, Triantafillopoulos A, Bates JHT, Hoidal JR, Cosio MG (2002) Alpha1-antitrypsin determines the pattern of emphysema and function in tobacco smoke-exposed mice: parallels with human disease. Am J Respir Crit Care Med 166(12 Pt 1):1596–1603
6. Therien AG, Bernier V, Weicker S, Tawa P, Falgueyret J-P, Mathieu M-C, Honsberger J, Pomerleau V, Robichaud A, Stocco R, Dufresne L, Houshyar H, Lafleur J, Ramachandran C, O'Neill GP, Slipetz D, Tan CM (2008) Adenovirus IL-13-induced airway disease in mice: a corticosteroid-resistant model of severe asthma. Am J Respir Cell Mol Biol 39(1):26–35
7. Amatullah H, North ML, Akhtar US, Rastogi N, Urch B, Silverman F, Chow C-W, Evans GJ, Scott JA (2012) Comparative cardiopulmonary effects of size-fractionated airborne particulate matter. Inhal Toxicol 24(3):161–171
8. Bates JHT (2009) Lung mechanics, an inverse modeling approach. Cambridge University Press, New York, p 220
9. What would you like to measure? http://www.scireq.com/science/measurements/. Accessed 9 Mar 2012
10. Hartney, JM, Strauch, P, Torres, RM (2011) Assessment of airway reactivity in C57BL/6 and BALB/c wild type mice with ova induced allergic lung disease. Unpublished work
11. Cook MJ (1965) The anatomy of the laboratory mouse. Elsevier, London. p 143

Chapter 17

Bilateral Vagotomy as a Tool for Determining Autonomic Involvement in Airway Responses in Mouse Models of Asthma

Jaime M. Cyphert

Abstract

This chapter describes the use of bilateral vagotomy as a tool for determining autonomic regulation of airway responses to the exogenous bronchoconstrictor thromboxane mimetic U46619 in an acute model of asthma in the mouse. Mice receive a sensitization of ovalbumin (OVA) and adjuvant followed by 3 days of OVA aerosol to induce allergic airway disease characterized by bronchoalveolar lavage (BAL) eosinophilia, increased mucus production, and elevated IgE and IL-13. Using a small animal ventilator (Flexi-vent) and the forced oscillatory technique fit to the constant phase model of the lung, a variety of features associated with human asthma can be evaluated in mouse models. For example, this protocol describes the methods to evaluate central and peripheral airway mechanics, airway resistance (R_{aw}) and tissue damping (G), and tissue elastance (H) in response to U46619. The contribution of autonomic nerves in this response is determined by severing both the left and right vagus nerves prior to aerosol challenge.

Key words Vagus nerve, Autonomic nervous system, Lung mechanics, Asthma

1 Introduction

Asthma is one of the most common respiratory diseases, affecting approximately 300 million adults and children worldwide [1]. Phenotypically, asthma is a heterogenous disease manifesting in many subtypes and is affected by interactions of both environmental and genetic factors. This disease is typically characterized by three principal characteristics: chronic airway inflammation; airway hyperresponsiveness (AHR); and reversible airflow obstruction [2]. Airway smooth muscle (ASM) plays a central role in regulating bronchomoter tone; however, ASM can constrict in response to many agents, either directly via receptors on the muscle, or indirectly through the activation of immune cells or nerves.

Sensory and parasympathetic nerves extending into the lungs may contribute significantly to airway obstruction and hyperreactivity

Irving C. Allen (ed.), *Mouse Models of Allergic Disease: Methods and Protocols*, Methods in Molecular Biology, vol. 1032, DOI 10.1007/978-1-62703-496-8_17,

in the diseased lung through the release of neurotransmitters that can elicit effects on further neurotransmission, mucus secretion, ASM, epithelial cells, and inflammatory cells [3–7]. Furthermore, dysregulation of these neurotransmitters, airway receptors, or the response of nerves during a disease state may lead to an alteration of normal airway tone or an increase/decrease in nerve excitability and signal transduction. One hypothesis is that asthma represents an imbalance or dysregulation of the autonomic nervous system.

The vagus nerve contains the majority of airway sensory afferents (reviewed in [8]), approximately 75 % of which are unmyelinated C-fibers, which span the entire respiratory tract from trachea to the central airways to the parenchyma [9]. While typically quiescent during tidal breathing, C-fiber activation provides excitatory input to neuronal pathways driving autonomic output to the airways, resulting in bronchoconstriction, mucus secretion, and vasodilation [10, 11]. Additionally, the vagus nerve also contains parasympathetic (or cholinergic) nerves, which are the primary controllers of human and animal airways. Specifically, the vagus nerve carries efferent cholinergic fibers that synapse in small ganglia within the airway wall, from which short postganglionic fibers innervate airway smooth muscle and submucosal glands [12]. Therefore, the vagus nerve contains the vast majority of nerves that are responsible for both sampling and controlling the airways.

Due to the complex nature of the disease and the limitations of mechanistic studies in humans, animal models are crucial for the study of neural involvement in the asthmatic response. By conducting a bilateral vagotomy prior to measuring airway responses to an inhaled or intravenous stimulus, one can assess the contribution of airway nerves/neurotransmitters to that response. The mouse is an ideal model for this assessment, as models of asthma, methods of in vivo airway mechanistic monitoring, and genetic manipulation are all well established. Here, we describe the use of bilateral vagotomy as a tool for determining autonomic regulation of airway responses to an exogenous bronchoconstrictor in an acute model of asthma in the mouse.

2 Materials

2.1 Equipment and Supplies

1. Computer/monitor.
2. Flexi-vent system (Scireq respiratory equipment) including the following pieces of equipment: Base Unit; EC controller unit; XC accessories controller; Module M1; Scireq Aeroneb plug-in; Scireq EKG plug-in (*see* **Note 1**); Manometer; and PEEP trap.
3. Scireq FV-AN-A1 aerosol base.
4. Aeroneb pro aerosol cup.

5. Tygon tubing.
6. Luer connector kit (Harvard apparatus).
7. Flexi-vent 5.1 (or newer) software.
8. Heating pad (*see* **Note 2**).
9. Ultrasonic nebulizer (DeVillbiss Health Care).
10. Forceps: Two sets small curved forceps (45–90°) and one set fine, curved Dumont #7 forceps.
11. Scissors: Straight and angled (45–90°).
12. 1 cm^3 syringe for injecting/anesthetizing animals.
13. 26 G 3/8″ needles for injecting animals.
14. 4-0 Silk Suture thread (Ethicon), 2 pieces/mouse.
15. 1.0 mm × 20 mm endo-tracheal tube (Harvard apparatus) with attached luer adaptor.
16. p200 and p1000 pipettes.
17. Reditip general-purpose pipette tips (200 and 1,000 μl).
18. Kim wipes.
19. Lab tape.
20. 15 ml conical tubes.
21. 1.5 ml Eppendorf tubes.
22. 500 ml glass beaker.
23. 100 ml graduated cylinder.
24. 100 ml glass solution jar.
25. 100 ml crimp-top glass injection vials.
26. Aluminum foil.

2.2 Chemical Reagents and Supplies

1. 100 % EtOH.
2. 70 % EtOH.
3. 0.9 % Saline (in non-sterile bottle and 20 ml sterile injection vials).
4. Urethane (Sigma).
5. Pancuronium bromide (Sigma).
6. Grade V Ovalbumin (≥98 %) (Sigma).
7. Alhydrogel (Brenntag).
8. U46619 (Cayman Chemical, 10 mg/ml).

2.3 Reagent Preparation

1. 1 % Ovalbumin (OVA): Mix 1 g of OVA in 100 ml of 0.9 % saline. Filter the solution.
2. Urethane—anesthetic (500 mg/ml stock solution): Weigh out 50 g of urethane crystals into a large graduated beaker (*see* **Note 3**). Add pre-warmed (not boiling) distilled water and bring the solution up to 100 ml. Continue to heat on low

heat and stir until the crystals are completely in solution. Cool the solution to room temperature. Dilute 1:4 in distilled water for 125 mg/ml working solution. Place into glass injection vials (with crimp tops) and wrap in aluminum foil to protect from light.

3. Pancuronium bromide—paralytic agent (8 mg/ml stock solution): Add 50 mg of pancuronium bromide powder to 6.25 ml of 0.9 % saline in a 15 ml conical tube. Cover with aluminum foil to protect from light and keep the stock refrigerated. To prepare working stock, dilute stock 1:100 in 0.9 % saline to make a 0.08 mg/ml working solution by injecting 200 μl of stock directly into a 20 ml, 0.9 % saline injection vial. Keep the working solution on ice.
4. U46619 (thromboxane analog, 10^{-2} M stock) (*see* **Note 4**): Add 100 μl of U46619/methyl acetate solution into an Eppendorf tube and slowly evaporate off the methyl acetate using nitrogen. Add 200 μl of 100 % EtOH and resuspend the oil residue to make a 10^{-2} M stock. Dilute the stock 1:10 in 0.9 % PBS to make a 10^{-3} M dose. Dilute the 10^{-3} M dose 1:10 in 0.9 % PBS to make a 10^{-4} M dose. Dilute the 10^{-4} M dose 1:10 in 0.9 % PBS to make a 10^{-5} M dose.

2.4 Mice

1. Adult mice, 6–12 weeks old (*see* **Note 5**).

3 Methods

3.1 Mouse Model of Allergic Airway Disease

1. Add 200 μl of 1 % OVA solution to 10 ml of alhydrogel and mix well.
2. Sensitize mice on day 1 by i.p. injection with 200 μl of OVA + alhydrogel.
3. On days 14–16 challenge mice with aerosolized 1 % OVA for 1 h/day using an exposure chamber equipped with an ultrasonic nebulizer.
4. On day 17 proceed with airway evaluations.

3.2 Flexi-Vent Calibration (See Note 6)

1. Fill the PEEP trap with distilled water, and set the interior tube 2–3 cm below the surface.
2. Open the Flexi-vent 5.1 software.
3. Select "Start new experiment from template" from the pop-up menu.
4. Choose the appropriate template from the pop-up menu (*see* **Note 7**).
5. When prompted, name your experiment.
6. When prompted, record the operator name.

7. Enter first subject information in order to proceed with calibration (identifier, strain, group, weight, gender).
8. Follow directions given by the calibration wizard to prime the nebulizer.
9. In the "Channel Selection" pop-up window select both Cylinder Pressure and Airway Pressure. To calibrate the transducers measuring cylinder and airway pressures, connect the transducers to a manometer so that a known pressure can be applied to both transducers. The pressure calibration wizard will guide you through the steps required to properly calibrate the pressure channels and will warn you if they were not calibrated correctly (click the Help button on the wizard for more detailed instructions).
10. Next select "EKG" and proceed with "known full-scale values" set as −3 to +1 mV.
11. Dynamic tube calibration: This allows you to perform all dynamic calibration measurements required to characterize the ventilator compartment in a single step. This must be completed before ventilating the subject. The Tube Calibration wizard will automatically display at the beginning of a new measurement after autocalibration and pressure calibration have been completed. Before starting the dynamic tube calibration make sure that the endotracheal tube (ETT) is attached to the Flexi-vent. Follow the instructions supplied by the wizard.
12. Start default ventilation and prepare to connect the mouse.

3.3 Intubation and Vagotomy Preparation

1. Turn on the 37 °C water bath heating pad.
2. Weigh each mouse.
3. Anesthetize a single mouse by IP injection of 1 g/kg of urethane (weight in grams × 16 = μl of working solution).
4. Once the mouse is fully anesthetized (as assessed by toe pinch), secure it to the heating pad using lab tape.
5. Spread 70 % EtOH on the throat of the mouse to wet the fur. Lift the skin to make a vertical cut on the throat to expose salivary glands. Separate the salivary glands with forceps to visualize the muscle surrounding the trachea. Lift the muscle and cut with straight scissors to expose the trachea.
6. Isolate the right and left vagus nerve and tease away from carotid artery using small, curved forceps.
7. Pass fine, curved Dumont forceps underneath the left vagus nerve and slowly open forceps to separate the nerve fiber from the surrounding tissue. Repeat for the right vagus nerve.
8. Pass suture string underneath both the left and right vagus nerve (*see* Fig. 1).

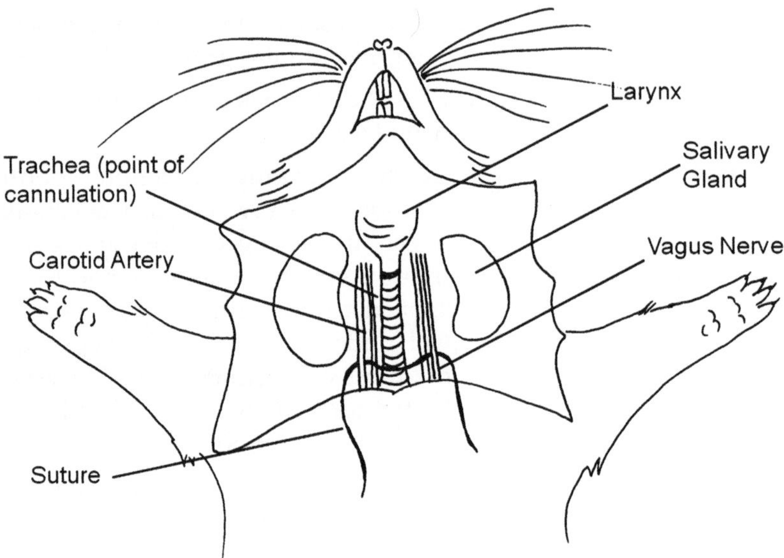

Fig. 1 Drawing depicting the preparation of the suture for bilateral vagotomy. Control sham operations are simulated by lifting and releasing of the suture. Bilateral vagotomy is conducted by lifting the nerves with the suture and then severing both the left and right vagus nerves

9. Make a horizontal incision between the second and third tracheal rings using angled scissors and insert the ETT.
10. Pass suture thread underneath the trachea using the ETT for support. Tie the suture thread tightly to secure the ETT in place.

3.4 Measuring Airway Responses in Mice

1. Attach the mouse to the Flexi-vent via the ETT (with default ventilation equal to 150–200 breaths/min).
2. Attach EKG leads to the mouse in the Lead II configuration.
3. Inject 0.8 mg/kg of pancuronium bromide (weight in g × 10 = μl of working solution to inject).
4. Wait 5 min for the paralytic drug to take effect before starting the experiment.
5. Double click on the desired script (*see* **Note 8**) on the lower right-hand side of the screen to start the experiment. The Experiment wizard will automatically display and guide you through the experiment.
6. Record baseline parameters.
7. Simultaneously sever both the left and right vagus nerves by lifting up on the suture string and cutting the nerves with straight scissors. Alternatively, a surgical sham for control animals is conducted by simply lifting the nerves via the suture string and releasing them intact.
8. Repeat baseline measurements (*see* **Note 9**).

9. When prompted, add 100 μl of 10^{-5} M U46619 to the nebulizer cup, record the concentration on the wizard window, and continue with the experiment (*see* **Note 10**).
10. After aerosolization is complete, remove excess liquid from the nebulizer cup by gently dabbing the membrane with an absorbent wipe.
11. Repeat **steps 9** and **10** for the 10^{-4} and 10^{-3} M doses of U46619.
12. When the script is complete, remove the mouse from the ventilator, stop ventilation, and select "switch subjects" from the toolbar.
13. Enter the next animal's information into the pop-up window and repeat the protocol.

3.5 Calculations

1. Scireq Flexi-vent 5.1 software automatically fits the data to the constant phase model and calculates airway mechanics parameters (R_{aw}, G, and H) from the recorded raw data when the data is exported.
2. To export data from the Flexi-vent software, select "File" from the top left of the screen and then select "export data" from the drop-down menu. An export wizard will direct the saving of the exported data in a folder or a disk of your choice.
3. The final data is typically expressed as percent change from baseline. To calculate this, the raw data is transferred to an excel spreadsheet and the dose–response of each animal is divided by its average baseline and then multiplied by 100 for each parameter of interest. Excluded data points (automatically detected by the system and denoted with a minus sign when exported) are manually removed before calculations.

4 Notes

1. The EKG plug-in is not required, but it is recommended for monitoring the heart rate in order to evaluate the depth of anesthesia and to ensure that the mouse is still alive during measurement of airway responses.
2. A water bath heating pad is recommended for precise body temperature regulation. If a commercial heating pad is used, monitoring of the animal's body temperature is recommended. Body temperature should be kept at or below 37 °C.
3. Urethane is a toxicant and should only be opened and weighed out in a chemical fume hood.
4. Make U46619 stock and dilutions fresh daily: do not store. It is recommended to purchase U46619 in methyl acetate and

to store it as 100 μl aliquots. One aliquot is sufficient for up to 18 mice.

5. The weight of the mice should be approximately 20 g, although the M1 module is capable of measuring airway parameters in subjects from 15 to 40 g. Female mice tend to be smaller than male mice, so it is recommended to either normalize mixed-sex experiments by weight (requiring a larger range of ages) or conduct single-sex experiments normalized by age.
6. In order to obtain good data, it is crucial to perform pressure, flow, and auxiliary channel calibrations before you start an experiment. Scireq recommends performing a calibration at least once a day before experiments.
7. The template should be created using the Template wizard with the following parameters: Mode: Quasi-sinusoidal; Tidal Volume: 10 ml/kg; Pressure Limit: 30 cm H_2O; Frequency: 150–200 breaths/min for adult mice. Typical perturbations used for FOT measurements are total lung capacity (TLC) and Quick Prime-3. Scireq technical support can also provide a Guide to Flexi-vent Template Creation.
8. Several default scripts are included with the software; however, we suggest modifying those scripts (in Microsoft Notepad™) so that the mouse is subjected to 1–2 TLC maneuvers prior to baseline measurements to ensure normalized lung resistance. At least 3 Quick Prime-3 measurements, separated by 10 s, should be conducted for baseline parameters (both before and after vagotomy/sham). Following baseline measurements, we recommend aerosolizing for 20 s at 50 %, then recording Quick Prime-3 every 10 s for 3 min, and then prompting for a loop back to aerosolize the next dose. This can be repeated for as many doses as desired.
9. A slight drop in baseline parameters can be seen following vagotomy due to the loss of intrinsic airway tone that is generally maintained by constitutive, low-level release of acetylcholine from parasympathetic nerves [13].
10. Alternatively, other bronchoconstricting agents or antigens can be used (i.e., OVA, histamine, serotonin). Additionally, intravenous challenge can replace the aerosol challenge when appropriate.

References

1. Masoli M, Fabian D, Holt S, Beasley R (2004) The global burden of asthma: executive summary of the GINA Dissemination Committee report. Allergy 59:469–478
2. Busse WW, Lemanske RF Jr (2001) Asthma. N Engl J Med 344:350–362
3. Myers AC, Undem BJ (1993) Electrophysiological effects of tachykinins and capsaicin on guinea-pig bronchial parasympathetic ganglion neurones. J Physiol 470:665–679
4. Watson N, Maclagan J, Barnes PJ (1993) Endogenous tachykinins facilitate transmission

through parasympathetic ganglia in guinea-pig trachea. Br J Pharmacol 109:751–759
5. Dakhama A, Kanehiro A, Makela MJ, Loader JE, Larsen GL, Gelfand EW (2002) Regulation of airway hyperresponsiveness by calcitonin gene-related peptide in allergen sensitized and challenged mice. Am J Respir Crit Care Med 165:1137–1144
6. Veres TZ, Rochlitzer S, Shevchenko M, Fuchs B, Prenzler F, Nassenstein C, Fischer A, Welker L, Holz O, Muller M et al (2007) Spatial interactions between dendritic cells and sensory nerves in allergic airway inflammation. Am J Respir Cell Mol Biol 37:553–561
7. Barnes PJ (1992) Modulation of neurotransmission in airways. Physiol Rev 72:699–729
8. Groneberg DA, Quarcoo D, Frossard N, Fischer A (2004) Neurogenic mechanisms in bronchial inflammatory diseases. Allergy 59:1139–1152
9. Agostoni E, Chinnock JE, De Daly MB, Murray JG (1957) Functional and histological studies of the vagus nerve and its branches to the heart, lungs and abdominal viscera in the cat. J Physiol 135:182–205
10. Canning BJ, Fischer A (2001) Neural regulation of airway smooth muscle tone. Respir Physiol 125:113–127
11. Mazzone SB, Canning BJ (2002) Evidence for differential reflex regulation of cholinergic and noncholinergic parasympathetic nerves innervating the airways. Am J Respir Crit Care Med 165:1076–1083
12. Barnes PJ (1986) Neural control of human airways in health and disease. Am Rev Respir Dis 134:1289–1314
13. Allen IC, Hartney JM, Coffman TM, Penn RB, Wess J, Koller BH (2006) Thromboxane A2 induces airway constriction through an M3 muscarinic acetylcholine receptor-dependent mechanism. Am J Physiol Lung Cell Mol Physiol 290:L526–L533

Chapter 18

Clara Epithelial Cell Depletion in the Lung

Sanchaita S. Sonar and Jan C. Dudda

Abstract

The bronchial epithelium has been increasingly recognized as an important immunomodulatory compartment in asthma and other lung diseases. Clara cells, which comprise the nonciliated secretory epithelial cells, are an important epithelial cell type with functions in the regulation of lung homeostasis and inflammation. Using naphthalene, Clara cells can be depleted within 24 h and regenerate by 1 month, hence, providing an easy method to study the impact of Clara cells on lung inflammation.

Key words Clara cells, Airway epithelium, Naphthalene, Asthma

1 Introduction

The airway epithelium comprises ciliated and secretory cells arranged in a continuous stratified structure. In mouse and other species, nonciliated bronchiolar Clara cells (CC) are the predominant epithelial cell type secreting both pro- and anti-inflammatory factors [1–3]. It accounts for 70–90 % of the cells in distal airways of many species including mice [4]. In humans, CC represent about 20 % of epithelial cells and have been shown to contribute to cell renewal in the normal conducting airway epithelium [5, 6]. CC respond to activated Th2 cells via the IL-4 receptor-α [7], can differentiate to mucus-producing goblet cells [8], and secrete anti-inflammatory factors such as Clara cell secretory protein (CCSP/CC-10) and eotaxin [9]. CCSP has been shown to counter-regulate the Th2 response in asthma [10]. Moreover, CC are also able to metabolize and detoxify xenobiotics and toxic compounds, such as naphthalene (NA), present in cigarette smoke [11, 12]. Therefore, CC of the airways are uniquely susceptible to injury by metabolizing chemicals into toxic intermediates.

NA is a prominent component of sidestream, whole, and filtered cigarette smoke [7]. For compounds like NA, toxicity is highly dose dependent and cell type and site selective [4, 13]. The toxicity

Irving C. Allen (ed.), *Mouse Models of Allergic Disease: Methods and Protocols*, Methods in Molecular Biology, vol. 1032, DOI 10.1007/978-1-62703-496-8_18,

of NA requires metabolic activation, catalyzed by cytochrome P450 monooxygenases that cause airway CC swelling, vacuolization, and exfoliation into the lumen of the airways 24 h after injury is initiated [14]. Susceptibility correlates with the presence of cytochrome P450 2F2 (CYP2F2) within CC. Therefore, murine CC are more susceptible to NA-induced cytotoxic injury than other types of airway epithelial cells. CC present in the distal airway are more susceptible at very low doses, with susceptibility extending to proximal airways with higher doses. Detailed time kinetics of NA-induced CC cytotoxicity has been elegantly shown previously [14].

2 Materials

2.1 Mice

1. 8–10-week-old C57BL/6, BALB/c mice or Swiss Webster mice.

2.2 Naphthalene

1. Naphthalene, 20 mg/ml stock (Sigma Aldrich Chemical, Munich, Germany).
2. Corn Oil (Sigma Aldrich Chemical, Munich, Germany).
3. Pentobarbital sodium.

2.3 Reagents for Immunohistochemistry

1. 10 % formalin.
2. Xylene.
3. 100; 90; 80; and 70 % Ethanol.
4. Distilled water.
5. 0.3 % H_2O_2 in methanol.
6. 3 % citrate buffer (pH 6.0).
7. 1 % bovine serum albumin.
8. CC10 antibody (Upstate, Millipore, MA).
9. DAPI (4′,6-diamidino-2-phenylindole) (Vector Laboratories, Burlingame, CA).
10. Hematoxylin.
11. Horseradish peroxidase (HRP) conjugated anti-rabbit secondary antibody (Santa Cruz Biotech, CA).
12. 3,3′ diaminobenzidine (DAB) (Vectastain Elite ABC Kit; Vector Laboratories, Burlingame, CA).

2.4 Reagents for OVA Sensitization and Challenge

1. 10 μg of endotoxin-free OVA (grade VI, Sigma-Aldrich) in 200 μl of 1× PBS per mouse.
2. 1 % OVA (grade V, Sigma Aldrich) in 1× PBS.

2.5 Microscope and Software

1. Light microscope (Olympus Europa GmbH, Hamburg, Germany).
2. Cell^F imaging software program (Soft Imaging System GmbH, Muenster, Germany).

3 Methods

3.1 Clara Cell Depletion in Naïve Animals

1. Prepare NA in a 50 ml falcon tube by dissolving 20 mg in 1 ml of corn oil (stock solution). Control animals should receive the same amount of corn oil i.p. It is best to make aliquots of corn oil and freeze to avoid contamination (*see* **Note 1**).
2. Inject animals with either 200 mg/kg of NA dissolved in corn oil (CO) (10 μl of stock solution) or CO alone (10 μl) intraperitoneally (i.p.) (*see* **Note 2**).
3. Sacrifice animals using an overdose of pentobarbital sodium at the time of analysis. Maximal exfoliation of CC is seen from 24 to 48 h after application of NA + CO, with cell death occurring as early as 6 h. CC start regenerating by day 3 and by day 10, about 60 % of CC regenerate. For analysis of CC numbers, immunohistological analysis of the lung by CC staining should be performed.

3.2 Immunohistological Analysis

1. Perfuse the lung with PBS via the heart. Insert a cannula into the trachea and fix with a ligature. Inflate and fix the lungs via the cannula by gentle infusion with 10 % formalin. Remove the inflated lungs and store in 10 % formalin. Embed the fixed lung tissues into paraffin and cut into 3 μm sections.
2. Deparaffinize the tissues using xylene and rehydrate in 100–70 % ethanol (10 % steps) for 5 min/concentration and finally in 1× PBS. Remove endogenous peroxidase activity using 1 % hydrogen peroxide in methanol for 30 min. Antigen retrieval can be performed by microwave treatment in 3 % citrate buffer (pH 6.0). However, this step may be optional depending on the antibody. Cool the slides down to room temperature and rinse three times with 1× PBS.
3. After washing in PBS, incubate sections in 1× PBS containing 1 % bovine serum albumin for 30 min, followed by incubation with the polyclonal rabbit antibody directed against Clara cell-specific 10-kDa protein (CC10) in the same solution for 1 h at 37 °C (*see* **Note 3**).
4. Incubate sections with a peroxidase-conjugated anti-rabbit secondary antibody for 30 min at room temperature. Visualize using DAB as the chromogen according to the ABC method following the manufacturer's instructions. All sections may be counterstained with hematoxylin. Sections can be counterstained with DAPI (blue) for detection of all cells.
5. Negative controls without the primary antibody and normal rabbit IgG should be included.
6. Sections can be semiquantitatively analyzed for CC numbers using light microscopy. CC can be counted as CC10-positive cells with nuclear profiles surrounding the proximal or the

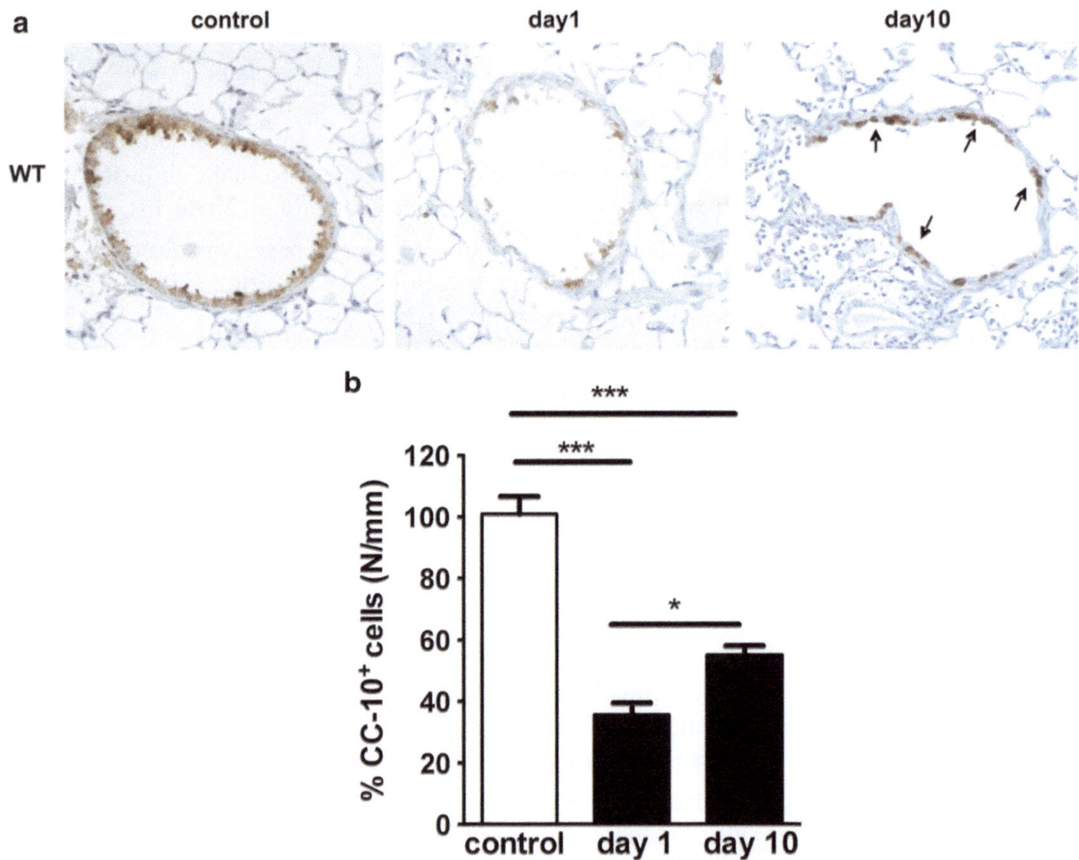

Fig. 1 Clara cell depletion. (**a**) CC10 staining was performed in lung sections of corn oil (control) and NA-treated mice (day 1 and day 10). Mice were sacrificed 24 h post NA treatment for CC10 staining. The CC10-positive cells stained with anti-CC10 antibody are diaminobenzidine (DAB) positive (*brown*) against the hematoxylin counterstain (*blue*). (**b**) Quantification of CC10-positive cells in the airways of corn oil (control) and NA-treated animals at day 1 and day 10. The graph represents CC10-positive cells with nuclear profiles per mm of the basement membrane, normalizing CC in the control group as 100 %. Results represent the mean ± SEM of at least six animals. ***$P<0.001$. *$P<0.05$. These data are representative of three experiments. Figure 1b, reproduced with permission of the European Respiratory Society. Eur Respir J February 2012 39:429–438; published ahead of print August 4, 2011, doi:10.1183/09031936.00197810

distal airways/mm of the basement membrane (Fig. 1). At least ten similar airways are counted per mouse using the software Cell^F (or a similar software) linked to the light microscope (*see* **Note 4**).

3.3 Clara Cell Depletion in Asthma

1. Sensitize two groups of mice with subcutaneous (SC) injections of 10 μg of endotoxin-free OVA (grade VI) in 200 μl of PBS and in another two control groups with sham injections of PBS on days 0, 7, and 14 (*see* **Note 5**).
2. On day 16, i.p. inject one group of SC OVA-sensitized mice and one group of mice receiving sham injections of PBS with

200 mg/kg of NA dissolved in CO. The dose depends on the amount of desired Clara cell exfoliation (*see* **Note 6**).

3. On days 26, 27, and 28, subject the SC OVA-sensitized and PBS-injected mice for 20 min with either aerosolized 1 % OVA (grade V) or aerosolized PBS, as appropriate.
4. Sacrifice mice 24 h after the last challenge or, if performing airway hyperreactivity (AHR) measurements, 48 h after the last challenge.
5. Harvest the lungs and conduct the immunohistochemical analysis as described under Subheading 3.2.

4 Notes

1. NA is a toxic irritant and is flammable. Hence, care must be taken while handling NA by wearing gloves, lab coat, face mask, and eye protection. Solutions should be prepared in a chemical fume hood. Prepare a fresh solution every time. Perform mouse injections under the hood.
2. Usually 200 mg/kg should be optimal to efficiently denude CC in proximal and distal airways; however, quantities may be optimized for the experiment. Additionally, female and male mice have been shown to vary in response.
3. The precise dilution of CC10 antibody should be tested for each lot.
4. CC counted on the basis of immunohistochemistry by staining nuclear profiles positive for CC10 antigen revealed an ~65 % reduction in CC10+ cells at day 1 post NA+CO administration. This number went to 40 % after 10 days (Fig. 1b). However, doses and time points can be manipulated based on the experimental goals.
5. Although this method has been described for subcutaneous murine models of asthma, given the many other experimental protocols for induction of asthma, including the i.p. sensitization, the route of airway exposure, and the variety of antigens available for asthma induction, protocols may be changed to suit specific experimental goals. However, since NA is toxic to the mouse, a minimum rest period of 5–10 days should be included post NA application before challenge with allergen.
6. CC in the distal airways are more susceptible to NA than cells in the proximal airways. Additionally, sex-based differential responses to NA have also been reported. Ideally, a dose–response for the strain and sex of mice used should be established in the lab prior to beginning large-scale experiments.

References

1. Elizur A, Adair-Kirk TL, Kelley DG, Griffin GL, deMello DE, Senior RM (2007) Clara cells impact the pulmonary innate immune response to LPS. Am J Physiol Lung Cell Mol Physiol 293:L383–L392
2. Elizur A, Adair-Kirk TL, Kelley DG, Griffin GL, Demello DE, Senior RM (2008) Tumor necrosis factor-alpha from macrophages enhances LPS-induced clara cell expression of keratinocyte-derived chemokine. Am J Respir Cell Mol Biol 38:8–15
3. Park MS, Zhao B, Ramsay PL, Chang AS, Reardon MJ, DeMayo FJ (2000) Expression of inflammatory cytokines in a mouse transformed Clara cell line by tumor necrosis factor-alpha. Ann N Y Acad Sci 923:336–337
4. Plopper CG, Suverkropp C, Morin D, Nishio S, Buckpitt A (1992) Relationship of cytochrome P-450 activity to Clara cell cytotoxicity. I. Histopathologic comparison of the respiratory tract of mice, rats and hamsters after parenteral administration of naphthalene. J Pharmacol Exp Ther 261:353–363
5. Boers JE, Ambergen AW, Thunnissen FB (1999) Number and proliferation of clara cells in normal human airway epithelium. Am J Respir Crit Care Med 159:1585–1591
6. Shijubo N, Itoh Y, Yamaguchi T, Imada A, Hirasawa M, Yamada T, Kawai T, Abe S (1999) Clara cell protein-positive epithelial cells are reduced in small airways of asthmatics. Am J Respir Crit Care Med 160:930–933
7. Kuperman DA, Huang X, Nguyenvu L, Holscher C, Brombacher F, Erle DJ (2005) IL-4 receptor signaling in Clara cells is required for allergen-induced mucus production. J Immunol 175:3746–3752
8. Evans CM, Williams OW, Tuvim MJ, Nigam R, Mixides GP, Blackburn MR, DeMayo FJ, Burns AR, Smith C, Reynolds SD, Stripp BR, Dickey BF (2004) Mucin is produced by clara cells in the proximal airways of antigen-challenged mice. Am J Respir Cell Mol Biol 31:382–394
9. Sonar SS, Ehmke M, Marsh LM, Dietze J, Dudda JC, Conrad ML, Renz H, Nockher WA (2012) Clara cells drive eosinophil accumulation in allergic asthma. Eur Respir J 39: 429–438
10. Wang SZ, Rosenberger CL, Espindola TM, Barrett EG, Tesfaigzi Y, Bice DE, Harrod KS (2001) CCSP modulates airway dysfunction and host responses in an Ova-challenged mouse model. Am J Physiol Lung Cell Mol Physiol 281:L1303–L1311
11. Buckpitt A, Boland B, Isbell M, Morin D, Shultz M, Baldwin R, Chan K, Karlsson A, Lin C, Taff A, West J, Fanucchi M, Van Winkle L, Plopper C (2002) Naphthalene-induced respiratory tract toxicity: metabolic mechanisms of toxicity. Drug Metab Rev 34:791–820
12. Chichester CH, Buckpitt AR, Chang A, Plopper CG (1994) Metabolism and cytotoxicity of naphthalene and its metabolites in isolated murine Clara cells. Mol Pharmacol 45: 664–672
13. Buckpitt AR, Castagnoli N Jr, Nelson SD, Jones AD, Bahnson LS (1987) Stereoselectivity of naphthalene epoxidation by mouse, rat, and hamster pulmonary, hepatic, and renal microsomal enzymes. Drug Metab Dispos 15: 491–498
14. Van Winkle LS, Buckpitt AR, Nishio SJ, Isaac JM, Plopper CG (1995) Cellular response in naphthalene-induced Clara cell injury and bronchiolar epithelial repair in mice. Am J Physiol 269:L800–L818

Chapter 19

A Mouse Model for Evaluating the Contribution of Fibrocytes and Myofibroblasts to Airway Remodeling in Allergic Asthma

Matthias Schmidt and Sabrina Mattoli

Abstract

Airway remodeling is a term used to collectively indicate bronchial structural changes that may lead to irreversible airflow obstruction and progressive decline in lung function in asthmatic patients. Bronchial myofibroblasts contribute to airway remodeling by producing collagenous proteins in the subepithelial zone and by increasing the density of contractile cells in the bronchial wall. A substantial proportion of bronchial myofibroblasts in asthma differentiate from circulating mesenchymal progenitor cells known as fibrocytes. Here, we describe a mouse model of allergic asthma for evaluating the functional role of fibrocytes and myofibroblasts in this disease and the inhibitory effects of novel therapeutic candidates.

Key words Airway remodeling, Asthma, Fibrocytes, Mice, Myofibroblasts

1 Introduction

1.1 Airway Remodeling in Asthma and in the Animal Model of Allergic Disease

Asthma is a common disorder of the airways characterized by recurrent episodes of airflow obstructions of variable duration, which may be triggered by various stimuli such as the exposure to environmental allergens or viral infections in genetically predisposed individuals [1]. The main histopathologic abnormalities include a chronic inflammatory infiltrate of the bronchial mucosa and a series of structural alterations collectively referred to with the term "airway remodeling" [2, 3] (Fig. 1). Structural alterations such as the thickening of the lamina reticularis and the increase in the smooth muscle mass are characteristic features of asthma [4]. These alterations have become major targets for the development of new therapeutic agents because they may cause fixed airway narrowing and contribute to a progressive loss of lung function in patients with severe disease and frequent clinical exacerbations [2, 3]. The thickening of the lamina reticularis is particularly evident in

Irving C. Allen (ed.), *Mouse Models of Allergic Disease: Methods and Protocols*, Methods in Molecular Biology, vol. 1032, DOI 10.1007/978-1-62703-496-8_19, © Springer Science+Business Media, LLC 2013

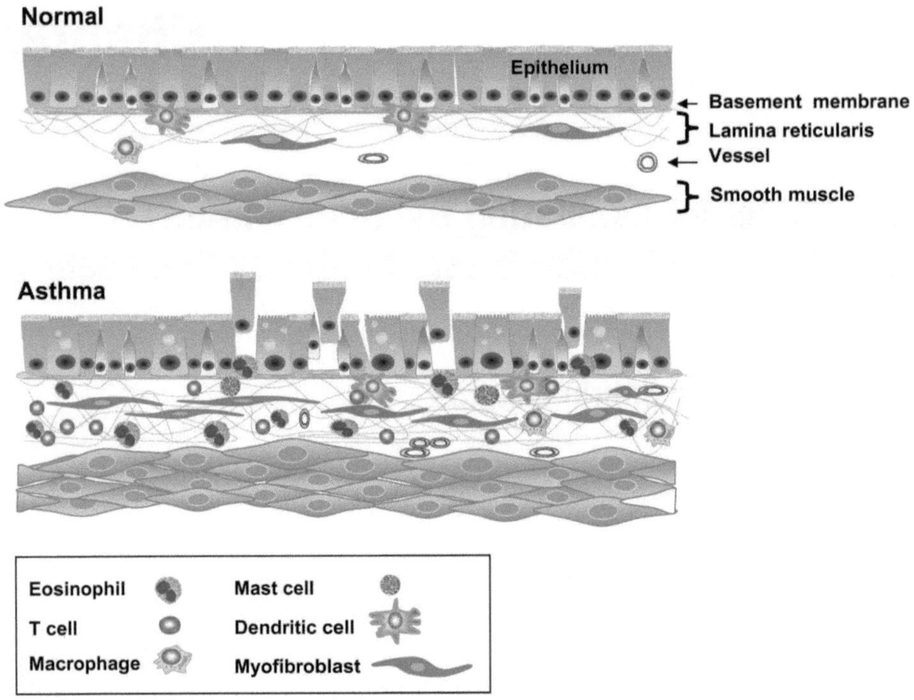

Fig. 1 Schematic illustration of the main inflammatory and structural changes that can be observed in the bronchial mucosa of patients with allergic asthma. Features of airway remodeling include hyperplasia and hypertrophia of the goblet cells, subepithelial fibrosis with thickening of the lamina reticularis, increased density of fibroblasts and myofibroblasts in the lamina propria, increased vascularity, and increased smooth muscle mass. Designed by using objects of the ScienceSlides 2005 software (VisiScience Corporation, Chapel Hill, NC, USA)

forms of asthma where the inflammatory infiltrate is predominantly composed of T helper type 2 (Th2) cells and eosinophils [5, 6] and reflects an increased deposition of collagen types I (COL1), III (COL3), and V (COL5), fibronectin, hyaluronan, various proteoglycans, and tenascin-C [7–11]. These changes in the composition of the lamina reticularis are collectively termed "subepithelial fibrosis" and are thought to be caused by the abnormal accumulation of fibroblasts and myofibroblasts in the lamina propria of the asthmatic bronchial mucosa [12, 13]. Like smooth muscle cells, bronchial myofibroblasts express the contractile protein α-smooth muscle actin (α-SMA) [12, 13]. Subepithelial fibrosis and the expansion of the population of contractile elements resulting from myofibroblast accumulation and increased smooth muscle mass in asthma may contribute to generate persistent airway narrowing by stiffening and contracting the bronchial wall [2, 3].

In allergic asthmatics, every exposure to the clinically relevant allergen can induce a further increase in the accumulation of fibroblasts and myofibroblasts in the lamina propria of their bronchial mucosa and further deposition of collagenous proteins in the subepithelial zone [14–16]. These features of ongoing airway remodeling persist after the resolution of the acute inflammatory response elicited by allergen inhalation [15]. In 2003, we provided the first evidence that a substantial proportion of the fibroblasts and myofibroblasts emerging in asthmatic airways between 4 and 24 h following allergen exposure have the phenotypic characteristics of fibrocytes [17]. The fibrocytes are circulating $CD45^{+}CD34^{+}COL1^{+}$ mesenchymal progenitor cells that constitutively produce extracellular matrix components relevant to asthma, in addition to COL1, and differentiate into myofibroblast-like cells upon stimulation with various growth factors and cytokines [18–21]. These cells also constitutively express CD11b, CD13, the class II major histocompatibility complex HLA-DR, the co-stimulatory molecules CD80 and CD86, the C-C motif chemokine receptors (CCRs) for the C-C motif chemokine ligand (CCL)5 (CCR3 and CCR5), CCL11 (CCR3 and CCR5), CCL24 (CCR3), and the C-X-C motif chemokine receptor (CXCR) for the C-X-C motif chemokine ligand (CXCL)12 (CXCR4) [18, 20]. In normal individuals, the frequency of circulating fibrocytes [22–25] and the density of fibrocytes in the bronchial mucosa [22, 26] are very low, although circulating cells can be isolated in long-term cultures of peripheral blood mononuclear cells under conditions that selectively favor their survival and proliferation [18–21]. Further studies on the role of fibrocytes in asthma, following our initial observations [17], have demonstrated an increased frequency of circulating fibrocytes in patients with allergen-exacerbated asthma [22, 23] and in those with persistently severe, treatment-refractory disease [24, 25]. In persistent asthma, fibrocyte infiltration of the lamina propria correlates with disease severity [24] and extent of subepithelial fibrosis [26]. Fibrocyte infiltration also involves the bronchial smooth muscle bundle [24], and most of the $CD34^{+}COL1^{+}$ cells detected in the bronchial wall of the asthmatic individuals express α-SMA and have an elongated, fibroblast-like shape [17, 24, 26].

The asthmatic bronchial epithelium and the bronchial smooth muscle produce chemokines and growth factors capable of inducing the recruitment of circulating fibrocytes and their local proliferation or differentiation into myofibroblast-like cells [17, 22–24, 27, 28] (Fig. 2). Th2 lymphocytes and eosinophils also release cytokines and growth factors that are known to promote the contractility and profibrotic function of fibrocytes [17, 20, 22], such as interleukin (IL)-4, IL-13, and transforming growth factor-β (TGF-β) (Fig. 2).

In order to evaluate the contribution of fibrocytes and fibrocyte-derived myofibroblast-like cells to airway remodeling in allergic asthma, we developed a murine model of human disease where animals were systemically sensitized to the antigen ovalbumin (OVA) and then subjected to repeat inhalation challenges with controlled levels of aerosolized OVA every week for up to 8 weeks. Following

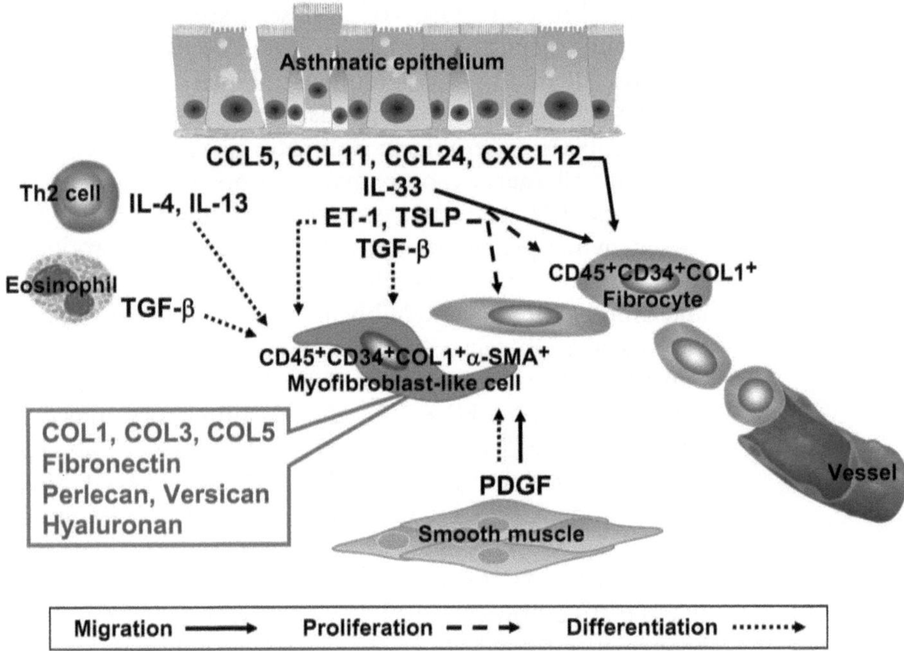

Fig. 2 Schematic illustrations of the factors that may induce the recruitment of circulating fibrocytes to the bronchial mucosa of asthmatic patients and promote their local proliferation and differentiation into myofibroblast-like cells. α-*SMA* α-smooth muscle actin, *CCL* C-C motif chemokine ligand, *COL1* type I collagen, *COL3* type III collagen, *COL5* type V collagen, *CXCL* C-X-C motif chemokine ligand, *ET-1* endothelin-1, *PDGF* platelet-derived growth factor, *TGF*-β transforming growth factor-β, *TSLP* thymic stromal lymphopoietin. Designed by using objects of the ScienceSlides 2005 software (VisiScience Corporation, Chapel Hill, NC, USA)

repeated exposures to the antigen for more than 4 weeks, the airway wall of these mice demonstrated many of the histopathologic abnormalities associated with the human condition. These abnormalities included sustained infiltration of the lamina propria and epithelium with eosinophils, the appearance of fibrocytes and myofibroblast-like cells below the epithelium, and a progressive thickening of the subepithelial zone, which reflected increased deposition of fibronectin and collagens [17] (Figs. 3 and 4). By tracking labeled circulating fibrocytes to the bronchial wall after an inhalation challenge with OVA at 6 weeks of repeated exposures, we provided direct evidence that these cells were recruited to areas of ongoing subepithelial fibrosis [17]. The recruited fibrocytes produced higher levels of intracellular COL1 than circulating fibrocytes and expressed α-SMA within 24 h following their migration at the tissue site [17]. We describe below the protocol for the specific evaluation of fibrocytes and myofibroblasts in this model of chronic allergic asthma. Various studies from other groups have recently confirmed the development and persistence of features of airway remodeling relevant to asthma in sensitized mice that are subjected to repeat allergen

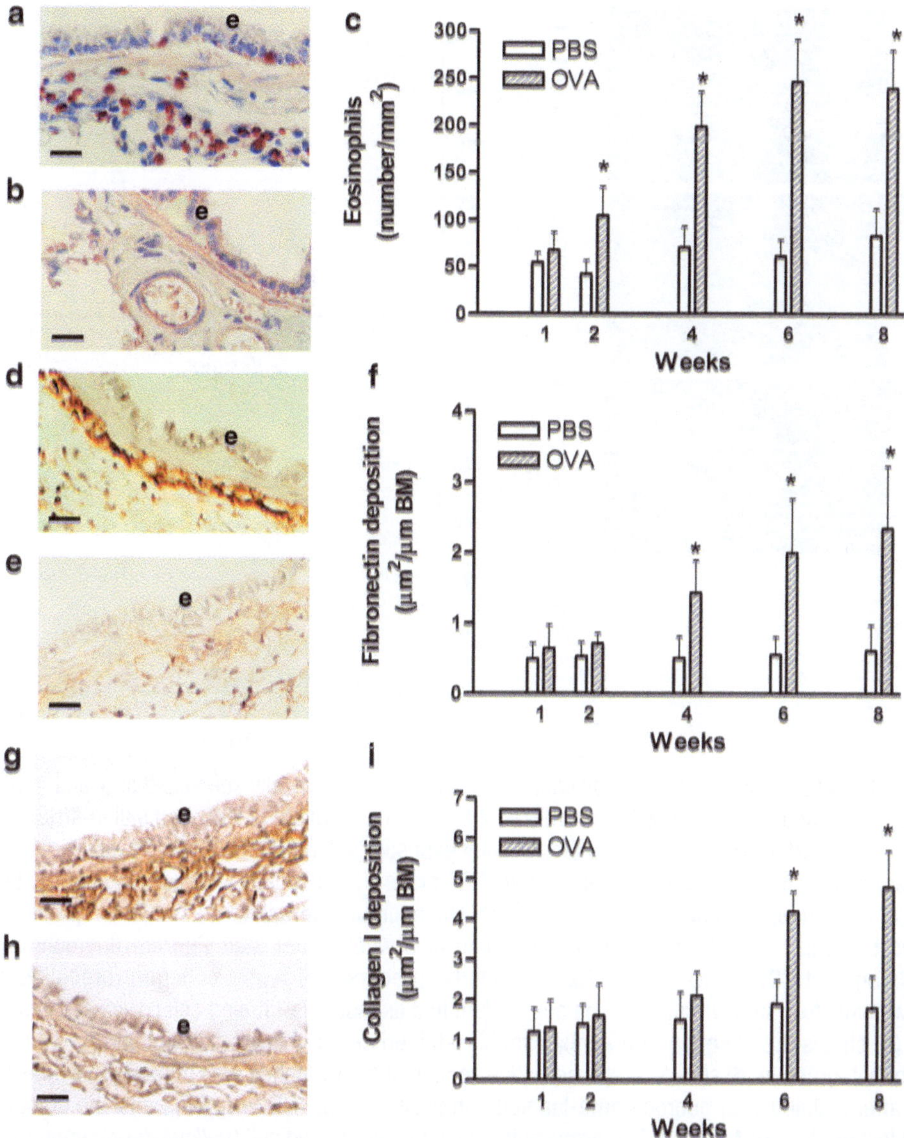

Fig. 3 Airway eosinophilia (**a–c**), and progressive increase in the deposition of fibronectin (**d–f**) and collagen type I (**g–i**) in the bronchial wall of BALB/c mice systemically sensitized to ovalbumin (OVA) and subjected to repeated challenges with aerosolized 2.5 % OVA in phosphate-buffered saline (PBS) three times a week over a period of 8 weeks, using a whole-body exposure system. Control mice systemically sensitized to OVA were subjected to repeated challenges with PBS alone. The response was assessed at the time-points indicated in (**c**), (**f**), and (**i**), 24 h after the last challenge. The microphotographs in (**a**) and (**b**), respectively, show the infiltration with eosinophils (*red* cells) of the lamina propria and epithelium of an OVA-exposed mouse at 2 weeks and the absence of a similar infiltration in the bronchial wall of a control mouse. The microphotographs in (**d**) and (**g**), respectively, show thickening of the subepithelial zone with increased deposition of fibronectin and type I collagen (*brown* stain) in the bronchial wall of OVA-exposed mice at 6 weeks. Less marked changes were observed in the bronchial wall of OVA-exposed mice at 2 (**e**) or 4 (**h**) weeks. Quantitative results are reported in (**c**), (**f**), and (**i**) and the data are expressed as the means and standard error. Significant differences between groups of mice are indicated by an *asterisk*. *BM* basement membrane, *e* epithelium. Scale bar = 50 µm. Reproduced with permission from ref. 17. Copyright 2003. The American Association of Immunologists, Inc

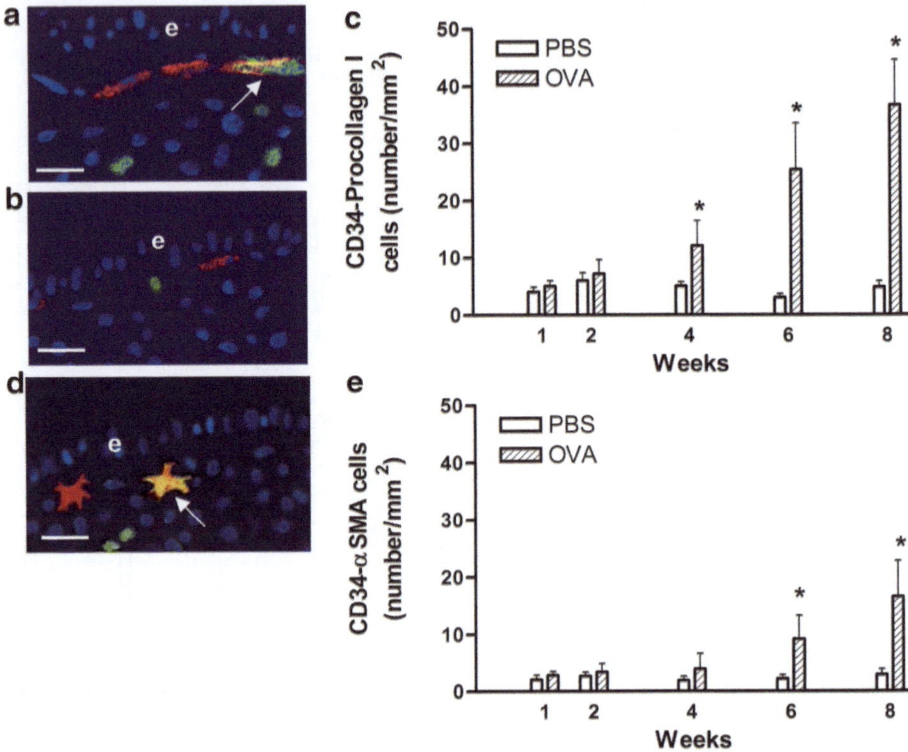

Fig. 4 Detection of fibrocytes in the airway wall of BALB/c mice systemically sensitized to ovalbumin (OVA) and subjected to repeated challenges with aerosolized 2.5 % OVA in phosphate-buffered saline (PBS) three times a week over a period of 8 weeks, using a whole-body exposure system. Control mice systemically sensitized to OVA were subjected to repeated challenges with PBS alone. The response was assessed at the time-points indicated in (**c**), and (**e**), 24 h after the last challenge. The microphotograph in (**a**) shows a representative section of the bronchial wall of an OVA-exposed mouse at 6 weeks after staining with fluorochrome-labeled antibodies against CD34 (*green*) and the intracellular precursor of type I collagen (procollagen I) (*red*). The *arrow* points to a fibrocyte that can be easily identified as a double-labeled cell (*yellow*). The microphotograph in (**b**) shows the absence of a similar double-stained cell in the bronchial wall of a control mouse. The microphotograph in (**d**) shows a representative section of the bronchial wall of an OVA-exposed mouse at 6 weeks after staining with fluorochrome-labeled antibodies against CD34 (*green*) and the smooth muscle/myofibroblast marker α-SMA (*red*). The *arrow* points to a double-labeled cell (*yellow*), representing a fibrocyte-derived myofibroblast. In all sections, nuclei were counterstained blue with DAPI. Quantitative results are reported in (**c**) and (**e**) and the data are expressed as the means and standard error. Significant differences between groups of mice are indicated with an *asterisk*. *e* epithelium. Scale bar = 50 μm. Reproduced with permission from ref. 17. Copyright 2003. The American Association of Immunologists, Inc

challenges every week for at least 5 weeks, irrespective of the method used for delivering the allergen to the airways [29–33]. Two of these studies [29, 30] evaluated the presence of myofibroblasts and myofibroblast-like cells in the bronchial wall and demonstrated an allergen-induced accumulation of COL1$^+$α-SMA$^+$ myofibroblasts

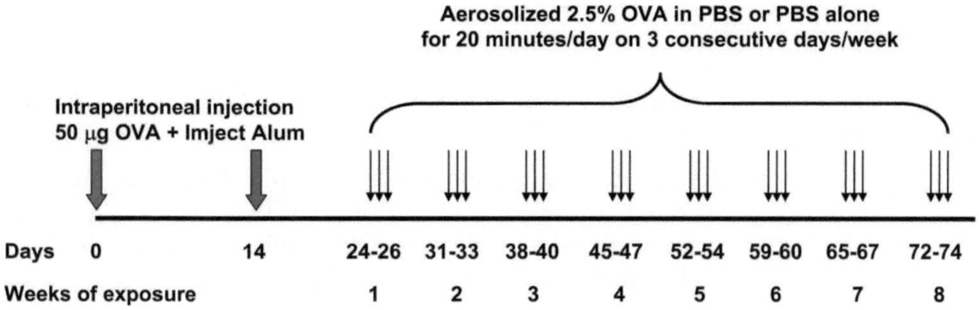

Aerosolized 2.5% OVA in PBS or PBS alone
for 20 minutes/day on 3 consecutive days/week

Intraperitoneal injection
50 μg OVA + Imject Alum

Days 0 14 24-26 31-33 38-40 45-47 52-54 59-60 65-67 72-74

Weeks of exposure 1 2 3 4 5 6 7 8

Fig. 5 Schematic illustration of the experimental procedures and timelines for systemic sensitization to ovalbumin (OVA) and repeated challenges with aerosolized 2.5 % OVA in phosphate-buffered saline (PBS) or PBS alone as control

and α-SMA⁺ myofibrocytes in concomitance with the development of subepithelial fibrotic changes. Interestingly, the administration of a low-molecular-weight antagonist of CCR3, a receptor expressed by eosinophils [34] and fibrocytes [20, 28], not only reduced the eosinophilic inflammation but also prevented the increased accumulation of myofibrocytes beneath the epithelium and the excessive subepithelial deposition of collagens that were elicited by repeated challenge with aerosolized OVA for at least 8 weeks [30].

1.2 Overview of the Experimental Procedures and Timelines

Pathogen-free, 6–8-week-old female or male BALB/c mice should be employed in all experiments because these mice develop a good Th2-biased immunological response and produce higher levels of allergen-specific IgE antibodies than other strains upon repeated exposure to OVA following systemic sensitization to this antigen [35–37]. Sensitization to OVA is achieved by repeat intraperitoneal administrations of the antigen absorbed to an adjuvant, such as alum, which boosts the immune response and promotes the production of Th2-derived cytokines. Two intraperitoneal injections of 50 μg OVA with sterile alum solution are performed at a distance of 14 days (Fig. 5). Starting on day 24, sensitized mice are then challenged with an aerosolized solution of 2.5 % OVA in phosphate-buffered saline (PBS) in a whole-body exposure chamber for 20 min/day on three consecutive days of each week over a period of 8 weeks (Fig. 5). Control mice are challenged with an aerosolized solution of PBS alone in the same way and for the same period of time (Fig. 5). Assessment of the response to repeat inhalation challenges with aerosolized OVA or PBS is conducted every week for the first 2 weeks and every 2 weeks thereafter, 24 h following the end of the last OVA or PBS challenge. Different subgroups of mice subjected to the same experimental procedure are sacrificed at each time point (e.g., on days 27, 34, 48, 61, and 75).

2 Materials

2.1 Reagents for Systemic Sensitization

1. Grade V, ≥98 % pure chicken egg OVA (Sigma-Aldrich, St. Louis, MO, USA).
2. 10× stock solution of PBS, 1 l, pH 7.4 ± 0.05: Add 80 g of NaCl, 2 g of KCl, 11.5 g of $Na_2HPO_4 \cdot 7H_2O$, 2 g of KH_2PO_4 to a graduated cylinder. Add distilled water to the 1-l mark. Dilute the stock solution in distilled water.
3. Imject Alum (Thermo Fisher Scientific/Pierce Biotechnology, Rockford, IL, USA).
4. 15-ml conical tubes.
5. 0.45 μm filters.
6. Sterile 100-ml graduated flask.
7. Sterile stir bar.
8. Stir plate.
9. Sterile gloves.
10. 1-ml syringe.

2.2 Equipment for Whole-Body Exposure

1. A whole-body exposure system for mice, equipped with components (**items 2–14**; Fig. 6) from ToxoRes Technologies (Dublin, Ireland) if not otherwise specified (*see* **Notes 1** and **2**).

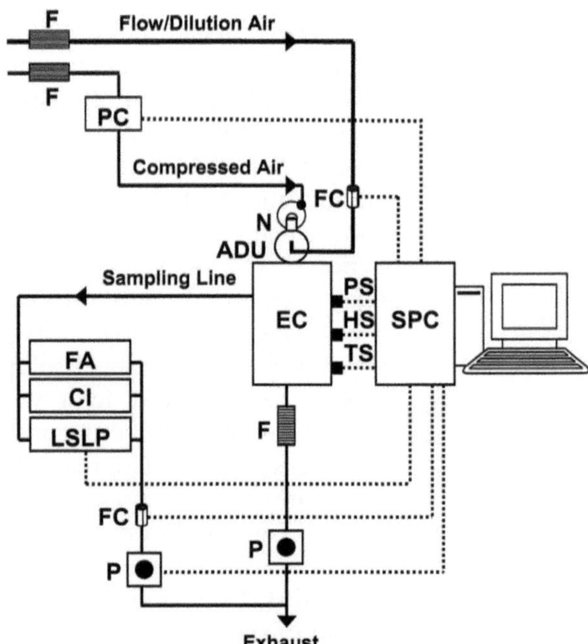

Fig. 6 Overview of the whole-body exposure system. *ADU* aerosol dilution unit, *CI* cascade impactor, *EC* exposure chamber, *F* filter, *FA* filter analyzer, *FC* flow control, *HS* humidity sensor, *LSLP* light-scattering laser photometer, *N* nebulizer, *P* pump, *PC* pressure control, *PS* pressure sensor, *SPC* signal-processing cabinet, *TS* temperature sensor

2. Stainless steel 0.3 m^3 whole-body exposure chamber with front safety glass for animal observation, a front air inlet, a side outlet for aerosol sampling, and back exhaust.
3. Wire flow-through cage with stainless steel cage support and body restraint.
4. Two lines for air supply to the exposure chamber and to the nebulizer with in-line flow controllers.
5. Line for exhaust air.
6. High-efficiency particulate air (HEPA) filters.
7. Air compressor with compressor control.
8. 3-jet Collison nebulizer (BGI, Waltham, MA, USA).
9. Aerosol diluting unit.
10. Sensors for recording the temperature and humidity in the exposure chamber.
11. Two high-volume pumps (Emerson, St. Louis, MO, USA).
12. Line for aerosol sampling.
13. Filter analyzer, multi-jet cascade impactor, and light-scattering laser photometer (TSE Systems, Bad Homburg, Germany) with the associated software for real-time and off-line measurement of aerosol mass concentration, aerosol particle size, and particle size distribution.
14. Exposure control cabinet for signal processing with real-time analysis of airflow, back-pressure, and airflow supply to the nebulizer; pressure, humidity, and temperature in the exposure chamber; aerosol mass concentration; and particle size distribution.

2.3 Reagents for Whole-Body Exposure

1. Grade V, ≥98 % pure chicken egg OVA (Sigma-Aldrich).
2. 1× PBS.
3. Sterile 50-ml conical tubes and flasks.
4. 0.45 μm filters.

2.4 Materials for Lung Tissue Processing

1. Anesthetic for intraperitoneal injection (e.g., 60 mg/kg of sodium pentobarbital or a combination of 10 mg/ml of ketamine and 1 mg/ml of xylazine).
2. 1-ml syringe.
3. Gloves, goggles, and protective clothing.
4. Blunt-ended needles.
5. Infusion apparatus.
6. 4 % paraformaldehyde solution: Add 8 g of reagent-grade, crystalline paraformaldehyde (Sigma-Aldrich) to 100 ml of tap water. Heat to 60 °C in a fume hood. Add a few drops of 1 N NaOH to help dissolve. When the solid has completely dissolved, let the solution cool to room temperature. Add 100 ml of 2× PBS

and adjust the pH to 7.4 with 1 N NaOH. This solution should be prepared fresh on the same day as the fixation.

7. 30 % sucrose in PBS for cryoprotection: Add 30 g of sucrose to a 500-ml graduated cylinder. Add 1× PBS to the 100 ml mark. Stir vigorously with a stir bar and store the solutions in a refrigerator.
8. Tissue-Tek optimal-cut-temperature (OCT) embedding compound (Miles Laboratories, Naperville, IL, USA).
9. Beakers.
10. Insulated thermos.
11. Long forceps.
12. Liquid nitrogen, in an appropriate storage tank (−196 °C).
13. Mounting blocks.
14. Freezer (−70 °C).
15. Zip-lock bags.
16. Isopentane.

2.5 Materials for Preparation of Frozen Tissue Sections

1. Gloves, goggles, and protective clothing.
2. Cryostat.
3. Clean glass slides.
4. 0.1 % poly-L-lysine solution (Sigma-Aldrich).
5. Staining racks and dishes.
6. Oven.
7. Freezer (−70 °C).

2.6 Materials for Immunohistochemical Analysis

1. Gloves, goggles, and protective clothing.
2. Staining racks and dishes.
3. Coplin jars.
4. Pipettes.
5. Humid chamber for incubations.
6. PBS.
7. Normal goat serum (Dako, Carpinteria, CA, USA) diluted 1:10 and 1:100 in PBS.
8. BLOXALL Blocking Solution (Vector Laboratories, Burlingame, CA, USA).
9. Fc Receptor Blocker (Innovex Biosciences, Richmond, CA, USA).
10. Rabbit antibody (IgG) against mouse COL1 (Merck Millipore, Darmstadt, Germany).
11. Rabbit antibody (IgG) against mouse fibronectin (Merck Millipore).

12. Rabbit antibody (IgG) against mouse collagen III (Abcam, Cambridge, United Kingdom).
13. VECTASTAIN Elite ABC Kit for rabbit IgG (Vector Laboratories).
14. Absolute alcohol, 95 % ethanol, and xylene.
15. VectaMount (Vector Laboratories).
16. Irrelevant antibodies raised in the same species as the primary antibodies listed above.
17. Glass coverslips.
18. Light microscope and image analysis system.

2.7 Materials for Immunofluorescence Analysis

1. Gloves, goggles, and protective clothing.
2. Staining racks and dishes.
3. Coplin jars.
4. Pipettes.
5. Humid chamber for incubations.
6. Dulbecco's phosphate-buffered saline (DPBS) without calcium and magnesium.
7. Fc Receptor Blocker (Innovex Biosciences, Richmond, CA, USA).
8. Normal donkey serum diluted 1:10 and 1:100 in PBS.
9. 0.1 % saponin (Sigma-Aldrich).
10. Fluorescein isothiocyanate (FITC)-conjugated anti-mouse CD34 monoclonal antibody (Cederlane, Burlington, ON, Canada).
11. Cyanine(Cy)3-conjugated antibody against α-SMA, clone 1A4 (Sigma-Aldrich).
12. Goat antibody (IgG) against mouse intracellular COL1 precursor, recognizing the N-terminus of procollagen I, α2 chain (Santa Cruz Biotechnology, Santa Cruz, CA, USA).
13. Rhodamine Red-X-AffiniPure or Cy3-AffiniPure and FITC-AffiniPure F(ab′)2 fragment donkey anti-goat IgG (Jackson ImmunoResearch, West Grove, PA, USA).
14. Irrelevant antibodies raised in the same species as the primary antibodies listed above.
15. ProLong Gold Antifade Reagent with DAPI (Life Technologies/Invitrogen, Paisley, United Kingdom).
16. Glass coverslips.
17. Wide-field fluorescence microscope connected to a laser scanning confocal system with appropriate filters.

2.8 Materials for Determination of Serum OVA-Specific IgE and IgG Levels

1. Serum-separator tubes.
2. Centrifuge.
3. Adjustable pipettes and repeat pipettor.
4. Distilled or deionized water.
5. Mouse total IgE assay kit (Chondrex, Redmond, WA, USA).
6. Mouse serum anti-OVA IgE antibody assay kit (Chondrex).
7. Anti-Ovalbumin IgG_1 (mouse) EIA kit (Cayman Chemical Company, Ann Arbor, MI, USA).
8. Plate reader capable of measuring absorbance at 450 nm, possibly using a dual beam at 450/630 nm.

3 Methods

3.1 Animal Housing and Care

1. Mice should be housed in conventional autoclaved cages, in a pathogen-free and air-conditioned room at 21–23 °C, with relative humidity of 55–65 %, and subjected to a 12-h light/dark cycle.
2. Provide free access to irradiated OVA-free food and acidified water, except when the mice are in the exposure chamber.
3. Permit acclimatization to the exposure chamber for at least 1 h/day during the week preceding the actual exposure (*see* **Note 3**).

3.2 Systemic Sensitization

1. Pour 2.5 mg of OVA into a 15-ml conical tube.
2. Add 5 ml of 1× PBS. The OVA concentration will be 0.5 μg/μl.
3. Vortex the tube three to four times.
4. Pass the solution through a 0.45 μm filter into a new 15-ml conical tube (*see* **Note 4**).
5. Place the 100-ml flask on the stir plate and start the stir bar.
6. Shake the capped bottle of Imject Alum well.
7. Pour the OVA solution into the flask, take 5 ml of Imject Alum out of the bottle, and add the solution dropwise to mix the OVA and Alum in a 1:1 ratio (vol:vol).
8. Continue stirring for at least 30 min after the addition of the entire 5 ml of Imject Alum.
9. Take the mixture into a 1-ml syringe and inject 0.2 ml containing 50 μg of OVA plus Imject Alum into the mouse peritoneal cavity (*see* **Notes 5** and **6**).

3.3 Whole-Body Exposure

1. Prepare a PBS solution containing 2.5 % OVA (*see* **Note 7**).
2. Pass 100 ml of this solution and 100 ml of PBS alone through a 0.45 μm filter into separate sterile flasks.

3. Depending on whether the experiment involves mouse exposure to OVA or PBS alone, pour the appropriate solution into the nebulizer (*see* **Note 8**).
4. Place the selected mouse in the exposure cage and insert the cage into the chamber. The nose of the mouse must be oriented toward the front air/aerosol inlet of the chamber and the animal must be fixed in that position with the body restraint.
5. Draw filtered aerosol diluting air through the chamber at a flow rate of 180 l/min with the mouse inside the chamber (*see* **Notes 9**).
6. Turn on the nebulizer by delivering compressed air at a pressure of 179 kPa and a flow rate of 10 l/min and allow the aerosol to equilibrate in the chamber for 5 min.
7. Check the aerosol concentration and reduce or increase the air supply to the nebulizer via the pressure control to obtain and maintain an aerosol concentration of 10–20 mg/m^3 (*see* **Note 10**), taking into account that the 3-jet Collison nebulizer requires a minimum airflow of 6 l/min.
8. Keep the temperature and relative humidity inside the exposure chamber at 21–23 °C and 40–50 %, respectively (*see* **Note 11**).
9. Expose the mice to controlled aerosol concentrations for 20 min.
10. Turn off the nebulizer and let fresh diluting air run into the chamber to flush the system for 5 min.
11. Stop the air supply and remove the animals from the chamber.

3.4 Lung Tissue Processing

1. Deeply anesthetize the animal via intraperitoneal injection of the anesthetic.
2. Arrange the animal on the dissection tray and secure the limbs.
3. Wash fur with 70 % alcohol.
4. Make a midline incision through the skin to expose the abdomen, thorax, and neck.
5. Expose the posterior abdominal aorta, and kill the animal by exsanguinations.
6. Expose the trachea and remove the ventral thoracic wall.
7. Place two ligatures around the trachea, below the larynx.
8. Make a straight narrow incision in the inter-cartilaginous space between the larynx and the first cartilaginous tracheal ring.
9. Cannulate the trachea with a small blunt-ended needle connected to the tube of the infusion apparatus and secure with the bottom ligature.
10. Infuse the lung with 4 % paraformaldehyde solution for 1 min at 25 cm fluid height. Infusion height is measured as the distance

between the lungs and the meniscus of the fixative in the reservoir. The volume of fixative used to fill the adult mouse lung will be 1–1.4 cm^3.

11. Withdraw the cannula and tie off the trachea with the upper ligature. Cut the trachea below the upper ligature.
12. Dissect the lungs out of the thorax and immerse the trachea and the lungs in cold fixative (20× the volume of the tissue) for 24 h.
13. Isolate the left lung and perform a traverse section (*see* **Note 12**).
14. Rinse the trachea and lower half of the sectioned left lung in three changes of cold PBS (20× the volume of the tissue) for 10 min each.
15. Transfer to a cold solution of 30 % sucrose in PBS (20× the volume of the tissue) for 24–72 h.
16. Transfer to a 2:1 mixture of 30 % sucrose solution and OCT embedding compound for an additional 24 h.
17. Wear goggles and gloves.
18. Blot off excess liquid and quickly immerse the tissue in OCT embedding compound in mounting blocks using long forceps.
19. Insert a beaker into an insulated thermos. Place melting isopentane in the beaker and carefully fill the space surrounding the beaker with liquid nitrogen, always wearing goggles and gloves. The temperature of the isopentane will drop to −140 °C in about 2 min.
20. Plunge the mounting block with the tissue specimens in isopentane for 10 s to freeze the tissue, using the long forceps (*see* **Note 13**).
21. Mark specimen orientation (longitudinal orientation for the trachea) on each block.
22. Store in zip-lock bags at −70 °C.

3.5 Preparation of Frozen Tissue Sections

1. Place clean glass slides in a staining rack.
2. Immerse the slides for 30 min in a large staining dish containing 1:10 dilution of 0.1 % poly-L-lysine solution in deionized water.
3. Remove the slides and oven dry for 1 h at 60 °C.
4. Fasten the mounting block to the block holder in the cryostat.
5. Align the knife to touch the surface of the tissue.
6. Set the section thickness to 4 μm.
7. Start cutting slowly until the section clings to the knife.
8. Bind the section to one of the poly-L-lysine-coated slides.
9. Allow the section to air-dry for 2–3 h at room temperature.

10. Repeat the steps above to prepare each additional section slide from the same frozen tissue sample and other samples.
11. Store the slides at −70 °C in slide boxes.

3.6 Immunohistochemical Analysis

1. Transfer the slides to a Coplin jar containing PBS and wash, dipping in and out of the solution, ten times.
2. Transfer the slides to another Coplin jar containing PBS for 5 min.
3. Quench endogenous peroxidase activity by incubating the slides in BLOXALL Blocking Solution for 10 min.
4. Wash slides in PBS for 5 min.
5. Cover sections with 3–6 drops of Fc Receptor Blocker to block the nonspecific binding of each primary antibody (rabbit anti-mouse IgG) to the Fc receptor present on the surface of several types of inflammatory cells and tissue macrophages. Incubate for 30 min at room temperature in the humidified chamber.
6. Rinse in PBS.
7. Cover sections with a solution containing 10 % normal goat serum in PBS and incubate for 15 min at room temperature in the humidified chamber.
8. Blot off excess serum from sections by placing one margin of the slightly angled slide on an absorbent paper towel.
9. Incubate replicate sections with each primary antibody or with the negative control antibody, all rabbit anti-mouse IgGs diluted 1:100–1:800 in PBS containing 1 % normal goat serum, for 30 min at room temperature (or overnight at 4 °C) in the humidified chamber (*see* **Note 14**).
10. Wash the slides two times in PBS containing 1 % normal goat serum for 5 min.
11. Use the VECTASTAIN Elite ABC Kit for rabbit IgG to apply the secondary anti-rabbit antibody and reveal antibody-binding sites by the immunoperoxidase procedure according to the manufacturer's instructions. Extracellular deposits of fibronectin, COL1, and COL3 beneath the bronchial epithelium and in the peribronchial zone will stain brown (Fig. 19.3d, e, g, h).
12. Counterstain sections in hematoxylin, if desired.
13. Dehydrate the slides in three changes of 95 % alcohol and two changes of absolute alcohol, and clear in two changes of xylene.
14. Mount with VectaMount and apply a coverslip.
15. Analyze each slide under a light microscope, using an image analysis system according to the manufacturer's instructions (*see* **Note 15**).

3.7 Immunofluorescence Analysis

1. Transfer the slides to a Coplin jar containing DPBS and wash, dipping in and out of the solution, ten times.
2. Transfer slides to another Coplin jar containing DPBS for 5 min.
3. Cover the sections with 3–6 drops of Fc Receptor Blocker. Incubate for 30 min at room temperature in the humidified chamber.
4. Rinse in DPBS.
5. Cover the sections with a solution containing 10 % normal donkey serum in DPBS and incubate for 15 min at room temperature in the humidified chamber.
6. Blot off excess serum from sections placing one margin of the slightly angled slide on an absorbent paper towel.
7. Incubate replicate sections with the FITC-conjugated antibody against α-SMA or the FITC-conjugated isotype-matched control, all diluted 1:100–1:800 in DPBS containing 1 % normal donkey serum, for 30 min at room temperature (or overnight at 4 °C) in the dark, in the humidified chamber (*see* **Note 14**).
8. Wash five times with DPBS containing 1 % normal donkey serum.
9. Cover the slides with a DPBS solution containing 1 % normal donkey serum and 0.1 % saponin for 10 min at room temperature in the dark. Saponin is used to permeabilize the cells and allow the binding of the primary antibodies against procollagen I and α-SMA to their intracellular target antigens.
10. Blot off excess solution.
11. Incubate replicate slides with the unlabeled goat antibody against procollagen I, Cy3-conjuaged antibody against α-SMA, or the corresponding control antibodies for 30 min at room temperature in the dark. All antibodies should be diluted in DPBS solution containing 1 % normal donkey serum and 0.1 % saponin.
12. Wash five times in DPBS solution containing 1 % normal donkey serum and 0.1 % saponin in the dark.
13. Incubate the slides previously incubated with either the unlabeled antibody against intracellular procollagen I or the unlabeled control antibody with the Rhodamine Red-X-AffiniPure F(ab′)2 fragment donkey anti-goat IgG for 30 min at room temperature in the dark.
14. Wash five times in DPBS.
15. Use ProLong Gold Antifade Reagent with DAPI to counterstain the cell nuclei and mount the slides.
16. Apply the glass coverslips.

17. Analyze the sections using a wide-field fluorescence microscope connected to a laser scanning confocal system with appropriate filters for the employed fluorochromes (*see* **Notes 15** and **16**).

3.8 Determination of Serum OVA-Specific IgE and IgG Levels

1. Collect samples of the blood in serum separator tubes at the time the mice are sacrificed.
2. Allow samples to clot for 30 min at room temperature.
3. Centrifuge for 10 min at 1,000 × *g*.
4. Decant the serum and store samples at −70 °C.
5. Measure the serum concentrations of total IgE and OVA-specific IgE and IgG_1 using the commercially available kits according to the manufacturers' instructions (*see* **Note 17**).

4 Notes

1. Similar customized and preassembled whole-body exposure systems are currently provided by TSE Systems (European/Asian Headquarters: Bad Homburg, Germany; North America Headquarters: Chesterfield, MO, USA). The preassembled 12-port Small Animal Exposure System from InTox (Moriarty, NM, USA) allows the concomitant exposure to aerosols of at least six mice, placed into distinct whole-body mouse tubes. This system is similarly equipped with a jet nebulizer that can generate aerosol particles in the 1–3 μm range at an appropriate airflow rate and back-pressure. It may represent a valid alternative if the sampling line is connected to instruments for the real-time monitoring of aerosol concentrations (not currently provided by the manufacturer), such as the OptoPan or the SpectroPan from TSE and the DustTrack DRX from TSI (Shoreview, MN, USA). The latter instrument must be calibrated for aerosols made of liquid droplets rather than dust.
2. All instruments should be calibrated, operated, and maintained according to the manufacturers' or suppliers' instructions.
3. Number mice by toe clip and make sure that the toe clip number and the litter number are correct before starting any experimental procedure.
4. The OVA solution should be freshly prepared the day of the injection.
5. Insert the needle into the lower part of abdomen (e.g., near the groin) to avoid injecting the OVA–Alum mixture into the intestines.
6. Stop insertion as soon as you feel a sudden reduction in the resistance, indicating that the needle has penetrated through the abdominal wall.

7. The OVA solution should be freshly prepared the day of each whole-body exposure.
8. The liquid reservoir of the nebulizer can be refilled with fresh solutions of OVA or PBS alone while the experiment is running.
9. The parameters for delivering diluting air to the exposure chamber and for aerosol generation can vary depending on the whole-body exposure system used for the experiments. A working protocol should be established and validated in preliminary experiments.
10. Repeated exposures to aerosol concentrations lower than 10 mg/m^3 may cause sustained but slight airway remodeling changes, which almost exclusively consist of subepithelial fibrosis and epithelium hypertrophy and are predominantly localized to the trachea [38]. In our hands, repeated exposures to aerosol concentrations up to 100 mg/m^3 do not cause extensive and nonspecific inflammatory lesions of the parenchyma surrounding the conducting airways. However, measurements of the mass concentration of a given aerosol with instruments obtained from different manufacturers, or with different models of the same instrument, do not provide comparable results. The differences in the recorded values may vary from two- to five-fold. Thus, it is recommended that the initial experiments for the establishment of the working protocol for repeat allergen challenges be started with aerosol concentrations between 50 and 70 mg/m^3. The instrument for real-time monitoring of the aerosol concentrations should be calibrated for use with aerosols made of liquid droplets rather than dust.
11. Under these conditions, the particle sizes of the aerosol generated by the 3-jet Collison nebulizer within the breathing zone of mice will range from 0.5 to 7 μm, which is appropriate for preferential deposition in the bronchi, rather than in the upper airways (nose and trachea) [39–41].
12. Orientate the left lung to obtain a traverse section of the first-generation bronchus and the accompanying artery and vein.
13. The density of fibrocytes and other CD34$^+$ progenitor cells can be greatly underestimated in tissue sections from formalin-fixed and paraffin-embedded tissue because of the difficulties in retrieving the CD34 antigen on the cell surface. The protocol reported here for tissue fixation, cryoprotection, and freezing usually permits an excellent conservation of the tissue architecture.
14. In any immunohistochemical and immunofluorescence analysis, positive control sections should be used to test serial dilutions of each primary and secondary antibody for optimal staining.

Skin tissue and a traverse section of the thoracic aorta can be obtained, in addition to the lungs and trachea, at the time the mice are sacrificed. All tissue samples should be processed in an identical way. Sections of the skin tissue should be used as positive controls for the detection of extracellular matrix components (fibronectin, COL1, and COL3) and cells producing COL1 (fibroblasts and myofibroblasts will stain positively with antibodies against the intracellular COL1 precursor procollagen I). Sections of the thoracic aorta should be used as positive controls for tissue labeling with antibodies against α-SMA because the smooth muscle layer of the vessel will be stained positively.

15. Sections of the airway wall that are associated to adjacent vessels through connective tissue attachments should be excluded. On each section, the region of interest is a 20-μm subepithelial band that includes the extracellular matrix components and contractile elements (myofibroblasts and smooth muscle cells) of the bronchial wall. An appropriate image analysis system can estimate the area covered by the brown stain in different fields along the epithelial basement membrane. The mean area is calculated and expressed as square micrometers per length of basement membrane in micrometer (Fig. 3f, i).

16. $CD34^+$ cells will stain green. Cells producing the intracellular precursor of COL1 (procollagen I) will stain red. The cell nuclei will stain blue. Cells expressing α-SMA will also stain red. Cells double stained for CD34 and procollagen I or CD34 and α-SMA are fibrocytes and fibrocyte-derived myofibroblast-like cells, respectively, and will stain yellow (Fig. 4a, b, d). The density of fibrocytes and fibrocyte-derived myofibroblast-like cells present in the subepithelial zone along the epithelial basement membrane can be expressed as the number of cells per square millimeters of subepithelial bronchial mucosa (Fig. 4d, g). By double staining replicate sections with Cy3-conjugated antibody against α-SMA and unlabeled goat antibody against procollagen I, using the FITC-AffiniPure F(ab′)2 fragment donkey anti-goat IgG as secondary antibody, it is also possible to identify all myofibroblasts and myofibroblast-like cells [29].

17. To confirm the effectiveness of the systemic sensitization to OVA, anti-OVA antibody levels are usually measured in the serum or in the plasma. Both OVA-specific IgE and IgG_1 can now be assayed with commercially available kits. In general, elevated levels of anti-OVA IgE are indicative of successful sensitization to the antigen. The measurement of anti-OVA IgG_1 is commonly used for assessing the magnitude of the Th2-biased immune response [42, 43].

References

1. National Asthma Education Prevention Program (2007) Expert Panel Report 3 (EPR-3): guidelines for the diagnosis and management of asthma – summary report 2007. J Allergy Clin Immunol 120(5 Suppl):S94–S138
2. Pascual RM, Peters SP (2009) The irreversible component of persistent asthma. J Allergy Clin Immunol 124:883–890
3. Durrani SR, Viswanathan RK, Busse WW (2011) What effect does asthma treatment have on airway remodeling? Current perspectives. J Allergy Clin Immunol 128:439–448
4. Jeffery PK (2004) Remodeling and inflammation of bronchi in asthma and chronic obstructive pulmonary disease. Proc Am Thorac Soc 1:176–183
5. Wenzel SE, Schwartz LB, Langmack EL, Halliday JL, Trudeau JB, Gibbs RL, Chu HW (1999) Evidence that severe asthma can be divided pathologically into two inflammatory subtypes with distinct physiologic and clinical characteristics. Am J Respir Crit Care Med 160:1001–1008
6. Woodruff PG, Modrek B, Choy DF, Jia G, Abbas AR, Ellwanger A, Koth LL, Arron JR, Fahy JV (1995) T-helper type 2-driven inflammation defines major subphenotypes of asthma. Am J Respir Crit Care Med 180:388–395
7. Roberts CR (1995) Is asthma a fibrotic disease? Chest 107:111S–117S
8. Chu HW, Halliday JL, Martin RJ, Leung DY, Szefler SJ, Wenzel SE (1998) Collagen deposition in large airways may not differentiate severe asthma from milder forms of the disease. Am J Respir Crit Care Med 158:1936–1944
9. Wilson JW, Li X (1997) The measurement of reticular basement membrane and submucosal collagen in the asthmatic airway. Clin Exp Allergy 27:363–371
10. Huang J, Olivenstein R, Taha R, Hamid Q, Ludwig M (1999) Enhanced proteoglycan deposition in the airway wall of atopic asthmatics. Am J Respir Crit Care Med 160:725–729
11. Pini L, Hamid Q, Shannon J, Lemelin L, Olivenstein R, Ernst P, Lemièr C, Martin JG, Ludwig MS (2007) Differences in proteoglycans deposition in the airways of moderate and severe asthmatics. Eur Respir J 29:71–77
12. Brewster CE, Howarth PH, Djukanovic R, Wilson J, Hogate ST, Roche WR (1990) Myofibroblasts and subepithelial fibrosis in bronchial asthma. Am J Respir Cell Mol Biol 3:507–511
13. Gabbrielli S, Di Lollo S, Stanflin N, Romagnoli P (1994) Myofibroblasts and elastic and collagen fiber hyperplasia in the bronchial mucosa: a possible basis for the progressive irreversibility of airflow obstruction in asthma. Pathologica 86:157–160
14. Gizycki MJ, Adelroth E, Rogers AV, O'Byrne PM, Jeffery PK (1997) Myofibroblast involvement in the allergen-induced late response in mild atopic asthma. Am J Respir Cell Mol Biol 16:664–673
15. Kariyawasam HH, Aizen M, Barkans J, Robinson DS, Kay AB (2007) Remodeling and airway hyperesponsiveness but not cellular inflammation persist after allergen challenge in asthma. Am J Respir Crit Care Med 175: 896–904
16. Kelly MM, O'Connor TM, Leigh R, Otis J, Gwozd C, Gauvreau GM, Gauldie J, O'Byrne PM (2010) Effects of budesonide and formoterol on allergen-induced airway responses, inflammation, and airway remodeling in asthma. J Allergy Clin Immunol 125:349–356.e13
17. Schmidt M, Sun G, Stacey MA, Mori L, Mattoli S (2003) Identification of circulating fibrocytes as precursors of bronchial myofibroblasts in asthma. J Immunol 171:380–389
18. Bucala R, Spiegel LA, Chesney J, Hogan M, Cerami A (1994) Circulating fibrocytes define a new leukocyte subpopulation that mediates tissue repair. Mol Med 1:71–81
19. Chesney J, Metz C, Stavitsky AB, Baker M, Bucala R (1998) Regulated production of type I collagen and inflammatory cytokines by peripheral blood fibrocytes. J Immunol 160: 419–425
20. Abe R, Donnelly SC, Peng T, Bucala R, Metz CN (2001) Peripheral blood fibrocytes: differentiation pathway and migration to wound sites. J Immunol 166:7556–7562
21. Bianchetti L, Barczyk M, Cardoso J, Schmidt M, Bellini A, Mattoli S (2012) Extracellular matrix remodelling properties of fibrocytes. J Cell Mol Med 16:483–495
22. Bellini A, Marini MA, Bianchetti L, Barczyk M, Schmidt M, Mattoli S (2012) Interleukin (IL)-4, IL-13, and IL-17A differentially affect the profibrotic and proinflammatory functions of fibrocytes from asthmatic patients. Mucosal Immunol 5:140–149
23. Bianchetti L, Marini MA, Isgrò M, Bellini A, Schmidt M, Mattoli S (2012) IL-33 promotes the migration and proliferation of circulating fibrocytes from allergen-exacerbated asthma. Biochem Biophys Res Commun 426: 116–121
24. Saunders R, Siddiqui S, Kaur D, Doe C, Sutcliffe A, Hollins F, Bradding P, Wardlaw A, Brightling CE (2009) Fibrocyte localization to the airway smooth muscle is a feature of asthma. J Allergy Clin Immunol 123:376–384

25. Wang CH, Huang CD, Lin HC, Lee KY, Lin SM, Liu CY, Huang KH, Ko YS, Chung KF, Kuo HP (2008) Increased circulating fibrocytes in asthma with chronic airflow obstruction. Am J Respir Crit Care Med 178:583–591
26. Nihlberg K, Larsen K, Hultgårdh-Nilsson A, Malmström A, Bjermer L, Westergren-Thorsson G (2006) Tissue fibrocytes in patients with mild asthma: a possible link to thickness of reticular basement membrane? Respir Res 7:50
27. Oh MH, Oh SY, Yu J, Myers AC, Leonard WJ, Liu YJ, Zhu Z, Zheng T (2011) IL-13 induces skin fibrosis in atopic dermatitis by thymic stromal lymphopoietin. J Immunol 186:7232–7242
28. Isgrò M, Bianchetti L, Marini MA, Bellini A, Schmidt M, Mattoli S (2012) The C-C motif chemokine ligands CCL5, CCL11 and CCL24 induce the migration of circulating fibrocytes from patients with severe asthma. Mucosal Immunol. doi:10.1038/mi.2012.109
29. Miller M, Cho JY, McElwain K, McElwain S, Shim JY, Manni M, Baek JS, Broide DH (2006) Corticosteroids prevent myofibroblast accumulation and airway remodeling in mice. Am J Physiol Lung Cell Mol Physiol 290: L162–L169
30. Wegmann M, Göggel R, Sel S, Sel S, Erb KJ, Kalkbrenner G, Renz H, Garn H (2007) Effects of low-molecular-weight CCR-3 antagonist on chronic experimental asthma. Am J Respir Cell Mol Biol 36:61–67
31. Locke NR, Royce SG, Wainewright JS, Samuel CS, Tang ML (2007) Comparison of airway remodeling in acute, subacute, and chronic models of allergic airway disease. Am J Respir Cell Mol Biol 36:625–632
32. Di Valentin E, Crahay C, Garbacki N, Hennui B, Guéders M, Noël A, Foidart JM, Grooten J, Colige A, Piette J, Cataldo D (2009) New asthma biomarkers: lessons from murine models of acute and chronic asthma. Am J Physiol Lung Cell Mol Physiol 296:L185–L197
33. Olmez D, Babayigit A, Erbil G, Karaman O, Bagriyanik A, Yilmaz O, Uzener N (2009) Histopathologic changes in two mouse models of asthma. J Investig Allergol Clin Immunol 19:132–138
34. Murphy PM, Baggiolini M, Charo IF, Herbert CA, Horuk R, Matsushima K, Miller LH, Oppenheim JJ, Power CA (2000) International union of pharmacology. XXII. Nomenclature for chemokine receptors. Pharmacol Rev 52:145–176
35. Herz U, Braun A, Rückert R, Renz H (1998) Various immunological phenotypes are associated with increased airway responsiveness. Clin Exp Allergy 28:625–634
36. Brewer JP, Kisselgof AB, Martin TR (1999) Genetic variability in pulmonary physiological, cellular, and antibody responses to antigen in mice. Am J Respir Crit Care Med 160: 1150–1156
37. Boyce JA, Austen KF (2005) No audible wheezing: nuggets and conundrums for mouse asthma models. J Exp Med 201:1869–1873
38. Kumar RK, Herbert C, Kasper M (2004) Reversibility of airway inflammation and remodelling following cessation of antigen challenge in a model of chronic asthma. Clin Exp Allergy 34:1796–1802
39. Raabe OG, Al-Bayati MA, Teague SV, Raslot A (1988) Regional deposition of inhaled monodisperse coarse and fine aerosol particles in small laboratory animals. Ann Occup Hyg 32:53–63
40. Menache M, Miller F, Raabe O (1995) Particle inhalability curves for humans and small laboratory animals. Ann Occup Hyg 39: 317–328
41. Thomas RJ, Webber D, Sellors W, Collinge A, Frost A, Stagg AJ, Bailey SC, Jayasekera PN, Taylor RR, Eley S, Titball RW (2008) Characterization and deposition of respirable large- and small-particle bioaerosols. Appl Environ Microbiol 74:6437–6443
42. Hogan SP, Mould A, Kikutani H, Ramsay AJ, Foster SP (1997) Aeroallergen-induced eosinophilic inflammation, lung damage, and airway heperreactivity in mice can occur independently of IL-4 and allergen-specific immunoglobulins. J Clin Invest 99:1329–1339
43. Kennedy JD, Hatfield CA, Fidler SF, Winterrowd GE, Haas JV, Chin JE, Richards IM (1995) Phenotypic characterization of T lymphocytes emigrating into lung tissue and the airway lumen after antigen inhalation in sensitized mice. Am J Respir Cell Mol Biol 12:613–623

Chapter 20

Assessment of Airway Hyperresponsiveness in Murine Tracheal Rings

Jeremiah T. Herlihy, Iurii Semenov, and Robert Brenner

Abstract

Isolated tracheal rings have often been used to directly measure the contractile output of airway smooth muscle (ASM). Here, we describe the method for excising murine tracheas, mounting tracheal rings in organ baths, and measuring the isometric forces generated by the ASM when stimulated by drug additions or electric field stimulation. The apparatus for the setup and the pathways responsible for stimulation are detailed. Examples of the responses and analyses of two types of ASM stimulation are illustrated: (1) the carbachol concentration–response curve and (2) the frequency–response curve elicited by electric field stimulation.

Key words Airway smooth muscle, Tracheal rings, Isometric force, Electric field stimulation, Concentration–response curves, Hyperresponsiveness

1 Introduction

Airway hyperresponsiveness (AHR) occurring in asthma is characterized by an excessive narrowing of the airways leading to an elevated resistance to airflow and, at times, complete obstruction of the airway lumen [1–5]. It is generally believed that the basis for AHR is complex and multifaceted, involving inflammation, alterations in airway smooth muscle (ASM) function, remodeling of the structures of the airway wall (including the ASM itself), and asthma-induced production of various spasmogens. The active element in airway narrowing is, of course, the contraction and shortening of the ASM. What is not so clear is the extent to which the contractile function per se of the ASM is altered in asthma. It may be that the basic contractile function of the ASM is normal as in the healthy lung, but that other factors, such as airway remodeling, inflammation, or presence of other contractile agents, result in excessive narrowing. On the other hand, asthma may involve an enhanced responsiveness of the ASM itself and excessive shortening of the muscle leads to airway obstruction.

Irving C. Allen (ed.), *Mouse Models of Allergic Disease: Methods and Protocols*, Methods in Molecular Biology, vol. 1032, DOI 10.1007/978-1-62703-496-8_20,

The development of in vitro methods has been helpful in dissecting a direct role for changes in ASM responsiveness per se in asthma from an indirect role involving other factors. A number of articles have been devoted to these methods [6–11]. In this chapter, the apparatus used for isometric contractile measurements as well as the solutions necessary to maintain the tissue in a viable state are described in detail. Descriptions of the isolation and in vitro mounting of the mouse tracheal ring for measurement of isometric force development are presented. In addition, the preparation and administration of commonly used contractile agents as well as the method to electrically induce contraction of the ASM are presented. The chapter offers examples of contractile responses to pharmacologic agents and electric field stimulation, as well as insight into the analysis of the data.

The methods described here are confined to the isometric contractile response of larger airway segments such as the trachea or primary bronchi. It is the most commonly used and easiest approach to measure the contractile output of ASM, although it is not without its own pitfalls in interpretation. Other methods, such as isotonic contractions and lung slices, have also been utilized and these have their own particular advantages for addressing issues of airway function. For example, airway narrowing is produced only when the ASM shortens. Too few studies have employed isotonic or auxotonic contractions, rather than isometric contractions, to characterize the effects of asthma on ASM contractile function and the contribution of afterload to the response of the muscle. Lung slices [12] offer another approach for examining changes in ASM properties, especially with visualization at the cellular and subcellular levels. The isometric method described in this chapter represents a good first approximation for examining the contribution of ASM to asthma-induced AHR.

2 Materials

2.1 Solutions (See Note 1)

1. Normal physiological salt solutions (PSS) (2 l): 119 mM (13.91 g) of NaCl, 4.7 mM (0.7 g) of KCl, 1.18 mM (0.32 g) of KH_2PO_4, 1.17 mM (0.58 g) of $MgSO_4{\cdot}7H_2O$, 18.0 mM (3.02 g) of $NaHCO_3$, 0.026 mM (0.1 ml of 0.5 M) of EDTA (*see* **Note 2**), 11.0 mM (3.96 g) of glucose, 12.5 mM (8.56 g) of sucrose (*see* **Note 3**), 2.0 mM (400 ml of 10.0 mM $CaCl_2$ stock solution) of $CaCl_2$ (*see* **Note 4**). The solution is bubbled with 95 % O_2–5 % CO_2 (pH 7.4 at 37 °C) (*see* **Note 5**).
2. High K^+ PSS: This is the same as the normal PSS except that the NaCl and KCl are adjusted: 56.7 mM (6.628 g) of NaCl and 67 mM (9.99 g) of KCl.
3. Stock carbachol (carbamylcholine) solution consists of 10 mM carbachol in normal PSS (*see* Table 1).

Table 1
Drug solutions and additions for the cumulative concentration–response curve shown in Fig. 3

Stock volume (ml)	Stock concentration (mM)	Amount added (μmol)[a]	Final concentration (μM)[b]
0.01	0.01	0.0001	0.01
0.02	0.01	0.0002	0.03
0.007	0.1	0.0007	0.1
0.02	0.1	0.002	0.3
0.007	1.0	0.007	1
0.02	1.0	0.02	3
0.007	10	0.07	10
0.02	10	0.20	30

[a]Moles of drug added = (stock volume × stock concentration)

[b]Cumulative concentration = (amount added (μmol)/$10 \times 10^{+3}$ μl) + previous concentration. The bath volume is 10 ml

2.2 Trachea-Mounting Hardware (Fig. 1)

1. Ring mounting: The tracheal ring is mounted between two stainless steel rods (*see* **Note 6**). The upper rod is attached to a force transducer (*see* **Note 7**), while the bottom rod is attached to a micrometer used for setting length and adjusting the rest force. Both the micrometer and the force transducer are mounted on metal rods anchored either on a baseboard or on an upright board. The screw clamps allow adjustments to convenient heights.
2. Tissue bath: The tracheal ring and stainless steel mounts are immersed in the PSS contained in the inner compartment of a glass-jacketed tissue bath. Tissue baths can be obtained from several suppliers and are available in various sizes and configurations to accommodate the needs of the investigator. The bath has inlets and outlets for (1) heating fluid (jacket), (2) bathing fluid (PSS) changes (bath), and (3) gas bubbling. Most experiments are performed at 37 °C. Circulation of preheated water (*see* **Note 8**) through the tissue bath jacket assures that the PSS contained in the inner compartment that bathes the tissue remains at 37 °C. The input to the inner chamber is connected via Tygon tubing to a reservoir containing the PSS (also heated and gassed). The bathing PSS is refreshed by opening a clamp to the bath inlet of the inner chamber and allowing the heated PSS to be either pumped from the heated reservoir (not shown) or allowed to flow by gravity feed from the heated reservoir (not shown) located above the tissue bath (*see* **Note 9**). Gases are continuously bubbled through the input to the inner chamber via tubing connected to a pressure regulator controlling the flow of gas from the large stock gas tank.
3. Electric field stimulation (EFS) (Fig. 1b): The EFS of the tracheal ring is produced by two platinum plate electrodes

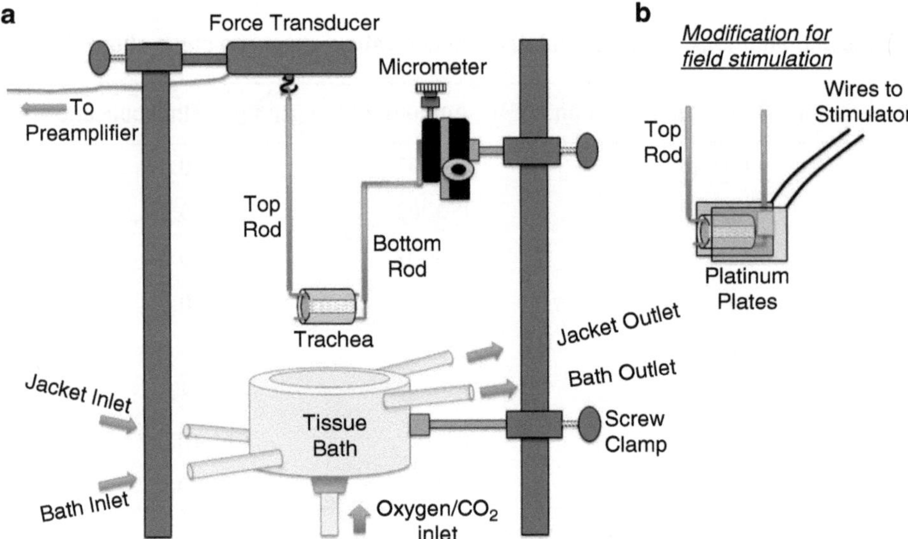

Fig. 1 Diagram of the apparatus used to measure the isometric contraction of isolated tracheal rings. (**a**) The jacketed tissue bath, force transducer, and micrometer are mounted on supporting rods. The use of screw clamps allows easy positioning of these elements. The trachea ring is mounted between the two stainless steel rods while the bath is in the lowered position. After the ring is mounted the bath (filled with heated, gassed PSS) is raised, thereby bathing the tissue. (**b**) Platinum electrodes connected to a stimulator are positioned side by side such that the tracheal ring lies between them. These electrodes should be mounted securely on the lower rod to insure that the distance between the electrodes does not change (reproduced from [10])

placed on either side of the mounted ring and connected to a Grass S88 stimulator (*see* **Note 10**).

4. Data acquisition: The signal from the force transducer is digitized using an A/D converter and amplifier and visualized on a personal computer (*see* **Note 11**). The system is calibrated each day prior to the commencement of the experiment (*see* **Note 12**).

3 Methods

3.1 Trachea Ring Isolation and Mounting

1. Prior to tissue isolation the force transducer is calibrated, the tissue bath is filled with normal PSS, and the airflow adjusted to obtain a light stream of O_2/CO_2.
2. Mice of approximately 2 months of age are deeply sedated with isoflurane and immediately sacrificed by cervical dislocation (*see* **Note 13**).
3. The skin (and fur) is removed from thorax to throat and the ribs are cut from the base of the sternum, laterally (on both sides) to the top of the heart. The sternum and ribs are then pulled forward to the throat to reveal the heart/lungs, thymus, trachea (ventral), and esophagus (attached to and dorsal to trachea).
4. The trachea is grasped via forceps above the pharynx and is excised by cutting below the bronchial bifurcation and above

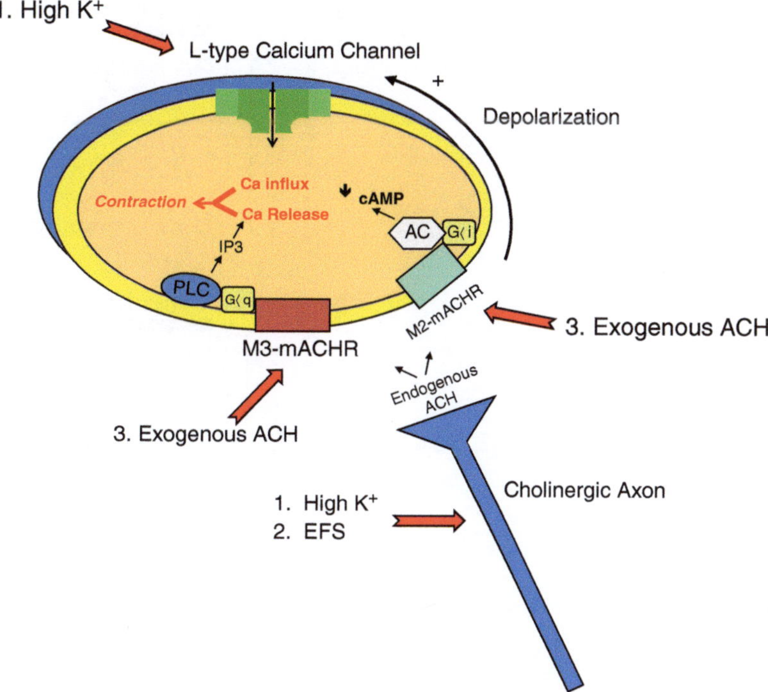

Fig. 2 Diagram of the major signaling pathways for an airway smooth muscle cell within the tracheal ring. Shown is L-type calcium channel activated by depolarization upon high K^+ stimulation (*1.*). M2 and M3 cholinergic receptors are activated by endogenous acetylcholine released from nerve endings (*1.* and *2.*) and exogenously applied acetylcholine (or cholinomimetic) (*3.*). The second messenger cascades leading to contraction are also shown. Not shown are other types of cells within the airway wall that may release other contractile and relaxing agents (reproduced from [10])

the forceps. The tracheal segment is placed in ice-cold oxygenated PSS where it is cleaned of loose connective tissue via fine scissors (*see* **Note 14**) and cut transversely into tracheal rings (*see* **Note 15**).

5. The tracheal ring is threaded over the two L-shaped stainless steel prongs (Fig. 1a) and the tissue bath is then raised so that the ring is immersed in PSS.
6. The micrometer is adjusted slowly to obtain a tension of ~1 g. Over the first 5–10 min, trachea passive tension (also called preload) tends to decline somewhat (stress-relaxation phenomenon) and the micrometer is used to adjust the passive tension at 1 g during equilibration (*see* **Note 16**). The trachea is allowed to equilibrate for at least 1 h before experimental challenges and the bathing PSS refreshed periodically.

3.2 ASM Stimulation (Fig. 2) (See Note 17)

1. High potassium contractions (Fig. 3a): The rings are challenged twice with the high K^+ PSS. The normal PSS is replaced by high K^+ PSS and the contraction is allowed to proceed until

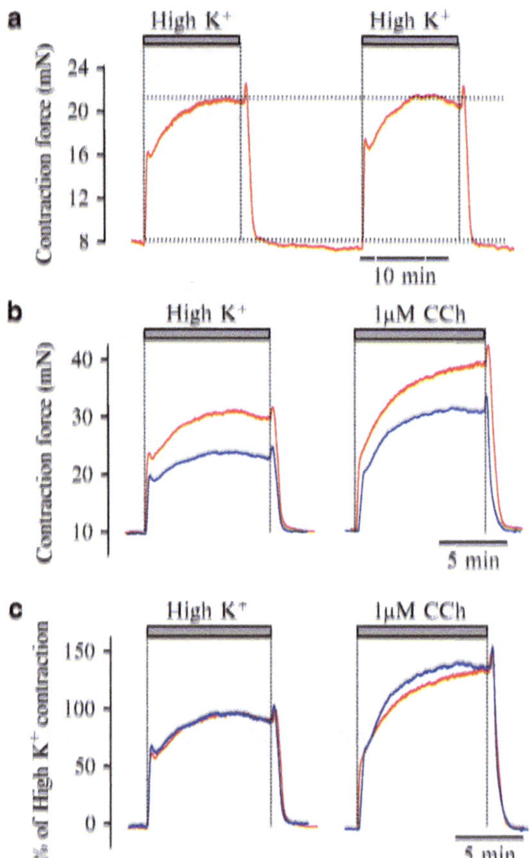

Fig. 3 Tracings of the contractile responses of tracheal rings to stimulation. (**a**) Duplicate contractile responses (mN) of a single ring as a function of time (min). Note the similarities of the sequential responses. (**b**) Tracings of the responses of two different rings to high K^+ (*left panel*) and 1.0 μM carbachol (CCh) (*right panel*). Note that one ring has a consistently larger response to both types of stimulation. (**c**) Normalization of the responses of the two rings to their respective maximum response to K^+ (100 %). Note the similarity between the two strips when the output is normalized to K^+ (reproduced from [10])

it plateaus out. The bath solution is exchanged with fresh PSS and the force allowed to return to baseline. The high K^+ challenge is then repeated a second time (*see* **Note 18**).

2. Pharmacologic stimulation (Fig. 4): Exogenous agents, such as ASM agonists and antagonists, can be added directly to the bath. In Fig. 4a, doses of carbachol stock were added to the tissue bath without rinsing between drug additions (cumulative addition), with each higher dose being added at the height of the contractile response from the previous addition. Figure 4b shows the composite log concentration (abscissa) vs. contractile response (ordinate) (*see* **Note 19**). Drugs can also be added to

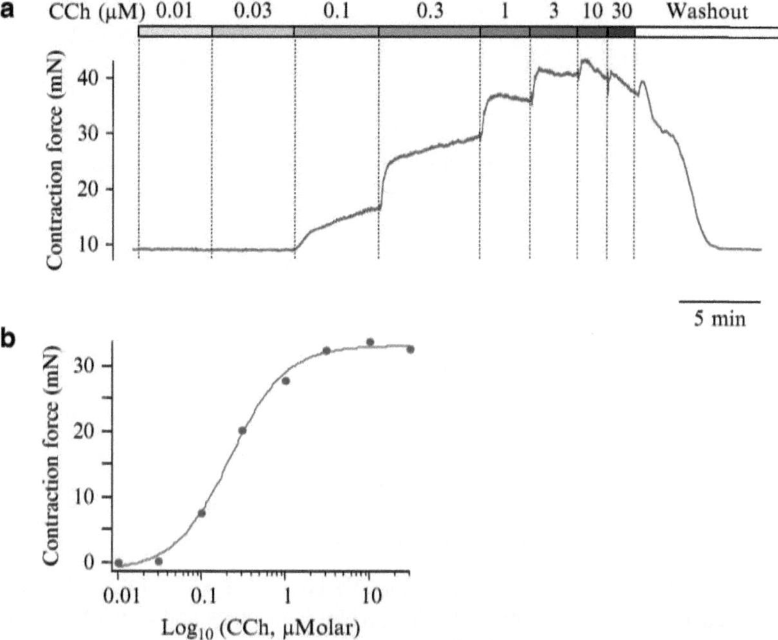

Fig. 4 Illustration of a cumulative concentration–response curve experiment. (**a**) Actual tracing of the contractile response to additions of carbachol. Numbers above the tracing indicate the concentration of carbachol in the bath after each succeeding addition. The protocol for making up the stock carbachol solutions and the appropriate volumes to be added are shown in Table 1. (**b**) Concentration–response curve for the data gained in (**a**). The maximum force developed for each carbachol concentration (mN) is graphed as a function of the log of the carbachol concentration (μM) (reproduced from [10])

the PSS prior to perfusion in the tissue bath. This can prove useful when a constant background of stimulation is required throughout the entire experiment. The normalization of the contractile output of a given tracheal ring presents some difficulty (*see* **Note 21**).

3. EFS: The stimulus parameters, such as voltage–response, frequency–response, etc., for a particular setup must be determined prior to beginning any series of experiments (*see* **Note 20**). The contractile response to increasing frequency (constant voltage, duration, and pulse width) during EFS is shown in Fig. 5a and the data are graphed in Fig. 5b as a frequency–response curve. The normalization of the contractile output of a given tracheal ring presents some difficulty (*see* **Note 21**).

3.3 Normalization and Data Analysis

1. Problems associated with setting the force or the length (between muscle clips) of the resting tracheal ring are discussed in **Note 16**. How to best to express the contractile output of a given ring also presents problems (*see* **Note 21**).

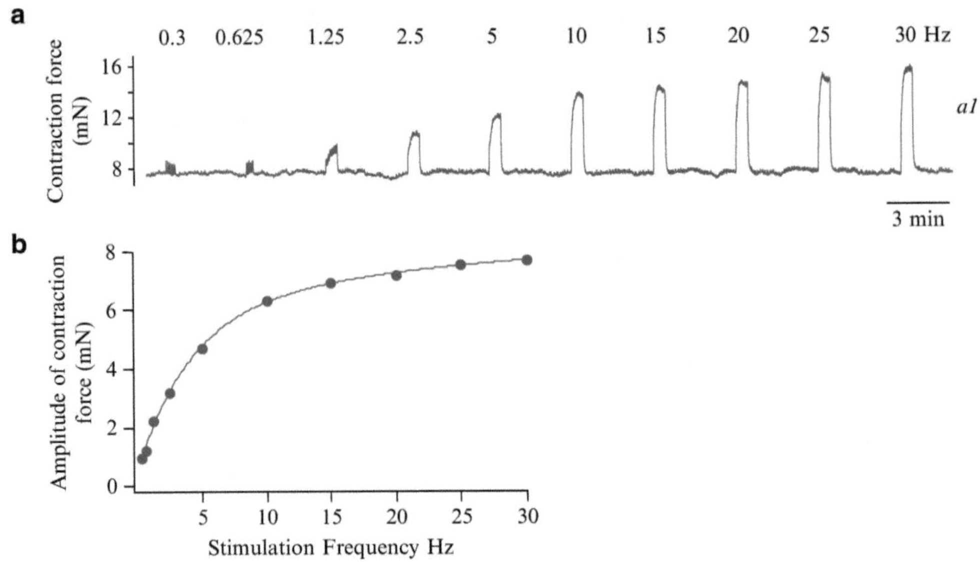

Fig. 5 Illustration of a force–frequency response curve experiment. (**a**) Actual tracings of the responses to different electrical frequencies (Hz) under conditions of 0.5 ms pulse and 40 V. The frequency, shown above the tracings, was varied from 0.3 to 30 Hz. (**b**) The contractile response to the EFS (mN) is graphed as a function of frequency (reproduced from [10])

4 Notes

1. The PSS are prepared at the beginning of each week using ultrapure water and are stored at 4 °C in a refrigerator. Solutions are utilized within 5 days of preparation and any unused solution after that time is discarded. The composition of the tissue bathing solutions varies widely among investigators. Not only do the concentrations of the common salts vary, but also the buffer types and other additional compounds differ.
2. EDTA is included to bind and minimize the effects of copper, iron, and other trace metals that catalyze the oxidation of certain susceptible pharmacological agents (e.g., catecholamines).
3. Sucrose is included to correct the osmolarity of the solution. The cell membrane is virtually impermeable to sucrose.
4. The stock $CaCl_2$ should be added to the stirred solution last and somewhat slowly. If added too quickly in the absence of CO_2, especially when the solution pH is high, a white precipitate will form that usually can be reversed upon the addition of CO_2.
5. Bicarbonate buffer is the most commonly used buffer for these types of experiments, but organic buffers also have been used. Because the CO_2 content of different gas tanks may vary from the nominal value (depending upon the accuracy of the vendor)

it is a good idea to set the pH of each stock solution with HCl or NaOH at 37 °C.

6. The inclusion of any metals containing iron, copper, etc. in the solutions or in contact with the tissue should be avoided. These metals break down releasing contaminants that can adversely affect the tissue. Stainless steel is preferred for use in biological fluids. Small Parts Inc., Miami Lakes, FL, is a good source for stainless steel rods and other useful items for fabrication of the mounting hardware.
7. Many different force transducers are commercially available. The FT.O3C Force Displacement Transducer (Grass Technologies, Warwick, RI) is widely used. It is rugged and reliable and offers ample sensitivity for use with mouse tracheal rings.
8. Many heating circulator pumps are available on the market. We have tended to use those supplied by Haake Instruments or B. Braun.
9. Because of the tubing dead space between the reservoir PSS and the inner chamber of the tissue bath, the first fluid to flow into the chamber upon washing will not be at 37 °C, but at room temperature. This abrupt transient change in temperature can lead to a transient contractile response of the muscle (*see* Fig. 3).
10. The electrodes should be solidly mounted in the apparatus such that the distance between the electrodes does not change. The platinum electrodes can be attached to the bottom rod so that the distance between the plates is fixed (we use 4 mm). All wires and soldered connections are insulated from the bathing solution by coating with Sylgard (Silicone Elastomer; Dow Corning Corp., Midland, MI) to prevent leaching of deleterious metals into the tissue bath.
11. Two data-gathering systems are used in our laboratories: MacLab 8 A/D system, which is an older version of AD Instrument Powerlab hardware (ADInstruments, Inc., Colorado Springs, CO), and BIOPAC Systems (Goleta, CA). Macintosh computers are used to visualize the signals during acquisition and later during data analysis.
12. The complete system is calibrated prior to each experiment by hanging known weights (2–5 g) from the force transducer. Many studies report the force in grams or gram-weight, which is consistent with the calibration procedure. However, this expression is not formally correct. Force equals mass × acceleration and the correct quantity for force is the Newton (N). Since the acceleration due to gravity is 9.8 m/s, 1 g-weight is approximately 0.0098 N and is generally expressed as 9.8×10^{-3} N or 9.8 mN.

13. We have found that tracheas from mice that are 2 months old or older are easily mounted. Younger mice may be used, but the smaller tracheas become more difficult to mount on the stainless steel rods. Some anesthetics should be avoided. For example, we have observed that Avertin (Tribromoethanol) has strong relaxant effects on ASM. The depth of anesthesia is appropriate when a toe pinch with forceps is unable to elicit a response.
14. The cleaning and ring preparation should be done as quickly as possible with minimal touching or damage to the tracheal segment. This stage can be facilitated if performed in a petri dish filled with silicone. By pinning the trachea below and above the bifurcation and pharynx, respectively, the danger of damage from too much handling with the forceps will be minimized.
15. Attempts should be made to keep the lengths (axial length) of the tracheal rings uniform. The output of any given ring is proportional to the number of muscle cells contracting in parallel. So, a ring that is twice as long as another ring should develop twice the force as the narrower ring. In addition, the transverse cut should also be uniform, i.e., 90° to the long axis of the trachea. A change in the orientation of the rings could lead to different force development, as shown for vascular smooth muscle strips [13]. It should be noted here that if in the course of remodeling due to asthma the ASM changes orientation, then the force development would be affected by the new orientation. Thus, the angle of the cut, as well as, possible reorientation of the ASM within the wall should be taken into account when analyzing the force output.
16. Our laboratory sets the rest force at 1.0 g, which is appropriate for the width of the rings utilized in our experiments. Preliminary experiments revealed that this rest force placed the rings at or near the length at which maximum force development occurs. The question of which rest force or rest length the ring should be set is problematic mainly because of the adaptation of the airway wall with regard to the force–length curve of the ASM [14]. The adaptation can occur quite rapidly and is observed as a shift of the curve along the length axis. At present, no universally accepted normalization point for the rest length or preload is available [14].
17. Figure 2 depicts the complex pathways leading to ASM stimulation. The depolarization due to addition of high K^+ PSS opens voltage-dependent calcium channels in the muscle allowing calcium influx and contraction. High K^+ PSS also opens voltage-dependent calcium channels in the nerve endings, causing release of acetylcholine and cholinergic-evoked contraction. Activation of the major cholinergic receptors (M_2

and M_3) by exogenous acetylcholine or a cholinergic mimetic causes contraction via second messengers. Electrical stimulation of the tracheal ring activates cholinergic nerves in the airway wall and release of acetylcholine, which in turn causes contraction of the ASM. Not shown are adrenergic receptors (B_2) on the ASM. Also not shown are several different other cell types (e.g., epithelia) that are found in the airway wall and that can produce and release other spasmogens or relaxing agents.

18. The high K^+ challenges serve three purposes. First, examination of this response can give an indication of whether the tissue was damaged during excision, preparation, and mounting. If the contractile response appears different from the usual response, it should be discarded. Second, we think of the high K^+ challenge as a "wake-up call" after the equilibration period and this is always included in our protocol for every experiment. Finally, the contraction to high K^+ is used to normalize the response to other contractile agents (*see* **Note 21**).
19. Most often the contractile response of the ASM to a particular agent is examined over the total range of effective concentrations. Such a concentration–response curve is usually obtained in a cumulative fashion, i.e., the concentration of the drug in the tissue bath is increased in an additive fashion without rinsing the bath between the additions of the drug. A representative experiment is shown in Fig. 4 where carbachol is added cumulatively to the tissue bath. Note that the range of concentrations extends over several log units and proceeds not at one-half log units, but at one-third log units. The use of one-third instead of one-half is mainly for appearance, i.e., data points graphed one-third between log units appear nearly equi-spaced between the log units. Table 1 demonstrates the drug preparation and addition procedure for the experiment shown in Fig. 4. The total volume of additions should not exceed 2 % of the initial bath volume. When additives are dissolved in organic solvents, the total volume of additions should be limited even further (<0.1 %) and preliminary test should be run to determine if the solvent itself causes any untoward effects. Moreover, the concentrations of drug stock solutions (stock) should be chosen such that convenient volumes can be added to the tissue bath. Table 1 lists the concentrations of the stock drug solutions, the volumes added to the tissue bath, and the final drug concentrations to which the trachea is exposed. Because dose–response curves are performed over several log units, the use of geometric means in data analysis should be employed [15].
20. For EFS each setup has its own peculiarities and therefore the stimulus parameters should be characterized empirically prior

to initiating any series of experiments. Contractile responses to stimulus durations, frequencies, voltages (strengths), and pulse durations are measured and the optimal settings chosen. In our setup where the plate electrodes are separated by about 4 mm, the optimal stimulation strength, frequency, and pulse width were 44 V, 30 Hz, and 0.5 ms, respectively.

21. The contractile response of a tracheal ring is most accurately expressed as the force developed divided by the cross-sectional area of the smooth muscle within the ring, accounting for any change in ASM orientation. Because of differences between ring sizes attempts are often made to normalize force output to the ring size. However, in practical terms, laboratories have adopted a number of ways to express the contractile response and no uniformly agreed-upon normalization procedure is available. The following are the most commonly used approaches:
    (a) No normalization: This method presents the actual force development in either grams or in mN without any attempt toward normalization. The assumptions are that (1) the tracheal rings are cut at the same length and the same orientation and (2) the ASM mass and orientation have not varied from ring to ring.
    (b) Normalization to ring weight: To correct for differences in the length of the rings utilized, the rings are removed from the apparatus after the experiments and weighed, generally after light blotting. The force is then normalized to the wet weight. In our laboratory this approach was unsatisfactory because the variability using tracheas from smaller mice was too large. If the length of the ring between the mounting rods is known, the average cross-sectional area can be calculated using the density of the ring (e.g., 1.05 g/cm^3). Other laboratories normalize force output to dry weight or to protein content.
    (c) Normalization to a given contraction: Our laboratory normalizes force to the contraction obtained with high K^+ PSS (Fig. 3b, c). The tracings in Fig. 3b depict the contractile responses in mN of two different tracheal rings to high K^+ and carbachol stimulation, respectively. The outputs in mN between the two rings are different. However, as shown in Fig. 3c, the contractile responses are equivalent when the contractions are normalized to the respective maximum high K^+ contractions. Some laboratories normalize to the maximum response to cholinergic stimulation.

Acknowledgments

This work was supported by grants from the Center for Innovation in Prevention and Treatment of Airway Diseases (CIPTAD) and NINDS (NS052574) to R.B.

References

1. Seow CY, Fredberg JJ (2001) Historical perspective on airway smooth muscle: the saga of a frustrated cell. J Appl Physiol 91:938–952
2. An SS, Bai TR, Bates JH et al (2007) Airway smooth muscle dynamics: a common pathway of airway obstruction in asthma. Eur Respir J 29:834–860
3. Fredberg JJ (2004) Bronchospasm and its biophysical basis in airway smooth muscle. Respir Res 5:2. doi:10.1186/1465-9921-5-2
4. Oliver MN, Fabry B, Marinkovic A, Mijailovich SM, Butler JP, Fredberg JJ (2007) Airway hyperresponsiveness, remodeling, and smooth muscle mass: right answer, wrong reason? Am J Respir Cell Mol Biol 37:264–272
5. Meurs H, Gosens R, Zaagsma J (2008) Airway hyperresponsiveness in asthma: lessons from in vitro model systems and animal models. Eur Respir J 32:487–502
6. Garssen J, Van Loveren H, Van Der Vliet H, Nikamp FP (1990) An isometric method to study respiratory smooth muscle responses in mice. J Pharmacol Methods 24:209–217
7. Hulsmann AR, de Jongste JC (1993) Studies of human airways in vitro: a review of the methodology. J Pharmacol Toxicol Methods 30:117–132
8. Fedan JS, Van Scott MR, Johnston RA (2001) Pharmacological techniques for the in vitro study of airways. J Pharmacol Toxicol Methods 45:159–174
9. Cooper PR, McParland BE, Mitchell HW, Noble PB, Politi AZ, Ressmeyer AR, West AR (2009) Airway mechanics and methods used to visualize smooth muscle dynamics in vitro. Pulm Pharmacol Ther 22:398–406
10. Semenov I, Herlihy JT, Brenner R (2012) In vitro measurements of tracheal constriction using mice. J Vis Exp (64):pii:3703, doi:10.3791/3703
11. Wright D, Sharma P, Ryu M-H, Risse P-A, Ngo M, Maarsingh H, Koziol-White C, Jha A, Halayko AJ, West AR (2012) Models to study airway smooth muscle contraction *in vivo*, *ex vivo* and *in vitro*: implications in understanding asthma. Pulm Pharmacol Ther 26:24–36. doi:10.1016/j.pupt.2012.08.006
12. Sanderson MJ (2011) Exploring lung physiology in health and disease with lung slices. Pulm Pharmacol Ther 24:452–465
13. Herlihy JT (1980) Helically cut vascular strip preparation: geometrical considerations. Am J Physiol 238:H107–H109
14. Bai TR, Bates JH, Brusasco V et al (2004) On the terminology for describing the length-force relationship and its changes in airway smooth muscle. J Appl Physiol 97: 2029–2034
15. Hancock AA, Bush EN, Stanisic D, Kyncl JJ, Lin CT (1988) Data normalization before statistical analysis: keeping the horse before the cart. Trends Pharmacol Sci 9:29–32

Chapter 21

Use of the Cockroach Antigen Model of Acute Asthma to Determine the Immunomodulatory Role of Early Exposure to Gastrointestinal Infection

Carolyn G. Durham, Lisa M. Schwiebert, and Robin G. Lorenz

Abstract

The increased incidence of asthma over the last 50 years in developed countries has been associated with a decrease in infections acquired early in childhood. These early infections are thought to shape subsequent immune responses. Although there have been multiple clinical associations between gastrointestinal infections and decreased asthma incidence, it has been difficult to move beyond a simple correlation when studying human patients. This section describes an acute asthma model in C57BL/6 mice designed to specifically evaluate the effect of prior gastric *Helicobacter* colonization and inflammation in a murine model of cockroach allergen-induced asthma.

Key words Asthma, *Helicobacter*, Gastritis, Murine, Cockroach antigen, Hygiene hypothesis, Toll-like receptors, Neonatal

1 Introduction

In 1989, Strachan proposed the hygiene hypothesis to answer the growing epidemiological trend of the rise of industrialization, decline in infectious diseases, and subsequent increase in diseases associated with a T-helper 2 (Th2) cell response, including asthma [1]. Despite the growing evidence for this hypothesis, the immunological mechanism by which decreasing infection rates and increasing Th2 diseases occur has not been elucidated [2]. Numerous studies have shown a role for viruses in asthma incidence. In fact, Strachan et al. showed that newborns who were exposed to respiratory viruses had an increased incidence of asthma [3]. However, there is a growing body of research that suggests that immune system development, spurred by early colonization with bacteria, decreases the rate of asthma development later in life [2]. For example, studies have shown that children reared in a household with a dog or whose bedrooms had high endotoxin levels were at

Irving C. Allen (ed.), *Mouse Models of Allergic Disease: Methods and Protocols*, Methods in Molecular Biology, vol. 1032, DOI 10.1007/978-1-62703-496-8_21,

a lower risk for developing asthma [4, 5]. Additionally, numerous studies have shown that living on a farm dramatically reduces the risk for asthma, presumably because of the constant levels of bacterial exposure [6]. This clearly demonstrates the benefit of exposing young children to bacteria and bacterial components in reducing asthma incidence.

In developing countries, many of the infectious diseases are known to elicit a Th1 phenotype. One of these bacteria is *Helicobacter pylori*, which is endemic in many developing countries. As countries become more industrialized, antibiotic therapy is more widespread and these infectious diseases decline. This is especially noted when the incidence of infection is higher in adults, since they were young when the bacterial exposure was greater, than in children who were reared under more newly established standards of infection control [7]. Interestingly, the timing of bacterial exposure is critical in whether or not the microbial acquisition helps in shaping the immune system or causing a pathogenic problem. A study done with *Helicobacter pylori* infection in children and adults indicated that in children less than 10 years old, IL10 and IFNγ were significantly upregulated when compared to older children and adults [8]. The IL10 increase persisted past 10 years old and was higher than that of noninfected people, indicating that this early exposure promotes a Th1 immune response and that regulation of this response persists.

The bacterial exposure component of the hygiene hypothesis has gained acknowledgment and prompted members of the American Thoracic Society to set forth the notion that bacterial manipulation is a key factor in asthma prevention. Furthermore, they charge that bacterial exposure, especially through the gastrointestinal tract, is fundamental to properly developing a Th1-skewed immune system [2]. A key component of this immune system development is the body being able to detect the presence of the bacteria. Our lab has previously shown that, in C57BL/6 mice, toll-like receptors (TLRs) 2 and 4 are significantly upregulated 2 weeks after birth [9]. TLRs are pathogen-associated pattern receptors. TLRs 2 and 4 are specific for Gram-positive and Gram-negative bacterial ligands, respectively. However, in mice born to dames on a broad-spectrum antibiotic cocktail and that are then weaned onto this cocktail, this upregulation does not occur [9]. This indicates that the ability to sense bacteria is critical in immune system development. Our lab has also shown that mice that were born to parents that had been on broad-spectrum antibiotics and were, themselves, maintained on this regimen, had delayed Th1/17 development [9]. These data demonstrate the need for bacterial recognition and bacterial exposure in immune system development. To evaluate the role of bacteria in the hygiene hypothesis, we have developed a model where gastritis is induced by infection with the gastrointestinal bacteria *Helicobacter felis*; and subsequently asthma is induced using cockroach antigen (CRA).

Helicobacter pylori infection is endemic in most developing countries, affecting at least 70 % of the population and colonizing about 20 % of the US population. Physiologically, the presence of *H. pylori* in the gut has been shown to elicit a strong IFNγ response, which has been shown to downregulate Th2 cells [10]. Specifically, administering the neutrophil-activating protein of *H. pylori*, both systemically and mucosally, reduces characteristic Th2 cytokines, IgE, and eosinophilia by activating the Th1 pathway [11]. These studies show that this bacterial infection causes an overwhelming Th1 response, one that epidemiologically and physiologically has been shown to directly affect the response of the Th2 pathway. In recent years, the role of Th17 cells in *Helicobacter* infections has been shown to be critical in pathogenesis. Shi et al. demonstrated that the Th17 cells are critical in acute infection, where it works with IL8 to recruit neutrophils and decrease bacterial burden [12]. Depleting these cells leads to proliferation of bacteria. Interestingly, if there is no control mechanism in place, such as regulatory T cells, IL17 is upregulated to the point where it is ineffective in pathogen clearance [13]. Data from our lab shows that in germfree mice, IL17 levels continue to climb after 8 weeks, while *H. felis* is never cleared. With conventionally reared C57BL/6 mice, IL17 increases initially, but decreases after 8 weeks [14]. Th1 and Th17 adaptive immunity plays a significant role in *Helicobacter* infections, though both must be tightly regulated.

Human studies demonstrate that polymorphisms in the TLR2 and TLR4 genes affect the pathogenesis of *Helicobacter* gastritis [15, 16]. However, there have been conflicting in vitro reports about which of these TLRs are needed to recognize the bacteria. Many epidemiological studies have shown an inverse correlation with this pathogen and asthma susceptibility. Chen and Blaser demonstrated that asthma onset in children younger than 5 years old was inversely associated with seropositivity for *H. pylori* (OR, 0.58; 95 % CI, 0.38–0.88). In the same study, seropositivity for *H. pylori* in children 3–19 years old was significantly inversely correlated with having a current case of asthma (OR, 0.41; 95 % CI, 0.24–0.69) [17]. Interestingly, with the rise of asthma, there has also been an increase in administering broad-spectrum antibiotics in small children. This illustrates that, not only is there a dysregulation in global bacteria but also that the bacteria, such as *H. pylori*, that were acquired during childhood that could potentially shape the immune system are being eliminated before their physiological effects can be properly achieved [18]. Additionally, *H. pylori* is associated with decreasing the severity of gastroesophageal reflux disorder, which is a positive correlate of asthma [10]. Immunologically, asthma is characterized as a Th2 disease, as asthmatic patients have increased serum IgE, production of which is known to be initiated by IL-4, 5, and/or 13 [10]. Interestingly, IFNγ production has been shown to hinder Th2 cytokine production;

IFNγ is a downstream target of NFκB, the transcription factor induced by TLR2 and 4 activation. Thus, activating TLR2 and 4 by environmental exposure to bacterial ligands could elicit a more Th1- and Th17-skewed adaptive response and result in the down-regulation of the Th2 phenotype in asthma patients [19].

Because asthma is a complex disease, various mouse models are used to elucidate various facets of the disease. Since mice do not spontaneously get asthma, the mice must be sensitized with a specific allergen and subsequently challenged with that allergen. Many labs use BALB/c mice for their studies because these mice have a Th2-skewed immune system and a robust asthmatic response upon asthma induction. However, this model does not parallel typical human disease since most people do not have a strongly Th2-skewed immune system. Therefore, the use of C57BL/6 mice is a good model because it has a Th1 bias, which is more like the human immune system. Using C57BL/6 mice is also beneficial when studying the bacterial colonization and/or sensing in asthma, as these mice respond more strongly to bacteria than the BALB/c mice [20]. Likewise, the allergens used in asthma studies vary greatly. Historically, ovalbumin has been used to induce the asthmatic phenotype because of its ability to produce strong Th2 responses [21, 22]. However, this allergen does not have clinical application, as ovalbumin is not a common allergen in humans. Therefore, more clinically relevant allergens, such as house dust mite and cockroach extracts, are becoming more frequently used [23, 24]. There are two categories of asthma models: acute and chronic. The acute models are used to study the onset and beginning stages of asthma, whereas the chronic models are used to study the long-term effect of asthma, such as airway remodeling. The chronic model is also helpful in studying therapies for asthma patients, since most patients already have remodeling taking place in their lungs [24].

In this model, we chose CRA because the cockroach is a common household pest. However, this model has only previously been evaluated in adult mice, whereas we needed a model of childhood asthma induction if the effect of early gastrointestinal infections is to be adequately tested. Therefore, we utilized 2-, 4-, and 6-week-old mice to determine the induction of acute asthma by CRA. We concluded that, at 2 weeks, the newly weaned pups did not have a mature enough immune response to mount a Th2 acute asthma response. At 6 weeks, their immune reactions had switched to a more Th1/17 phenotype and the results were more variable. However, 4-week-old C57BL/6 mice had both a robust and consistent response to CRA and can now be established as an excellent model for acute sensitization and challenge with CRA to study the development and early stages of asthma (Figs. 1 and 2).

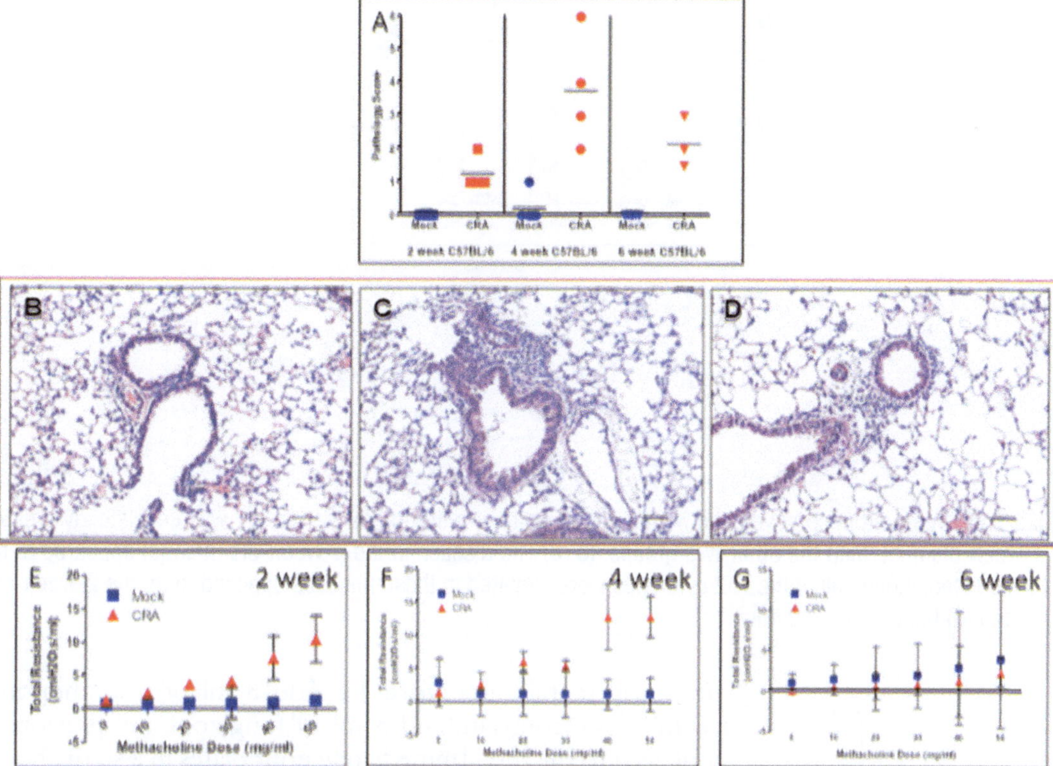

Fig. 1 Four-week-old mice have more robust pathology and airway resistance than 2- or 6-week-old mice. (**a**) Four-week-old mice developed more inflammation within their airways and vasculature. Although 6-week-old CRA-treated mice have moderate perivascular and peribronchial inflammation, the younger 4-week-old mice have much greater perivascular and peribronchial inflammation after asthma induction. The 2-week-old mice have only mild perivascular and peribronchial inflammation after CRA treatment. (**b–d**) Representative H&E images of the 2-week-old mice, 4-week-old mice, and 6-week-old mice, respectively. (**e**) Resistance (*R*) in the airways was consistently higher in the 4-week-old mice when compared with the mock-treated, as well as (**f**) the treated 2-week-old mice and (**g**) the treated 6-week-old mice

2 Materials

2.1 Helicobacter Components

1. C57BL/6 mice (Jackson Laboratory, Bar Harbor, ME).
2. *Helicobacter felis* ATCC 49179.
3. ATCC Medium 260 Plates: Trypticase soy agar, defibrinated calf blood (5 % v/v) (Colorado serum Company, Denver, CO), trimethoprim (1 mg/ml), vancomycin (10 mg/ml), fungizone (1 % v/v). Resuspend 20 g of Trypticase soy agar in 500 ml of ultrapure water (e.g., Milli-Q or an equivalent) and heat with frequent agitation to boiling for 1 min to completely dissolve the powder. This should be autoclaved for 15 min at 121 °C and then cooled to 55 °C in a water bath. When cooled, add 25 ml of the defibrinated calf blood using sterile technique and

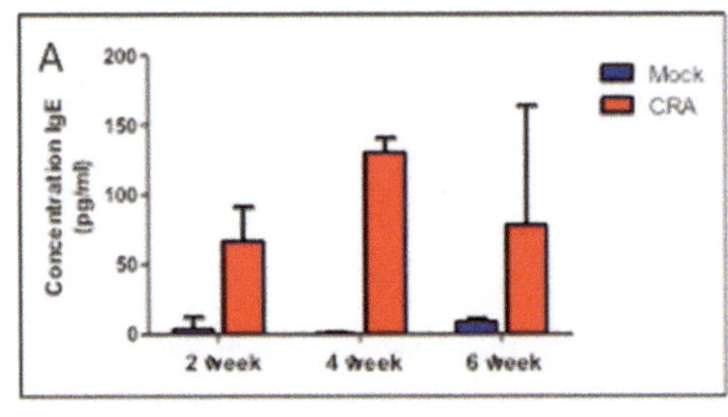

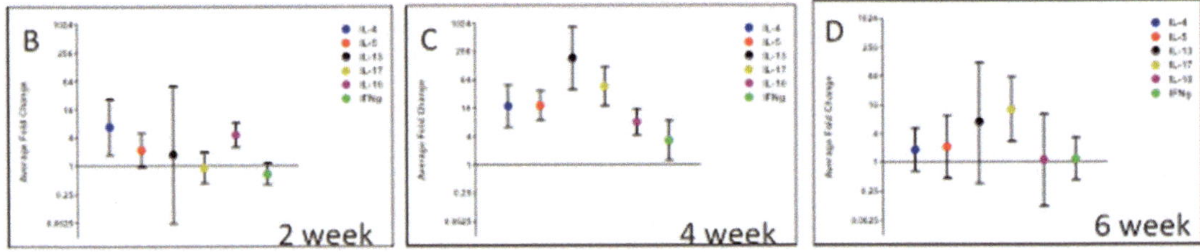

Fig. 2 Four-week-old mice developed higher serum asthma markers. (**a**) Serum IgE was consistently greater in 4-week-old mice than the other two groups. (**b–d**) The disease in the 4-week-old mice (**c**) appeared to be IL13 mediated, though all of the Th2 cytokines were elevated in these mice, as opposed to (**b**) the 2-week-old mice and (**d**) the 6-week-old mice

stir slowly to mix (*see* **Note 1**). Add 5 ml of trimethoprim, 1.5 ml of vancomycin, and 5 ml of fungizone (all previously sterilized) to the mix. Immediately pour plates in a sterile hood to approximately ½ full and flame the tops to get rid of any air bubbles. Allow the medium to solidify, and then store at 4 °C in a sealed container for no more than 1 month. This makes 20–25 plates.

4. Brain heart infusion (BHI) broth: Add 37 g of BHI broth to 1 L of deionized distilled water. Autoclave for 30 min on the liquid cycle. Let cool to 55 °C in a water bath and then add the following reagents: 3 μg/ml of vancomycin (3.0 ml of a 10 mg/ml stock); 10 μg/ml of trimethoprim (10.0 ml of a 1 mg/ml stock); 1 % fungizone (10 ml); and 5 % defibrinated fetal calf serum (50 ml).
5. BBL™ CampyPak™ Plus Microaerophilic System Envelopes with Palladium Catalyst (BD, San Jose, CA).
6. Histology sponges and cassettes.
7. Citrosolv (Fisher).
8. Pepsin (0.25 % in PBS).
9. Rabbit anti-*H. felis*/*H. pylori* antibody (Covance, Emeryville, CA).
10. Cy3 donkey anti-rabbit antibody (1:200 dilution, Jackson Immunoresearch, West-Grove, PA).
11. FITC-labeled lectin *N*-acetyl-D-glucosamine-specific *Griffonia simplicifolia* II (5 μg/mL, Invitrogen, Eugene, OR).
12. Hoechst 33258 (0.5 μg/ml of bis-Benzimide; Sigma, St. Louis, MO).

2.2 CRA Asthma Model Components

1. Cockroach antigen (Hollister-Stier, Spokane, WA) (*see* **Note 2**).
2. Incomplete Freund's adjuvant (IFA).
3. Phosphate-buffered saline (PBS).
4. 2-glass syringes (5 ml each).
5. Three-way stopcock.
6. 1 ml syringe with needle (32 G).
7. Eppendorf tubes (1.5 ml, one per mouse).
8. Isoflurane.
9. P20 and P200 pipette.
10. Plastic disposable pipette dropper (one per mouse).
11. 10 % buffered formalin.
12. Bouin's fixative solution: This is a picric acid–formalin–acetic acid mixture that can be either made within the lab (300 ml of saturated picric acid, 100 ml of formaldehyde, 20 ml of acetic acid) or purchased. This fixative allows better and crisper nuclear staining than 10 % neutral-buffered formalin. As picric acid is extremely explosive if allowed to dry out, it is usually safer to just purchase the Bouin's fixative solution.
13. RNAlater RNA Stabilization Reagent (Ambion, Austin, TX): This is an immediate RNA stabilization and protection reagent. It allows tissue archiving without the risk of RNA degradation.
14. Methacholine: Used in the methacholine challenge, in which the subject inhales aerosolized methacholine to determine the level of bronchial hyperreactivity.
15. Ketamine: Used for the induction and maintenance of general anesthesia.
16. Flexivent (Scireq, Montreal, Canada): This is a computer-controlled precision pump that controls mechanical ventilation while also obtaining measurements of respiratory mechanics.

2.3 ELISA Components

1. Immunlon 96 well plates (Thermo Fisher Scientific, Waltham, MA).
2. Goat Anti-Mouse IgE-UNLB (10 μg/ml; Southern Biotech, Birmingham, AL): For use in coating the ELISA plate.
3. Wash buffer (PBS, 0.5 % Tween-20).
4. Blocking buffer (PBS, 5 % bovine serum albumin (BSA)).
5. Diluent buffer (PBS, 1 % BSA).
6. Mouse IgE Standard (Southern Biotech).
7. Goat Anti-Mouse IgE-AP (Southern Biotech) (1:2,000 in diluent buffer): For detection of IgE in serum.
8. 3 N NaOH: 120 g in 1,000 ml of water.

9. SIGMA*FAST*™ *p*-Nitrophenyl phosphate Tablets (Sigma).
10. VERSAmax microplate reader (Molecular Devices, Sunnyvale, CA).

2.4 RNA and QPCR Components

1. Applied Biosystems Assays-On-Demand primer/probe sets.
2. TaqMan Universal PCR Mix (PE Applied Biosystems; Foster City, CA).
3. Trizol® (Life Technologies, Grand Island, NY).
4. Turbo DNase Kit (Ambion, Austin, TX).
5. Roche Transcriptor First Strand cDNA Synthesis Kit (Roche, Penzberg, Germany).
6. Stratagene MX3000P Real-Time Cycler (Agilent Technologies).

3 Methods

3.1 Growing Helicobacter felis

1. One vial of *H. felis* (ATCC 49179) is inoculated onto an ATCC Medium 260 plate (*see* **Note 3**).
2. Incubate at 37 °C for 2 days in an anaerobic jar with a CampyPak (activate CampyPak as per instructions with water). Make sure that the container has an airtight seal (*see* **Note 4**).
3. Check *H. felis* viability by dropping one drop of the bacterial suspension onto a microscope slide and covering with a standard coverslip. Using a 20× or 40× objective lens on a light microscope, focus on the bacteria. Make sure that the majority of them are motile by watching them swim through multiple viewing fields.
4. If motile, using the broth from the plate, inoculate BHI broth (100 ml) in a flask. Secure in an anaerobic jar with a CampyPak (*see* **Note 5**).
5. Incubate at 37 °C for 18–24 h, with gentle shaking.
6. Check viability, as outlined in Subheading 3.1, **step 3**.
7. Determine the optical density of the bacteria culture (OD_{450}; 1 $OD_{450} \cong 10^9$ bacteria) (*see* **Note 6**).
8. Harvest bacteria by centrifuging at 3,000 × *g* for 10 min, and then resuspend the pellet in glycerol:BHI freezing media (31 ml of glycerol:69 ml of BHI). Store aliquots of bacteria (2×10^9 CFU/ml) at −80 °C. The frozen stock should remain viable for ~4 months.

3.2 H. felis Inoculation

1. Days 0 and 3: Inoculate mice orally (per os (p.o.)) using a 200 μl pipette with 0.05 ml of *H. felis* (2×10^9 CFU/ml in glycerol:BHI) using a frozen aliquot.
2. Day 7: Inoculate mice p.o. as described in Subheading 3.2, **step 1**, using freshly grown *H. felis*. Use the same culture

technique as described above in Subheading 3.1, with the exception that a vial of frozen stock of *H. felis* can be used to start the culture instead of a new vial from ATCC (*see* **Note 7**).

3.3 Asthma Sensitization (Day 0)

1. CRA is resuspended in PBS to a final concentration of 4 mg/ml (*see* **Note 2**).
2. It is then put into one glass syringe. A second glass syringe is filled with an equal amount (v/v) of IFA.
3. Connect these two glass syringes to a 3-way stopcock, and then emulsify the IFA and CRA by syringe-extrusion (alternatively pushing the solution in each syringe through progressively smaller pore sizes in the stopcock) for 10–15 min (*see* **Note 8**).
4. The solution is finished emulsifying when a drop of the solution does not disperse on the top of ice-cold water. Use the solution immediately (*see* **Note 9**).
5. Using a non-tuberculin syringe and a 32G needle, inject the mice intraperitoneally (50 μl) and subcutaneously (50 μl).

3.4 Asthma Induction via Intranasal Challenge (Days 14, 18, 22, 26) (See Note 10)

1. Mix CRA with PBS (0.075 mg/ml) (*see* **Note 2**).
2. Anesthetize mice individually using isoflurane (*see* **Note 11**).
3. Using a P20 pipette, drop PBS:CRA solution (10 μl, which equals 0.75 μg) onto the nostril. Once the mouse inhales the solution, drop another 10 μl onto the nostril (*see* **Note 12**).

3.5 Asthma Induction via Intratrachial Challenge (Day 28)

1. Mix CRA with PBS (0.12 μg/ml) (*see* **Note 2**).
2. Anesthetize mice individually using isoflurane (*see* **Note 13**).
3. When the mouse begins to awaken and gasp using its diaphragm, instill PBS:CRA (50 μl, 6.0 μg) solution into the mouse's throat between gasps with a P200 pipette (*see* **Note 14**).

3.6 Sacrifice (Day 29)

1. Anesthetize mice using isoflurane.
2. Perform cervical dislocation.

3.7 Tissue Collection

1. Mice are euthanized using 5 ml of isoflurane for approximately 30 s and followed by cervical dislocation.
2. Blood is collected via heart puncture, allowed to clot for 20 min at room temperature (r.t.), centrifuged for 10 min at 16,200 × *g*, and the serum removed and stored at −20 °C until analysis.
3. The stomach is removed and quartered. Each quarter is fixed in Bouin's fixative for histology, frozen at −80 °C (two quarters) for protein analysis, or stored in RNAlater for RNA analysis, as per protocol.
4. Place 1 stomach quarter flat between two thin histology sponges in a histology cassette. Store the cassette in Bouin's fixative for 24 h at 4 °C. Bouin's fixative is replaced with 70 %

ethanol every 24 h for 48 h (*see* **Note 15**). The tissue can be embedded in paraffin along its long, cut edge in order to get a cross section of the epithelium. One 5 μm slide is stained with hematoxylin and eosin and scored for pathology. Other slides can be stained with various antibodies to determine *Helicobacter* infection rates, presence of inflammatory cells, differentiated epithelial cells, proliferation, and/or apoptosis, as needed.

5. Freeze stomach quarters 2 and 3 at −80 °C for protein extraction, if needed.
6. Store stomach quarter 4 in RNAlater and process as directed by the manufacturer's protocol for future quantitative real-time RT-PCR (qRT-PCR).
7. The lungs are removed above the main stem branch directly below the larynx. The lungs are then separated directly below the main stem branch. Using a 25G needle and a 3 ml syringe, the left lung is perfused with 1–2 ml of formalin through the main bronchus until it is expanded, but not overextended. Pressure must be maintained on the fluid in the lungs by gripping the forceps around the needle inserted into the bronchus while gently applying pressure to the syringe. This is held for 1–2 min. Then, the lung is removed from the needle and placed into a histology cassette and stored in formalin.
8. The tissue in the cassettes is stored in formalin for 24 h. The formalin is then replaced with 70 % ethanol once every 24 h for 2 days. The tissue can be embedded in paraffin and stained with hematoxylin and eosin. Lung sections are then scored for pathology.
9. The right lung is stored in RNAlater as directed by the manufacturer's protocol for future qRT-PCR.

3.8 Airway Hyperresponsiveness

1. Mice are anesthetized with 450 mg/kg of ketamine, and a tracheotomy tube (18 G) is inserted and connected to the inspiratory and expiratory ports of a ventilator (Flexivent). Mice are ventilated at a rate of 160 breaths per minute at a tidal volume of 0.2 ml with a positive end-expiratory pressure of 2–4 cm water.
2. Increasing concentrations of methacholine (0, 10, 20, 30, 40, and 50 mg/ml) are administered via aerosolization. From 20 s to 3 min after each aerosol challenge, detailed measurements should be recorded continuously. The measurements should include resistance (R), compliance (C), and elastance (E) (*see* **Note 16**).

3.9 IgE ELISAs

1. Immunlon 96 well plates are coated with Goat Anti-Mouse IgE-UNLB (10 μg/ml) in PBS, overnight at 4 °C.
2. The next day, the plate is washed with wash buffer five times. The nonspecific binding sites are blocked for >1 h using blocking buffer.

3. After washing the plates five times with wash buffer, the serum samples are added. The serum from mice that received CRA is diluted 1:2 with diluent buffer, and the mock-treated mice serum samples are used neat. Mouse IgE-UNLB is diluted to a start concentration of 2,000 pg/ml, and then diluted 1:2 seven more times for the complete standard curve. The standards and samples are incubated overnight at 4 °C.
4. The next day, the plate is washed five times with wash buffer. Goat Anti-Mouse IgE-AP (1:2,000 in diluent buffer) is added and incubated at r.t. for 2 h.
5. After washing the plate five times with wash buffer, SIGMA*FAST*™ *p*-Nitrophenyl phosphate Tablets are dissolved in 20 ml of deionized water and added to the plate. Plates are incubated for 30 min at r.t. in the dark.
6. 3 N NaOH is added to stop the reaction, and the plate is read at 405 nm on a microplate reader.

3.10 RNA and RT-PCR

1. RNA isolation: The Trizol® (phenol and guanidine isothiocyanate) method can be used to isolate the total RNA from one quarter of each stomach and the left lung [25].
2. Before making cDNA, the RNA is processed to remove contaminating DNA using the Turbo DNase Kit. cDNA is made using the Roche Transcriptor First Strand cDNA Synthesis Kit with mRNA (2 μg) from each sample. Quantitative real-time reverse transcription polymerase chain reaction (QPCR) is performed on each sample. Primers/probes used are from Applied Biosystems Assays-On-Demand. These are used with TaqMan Universal PCR Mix. All RNA data is analyzed using the $-2^{\Delta\Delta Ct}$ relative quantitation method, described in the Applied Biosystems manufacturer's protocol (*see* **Note 17**) [25–27].

3.11 Pathology Scoring

1. Stomach: One-quarter stomach from each mouse that was stained using hematoxylin and eosin should be scored on a scale of 0–3 in each of the three categories. The scores from the three categories are then added together for a total score, with 0 being the lowest and 9 being the highest possible scores (Table 1) [28].
2. Lung: Each section should be scored using a method derived from Curtis et al. in which the inflammation around the vasculature and the bronchial is evaluated and added together for a total inflammation score, with 0 being the lowest and 6 being the maximum (Table 2) [29].

3.12 H. felis Staining and Quantification (See Note 18) [30]

1. Deparaffinize an unstained tissue section as follows: Wash the slides two times for 10 min per wash with Citrosolv; next, wash the slides three times for 10 min with isopropyl alcohol; and finally, rinse the slides for 5 min with running deionized water.

Table 1
Stomach pathology scoring

Score	Longitudinal extent of inflammation	Vertical extent of inflammation	Histological changes
0	None	None	None
1	Patchy	Basal lamina propria only	Mild loss of differentiated epithelial cells
2	<50 %	Transmural	Moderate loss of differentiated epithelial cells
3	>50 %	Both mucosa and submucosa involved	Severe loss of differentiated epithelial cells

H&E-stained stomach sections are evaluated based on the longitudinal extent of inflammation, the vertical extent of inflammation, and histological changes. Each parameter is scored on a scale of 0–3

Table 2
Lung pathology scoring

Score	Vascular	Bronchial
0	No inflammation	No inflammation
1	Occasional cuffing	Occasional cuffing
2	Most vessels surrounded by a thin layer (1–5) of inflammatory cells	Most vessels surrounded by a thin layer (1–5) of inflammatory cells
3	Most vessels surrounded by a thick layer (>5) of inflammatory cells	Most vessels surrounded by a thick layer (>5) of inflammatory cells

H&E-stained lung sections are evaluated based on the extent of inflammation around the vasculature and airways. Each parameter is scored on a scale of 0–3

2. After rehydrating the tissue in PBS, pepsin (0.25 % in PBS) is incubated on the slides for 10 min at r.t.
3. After rinsing the slides in PBS, to block nonspecific binding sites and to permeabilize the tissue, add PBS blocking buffer (1 % bovine serum albumin, 0.3 % Triton X-100) to each slide and incubate for 1 h at r.t.
4. The slides are then washed in PBS and the tissue stained with undiluted rabbit anti-*H. pylori* antibody to semi-quantitate *H. felis* colonization. This antibody is known to cross-react with *H. felis*.
5. After washing the slides in PBS, Cy3 donkey anti-rabbit antibody (1:200 dilution) and FITC-labeled lectin *N*-acetyl-D-glucosamine-specific *Griffonia simplicifolia* II (5 μg/mL) are added to the tissue and incubated for 1 h at r.t. for detection of *H. felis* and mucous neck cells, respectively.
6. To counterstain the nuclei, the slides are incubated for 20 min at r.t. with Hoechst 33258 (0.5 μg/ml).

7. Colonization of the antrum with *H. felis* is evaluated on a scale of 0–4, where 0 = no bacteria per gland; 1 = 1–2 bacteria per gland; 2 = 3–10 bacteria per gland; 3 = 11–20 bacteria per gland; and 4 = ≥20 bacteria per gland.

4 Notes

1. Because the defibrinated calf blood is frozen, it must be thawed in a 37 °C water bath.
2. CRA is not stable after dilution. Therefore, all dilutions must be made fresh and used immediately.
3. The frozen aliquots of *H. felis* must be thawed at 50 °C.
4. When incubating the cultures, incubate with the solid agar on the bottom. Because the *H. felis* grows at the solid/liquid interface, turning the plate upside down will cause the liquid to spill and not be in contact with the solid media. This will result in no bacterial growth.
5. Because *H. felis* does not grow in colonies, remove the broth culture from the plate using a 5 ml pipette. Using a clean pipette, draw up 2 ml of BHI and put it on the used plate. Swirl the plate on a flat surface and then tilt it at a 45° angle to remove the liquid. Place this liquid into the fresh BHI broth. Repeat with a clean pipette and 2 ml of additional clean BHI.
6. If frequently taking aliquots for OD readings, replace the CampyPak microaerophilic packets every time you open the container.
7. In our lab, this infection scheme results in a 100 % infection rate.
8. During the emulsification process, the pore size in the 3-way stopcock must be made progressively smaller by closing the pore incrementally. This solution will be progressively more difficult to mix. This means that the emulsification is occurring.
9. If the solution is not completely emulsified, the antigen will disperse immediately after injection and will not induce the appropriate immune response.
10. The intranasal challenge causes proliferation of the CRA-specific T cells and elicits their migration into the airways, causing an asthmatic phenotype. Performing this procedure several days apart gradually builds up the asthmatic response in the mouse, similar to the development of asthma in children. The intratracheal challenge is designed to elicit a maximum number of T cells into the airways without causing the animal respiratory distress. The intratracheal challenge is much harder for the mouse to endure. Therefore, this route of administration is only conducted at the end of the procedure.

11. When performing the intranasal challenge, the mouse should only be exposed to the isoflurane for about 15 s, which should induce a low level of anesthesia.
12. The procedure must be done very quickly to get the "sniff" response to the drop of CRA, which ensures that it goes into their lungs and is not swallowed. During this procedure, the mouse will begin recovering from unconsciousness and the muscles will begin to tighten. Brace the lower jaw of the mouse with your thumb and the top of the mouse's head with your forefinger, wrapping your other fingers around its torso. In the event that the mouse awakens from the anesthesia before the procedure is complete, you will have a firm grip on the mouse.
13. The mouse should be exposed to the isoflurane for 30 s until completely limp with barely detectable breath movements in its chest. Wait to administer the challenge until the mouse begins to awaken and its diaphragm spasms.
14. The mouse should be held as previously mentioned upon being removed from the isoflurane through the entire procedure until it is fully awake. Often, if the mouse is not held it will die, possibly due to drop in body temperature. The pipette should be poised at the back of the throat, depressing the mouse's tongue. Ensure that the pipette is ready to deposit the antigen when the mouse awakens. The procedure goes very quickly and the mouse can awaken very rapidly, so care must be taken to continuously restrain the mouse while anesthetized and release the mouse if it awakens.
15. Tissue should not be fixed in Bouin's fixative for more than 24 h or pigments can begin to form. Excess fixative should be washed out of the tissue using the alcohol/water washes.
16. During this procedure, several measurements (including compliance and resistance) are taken; however, we only report the resistance measurement because this particular asthma induction protocol is not designed to dramatically affect other parameters, such as compliance. The acute nature of this model does not result in significant, long-term airway remodeling.
17. The housekeeping gene for comparison used in these experiments was the 18S gene because this gene has been determined to be relatively stable, even under inflammatory conditions [26, 31, 32]. This method uses the difference of the average crossing threshold (Ct) of the 18S gene from the average Ct of the target gene to determine the relative expression of the target gene within each group of animals (Ct). Next, the Ct is calculated determining the difference of the experimental Ct (*H. felis*-infected mice) from the control Ct (mock-infected mice). Finally, the average fold change of the gene is calculated with the following formula: $2^{-\Delta\Delta Ct}$. Using the standard deviation

of the Ct of the experimental group in the average fold change formula, the upper and lower limits are calculated.

18. A quarter of the stomach with the squamo-columnar junction and antrum from each mouse is deparaffinized, stained, and quantitated.

Acknowledgments

The authors would like to thank Kim Estell for assistance with airway hyperresponsiveness analysis and Ben Christmann for helping with the lung inflammation technique. We would also like to thank J. McNaught for slide preparation and M. Harris for animal husbandry, and members of the Lorenz lab for valuable advice. This study was supported in part by NIH grants R01 DK059911; P01 DK071176; the American Asthma Foundation grant 06-0167; and University of Alabama at Birmingham Digestive Diseases Research Development Center grant P30 DK064400. CGD is supported by the Howard Hughes Medical Institute Med into Grad Fellowship. Aspects of this project were conducted in biomedical research space that was constructed with funds supported in part by NIH grant C06RR020136.

References

1. Strachan DP (2000) Family size, infection and atopy: the first decade of the "hygiene hypothesis". Thorax 55(Suppl 1):S2–S10
2. Yoo J, Tcheurekdjian H, Lynch SV, Cabana M, Boushey HA (2007) Microbial manipulation of immune function for asthma prevention: inferences from clinical trials. Proc Am Thorac Soc 4(3):277–282
3. Strachan DP, Seagroatt V, Cook DG (1994) Chest illness in infancy and chronic respiratory disease in later life: an analysis by month of birth. Int J Epidemiol 23(5):1060–1068
4. Ownby DR, Johnson CC, Peterson EL (2002) Exposure to dogs and cats in the first year of life and risk of allergic sensitization at 6 to 7 years of age. JAMA 288(8):963–972
5. Braun-Fahrlander C, Riedler J, Herz U, Eder W, Waser M, Grize L, Maisch S, Carr D, Gerlach F, Bufe A, Lauener RP, Schierl R, Renz H, Nowak D, von Mutius E (2002) Environmental exposure to endotoxin and its relation to asthma in school-age children. N Engl J Med 347(12):869–877
6. Riedler J, Braun-Fahrlander C, Eder W, Schreuer M, Waser M, Maisch S, Carr D, Schierl R, Nowak D, von Mutius E (2001) Exposure to farming in early life and development of asthma and allergy: a cross-sectional survey. Lancet 358(9288):1129–1133
7. Kusters JG, van Vliet AH, Kuipers EJ (2006) Pathogenesis of Helicobacter pylori infection. Clin Microbiol Rev 19(3):449–490
8. Harris PR, Wright SW, Serrano C, Riera F, Duarte I, Torres J, Pena A, Rollan A, Viviani P, Guiraldes E, Schmitz JM, Lorenz RG, Novak L, Smythies LE, Smith PD (2008) Helicobacter pylori gastritis in children is associated with a regulatory T-cell response. Gastroenterology 134(2):491–499
9. Dimmitt RA, Staley EM, Chuang G, Tanner SM, Soltau TD, Lorenz RG (2010) Role of postnatal acquisition of the intestinal microbiome in the early development of immune function. J Pediatr Gastroenterol Nutr 51(3): 262–273
10. Blaser MJ, Chen Y, Reibman J (2008) Does Helicobacter pylori protect against asthma and allergy? Gut 57(5):561–567
11. Amedei A, Cappon A, Codolo G, Cabrelle A, Polenghi A, Benagiano M, Tasca E, Azzurri A, D'Elios MM, Del Prete G, de Bernard M (2006) The neutrophil-activating protein of

Helicobacter pylori promotes Th1 immune responses. J Clin Invest 116(4):1092–1101
12. Shi Y, Liu XF, Zhuang Y, Zhang JY, Liu T, Yin Z, Wu C, Mao XH, Jia KR, Wang FJ, Guo H, Flavell RA, Zhao Z, Liu KY, Xiao B, Guo Y, Zhang WJ, Zhou WY, Guo G, Zou QM (2010) Helicobacter pylori-induced Th17 responses modulate Th1 cell responses, benefit bacterial growth, and contribute to pathology in mice. J Immunol 184(9):5121–5129
13. Kao JY, Zhang M, Miller MJ, Mills JC, Wang B, Liu M, Eaton KA, Zou W, Berndt BE, Cole TS, Takeuchi T, Owyang SY, Luther J (2010) Helicobacter pylori immune escape is mediated by dendritic cell-induced Treg skewing and Th17 suppression in mice. Gastroenterology 138(3):1046–1054
14. Schmitz JM, Durham CG, Ho SB, Lorenz RG (2009) Gastric mucus alterations associated with murine Helicobacter infection. J Histochem Cytochem 57(5):457–467
15. Tahara T, Arisawa T, Wang F, Shibata T, Nakamura M, Sakata M, Hirata I, Nakano H (2008) Toll-like receptor 2 (TLR)—196 to 174del polymorphism in gastro-duodenal diseases in Japanese population. Dig Dis Sci 53(4):919–924
16. la Trejo-de OA, Torres J, Perez-Rodriguez M, Camorlinga-Ponce M, Luna LF, Abdo-Francis JM, Lazcano E, Maldonado-Bernal C (2008) TLR4 single-nucleotide polymorphisms alter mucosal cytokine and chemokine patterns in Mexican patients with Helicobacter pylori-associated gastroduodenal diseases. Clin Immunol 129(2):333–340
17. Chen Y, Blaser MJ (2008) Helicobacter pylori colonization is inversely associated with childhood asthma. J Infect Dis 198(4):553–560
18. Johnson CC, Ownby DR, Alford SH, Havstad SL, Williams LK, Zoratti EM, Peterson EL, Joseph CL (2005) Antibiotic exposure in early infancy and risk for childhood atopy. J Allergy Clin Immunol 115(6):1218–1224
19. Schaub B, Lauener R, von Mutius E (2006) The many faces of the hygiene hypothesis. J Allergy Clin Immunol 117(5):969–977, quiz 978
20. Gueders MM, Paulissen G, Crahay C, Quesada-Calvo F, Hacha J, Van Hove C, Tournoy K, Louis R, Foidart JM, Noel A, Cataldo DD (2009) Mouse models of asthma: a comparison between C57BL/6 and BALB/c strains regarding bronchial responsiveness, inflammation, and cytokine production. Inflamm Res 58(12):845–854
21. Pastva A, Estell K, Schoeb TR, Atkinson TP, Schwiebert LM (2004) Aerobic exercise attenuates airway inflammatory responses in a mouse model of atopic asthma. J Immunol 172(7):4520–4526
22. Hewitt M, Estell K, Davis IC, Schwiebert LM (2010) Repeated bouts of moderate-intensity aerobic exercise reduce airway reactivity in a murine asthma model. Am J Respir Cell Mol Biol 42(2):243–249
23. Epstein MM (2004) Do mouse models of allergic asthma mimic clinical disease? Int Arch Allergy Immunol 133(1):84–100
24. Nials AT, Uddin S (2008) Mouse models of allergic asthma: acute and chronic allergen challenge. Dis Model Mech 1(4–5):213–220
25. Chomczynski P, Sacchi N (1987) Single-step method of RNA isolation by acid guanidinium thiocyanate-phenol-chloroform extraction. Anal Biochem 162(1):156–159
26. Bas A, Forsberg G, Hammarstrom S, Hammarstrom ML (2004) Utility of the housekeeping genes 18S rRNA, beta-actin and glyceraldehyde-3-phosphate-dehydrogenase for normalization in real-time quantitative reverse transcriptase-polymerase chain reaction analysis of gene expression in human T lymphocytes. Scand J Immunol 59(6):566–573
27. Guide to performing relative quantitation of gene expression using real-time quantitative PCR. Part#: 4371095 Rev B. Accessed via Applied Biosystems website on 05-10-13: www.3.appliedbiosystems.com/cms/groups/mob_support/documents/generaldocuments/cms_042380.pdf
28. Roth K, Kapadia S, Martin S, Lorenz R (1999) Cellular immune responses are essential for the development of Helicobacter felis-associated gastric pathology. J Immunol 163(3):1490–1497
29. Curtis JL, Warnock ML, Arraj SM, Kaltreider HB (1990) Histologic analysis of an immune response in the lung parenchyma of mice. Angiopathy accompanies inflammatory cell influx. Am J Pathol 137(3):689–699
30. Brown JK, Pemberton AD, Wright SH, Miller HR (2004) Primary antibody-Fab fragment complexes: a flexible alternative to traditional direct and indirect immunolabeling techniques. J Histochem Cytochem 52(9):1219–1230
31. Ropenga A, Chapel A, Vandamme M, Griffiths NM (2004) Use of reference gene expression in rat distal colon after radiation exposure: a caveat. Radiat Res 161(5):597–602
32. Rubie C, Kempf K, Hans J, Su T, Tilton B, Georg T, Brittner B, Ludwig B, Schilling M (2005) Housekeeping gene variability in normal and cancerous colorectal, pancreatic, esophageal, gastric and hepatic tissues. Mol Cell Probes 19(2):101–109

Chapter 22

Expression Profiling to Identify Candidate Genes Associated with Allergic Phenotypes

Willie June Brickey

Abstract

Transcript profiling reveals valuable insights to molecular and cellular activity related to disease. Gene expression profiles provide clues as to how tissues or cells in a particular environment may respond to stimuli. Gene-targeted examination of transcript changes is accomplished by employing a quantitative PCR approach using cDNA prepared from isolated RNA.

Key words Transcript, Profiling, Quantitative PCR, Allergy

1 Introduction

Allergy is characterized by the presence and activity of many cell types, including eosinophils, mast cells, natural killer cells, macrophages, and neutrophils. In addition to leukocyte populations, additional specialized cell types also play a role during allergy-induced asthma, including smooth muscle cells, epithelia, and endothelia. Inflammatory factors, such as cytokines, chemokines, transcriptional regulators, cell surface markers, cell signaling activators, and mediators, influence allergic and immunogenic responses that may result in chronic inflammation, hyperactivity, and/or tissue remodeling. By examining cell- or tissue-specific molecular changes or profiles, mechanisms that initiate disease and/or propagate symptoms may be revealed. Additionally, gene expression profiling supports the identification of candidates for therapeutic targets that may either ameliorate or prevent disease.

Global transcript approaches in which >1,000 genes are assessed simultaneously include the use of genome-wide microarrays and direct sequencing from isolated nucleic acids or protein-bound DNA fragments. Common examples of these techniques include whole transcriptome shotgun sequencing or RNA sequencing (RNA-Seq) and chromatin immunoprecipitation (ChIP)-Seq.

Irving C. Allen (ed.), *Mouse Models of Allergic Disease: Methods and Protocols*, Methods in Molecular Biology, vol. 1032, DOI 10.1007/978-1-62703-496-8_22, © Springer Science+Business Media, LLC 2013

Additional levels of regulation may be discovered by analyzing alternatively spliced gene products and microRNA species. Overall, several reports utilizing technology-driven approaches and gene-targeted PCR applications have demonstrated the complexity of cellular interactions and responses to allergen and treatment in asthma and other allergic diseases [1–8]. As these high-throughput profiling methods require much more advanced technology, expensive equipment and reagents, expertise, and sophisticated data analysis capabilities, they will not be presented here.

Here, we present protocols for gene-targeted quantitative PCR (qPCR). These molecular approaches are utilized to obtain qualitative and quantitative data about gene expression in isolated cells or tissues. The first step in profiling gene expression is to obtain high-quality RNA. Next, reverse transcription (RT) is performed to produce complementary DNA (cDNA) that is used as a template for PCR amplification. Gene expression profiles or changes are determined by analyzing PCR products using sequence-specific probes plus forward and reverse primers (i.e., TaqMan®-mediated amplification) or the intercalation of a fluorescent molecule such as SYBR® Green with forward and reverse primers. These molecular approaches for gene analysis are relatively easy and straightforward to perform, which makes qPCR a critical technique for examining and validating potential therapeutic targets and/or diagnostic genes that are related to allergic disease.

2 Materials

1. Protective equipment: Fume hood or biological safety cabinet, gloves, goggles, lab coat.
2. Tissue or cell source.
3. Liquid nitrogen or dry ice plus a 95 % ethanol freezing bath.
4. Freezers: –80 and –20 °C.
5. RNaseZap® for surface decontamination.
6. Tissue disrupter: Homogenizer, tissue lyser, or bead mill with beads of appropriate size and density.
7. RNA isolation reagent: Phenol/guanidine thiocyanate, TRIzol®.
8. Alternative: RNA isolation kits or reagents; RNA*later*® for temporary tissue storage prior to RNA isolation.
9. Chloroform.
10. Isopropyl alcohol.
11. 70 % Ethanol.
12. 100 % Ethanol.
13. Sterile, deionized water (RNase-free).

14. Eppendorf tubes and cryovials.
15. Alternative: Spin columns.
16. Spectrophotometer (i.e., Nanodrop).
17. Pipettors (2, 10, 200, 1,000 μl).
18. 384-Well or 96-well PCR plate, depending on real-time PCR thermocycler used to evaluate expression; with optically transparent adhesive film for sealing of plate prior to loading into thermocycler.
19. 384-Well or 96-well thermocycler.
20. Enzymes: Reverse transcriptase, RNase inhibitor, Taq DNA polymerase.
21. Molecular reagents for reverse transcription: Primers [random hexamer and oligo d(T) nucleotide]; deoxynucleotide mix: 10 mM each of dGTP, dATP, dCTP, dTTP; 0.1 M dithiothreitol (DTT); 10× reaction buffer (supplied with enzyme from commercial sources or 500 mM KCl, 30 mM $MgCl_2$, 1 M Tris–HCl pH 9.3); reverse transcriptase.
22. Molecular reagents for qPCR: cDNA template; gene-specific primers (forward, reverse, probe); 10× PCR buffer supplied with DNA polymerase; SYBR® Green dye-containing PCR and enzyme reaction mix; dNTP mix: 10 mM each of dGTP, dATP, dCTP, dTTP.
23. Glycogen; amplicon-containing DNA plasmid to use as standardization control.

3 Methods

3.1 RNA Isolation

1. Dissect tissue from animal or isolate cells.
2. Flash freeze tissue or isolated cells and store at −80 °C (*see* **Note 1**).
3. Process tissue in phenol/guanidine thiocyanate reagent (*see* **Note 2**): Place 100–200 mg of frozen tissue in a 2 ml screw top cryovial with a ring in the cap; add beads (~25 % of space in cryovial) and 1 ml of TRIzol® reagent (Life Technologies). Then agitate for short pulses interspersed with periods of rest on ice, to prevent the heating of samples prior to complete tissue dispersal. (For example, with lung tissue: use 1.4 mm ceramic beads and shake in the bead mill for 40 s, rest for ≥20 s, and repeat with a 40 s pulse.) Transfer the homogenate to a fresh tube and continue with sample processing as directed by the manufacturer's protocol.
4. Follow the manufacturer's suggested protocol to isolate RNA from lysate by separating the aqueous from organic phases and

precipitating nucleic acid in isopropyl alcohol (*see* **Notes 3** and **4**).

5. Dissolve precipitated RNA in RNase-free water (or Tris–EDTA) and store RNA at −80 °C.
6. Assess spectral features (i.e., absorbance at 260 and 280 nm) to determine quantity and purity of RNA (*see* **Note 5**).

3.2 Production of cDNA by Reverse Transcription

1. Set up reactions by combining RNA, primer, RNase inhibitor, reverse transcriptase, deoxynucleotides, and reverse transcription buffer in an Eppendorf snap-cap tube (*see* **Note 6**).
2. Incubate according to the manufacturer's guidelines for the reverse transcriptase (*see* **Note 7**).
3. Store cDNA at −20 °C.

3.3 Quantitative PCR Amplification

1. Determine the gene or the gene targets of interest. Obtain commercially available primers or generate appropriate primers based on known gene sequences (*see* **Note 8**).
2. Set up reactions for qPCR by first aliquoting the template, which is usually diluted at least 2–5 fold in RNase-free water, into a PCR plate. Prepare the master mix for each target, containing primers plus Taq DNA polymerase in the reaction buffer. Aliquot the prepared master mix onto a PCR plate (*see* **Note 9**).
3. Perform PCR amplification using a 96-well or a 384-well thermocycler to determine either absolute or relative changes in expression. Include a melting curve step if using SYBR® Green dye incorporation. SYBR® Green dye is a useful way to assess the homogeneity of the amplified product, suggesting the production of a single species. Alternative multiplex profiling approaches using PCR profiling arrays can be performed (*see* **Note 10**).

3.4 Data Analysis

1. Determine the quantity of amplified product using the software package that is supplied with the thermocycler.
2. Utilize a plasmid standard that contains the amplified gene product to determine the absolute quantity of the target gene (*see* **Note 11**).
3. Simultaneously amplify an internal control target for each biological sample using primers to detect a housekeeping gene (*see* **Note 12**).
4. Determine the relative quantity using C_T analysis (*see* **Note 13**).

4 Notes

1. To preserve tissue, flash freeze in a cryovial in liquid nitrogen (or using ethanol plus a dry ice chilling bath). Store samples at −80 °C. Alternatively, RNA*later*® or a similar reagent can be

used to store fresh tissue prior to disruption. RNA*later*® rapidly permeates fresh tissue, inactivates RNases, and stabilizes RNA within tissues or cells, thereby eliminating the requirement for immediate freezing of biological samples during the harvest or the isolation. Tissue can be stored in RNA*later*® at 4 °C for 1 month or −20 °C indefinitely prior to tissue disruption.

2. Many alternatives exist for tissue/cell disruption. The first factor is the solubilizing extraction agent [9], which may include but is not limited to TRIzol® or TRIsure® (Bioline). A 1:5 volume ratio of tissue to extraction reagent is typically utilized. Alternatively, RNA isolation kits based on spin columns using affinity of nucleic acids to silica-based matrices and specific for nucleic acids of interest are commercially available. The second factor entails the physical disruption method. Tissue homogenizers with blades grind tissues, with adverse consequences of foaming, aerosol formation, and challenges with cleaning in between sample application. As an alternative, bead mills are used to disrupt samples and release nucleic acids by "cracking" specimens against glass, ceramic, or steel beads during vigorous agitation. Bead mills permit high-throughput processing with multiple samples in individual cryovials while minimizing foaming effects. The choice of beads depends on the density and fibrous nature of the tissue from which the RNA will be extracted. A third low-technology approach entails pulverizing frozen tissue in liquid nitrogen using a mortar and pestle. However, this approach requires the maintenance of the frozen state of samples and increased time for processing of individual samples.

3. Follow laboratory safety procedures by using hazardous chemicals in a fume hood. Always wear personal protective equipment (i.e., gloves, goggles, lab coat) when handling hazardous reagents such as phenol and chloroform.

4. Prior to RNA work, the lab bench area should be carefully cleaned and treated with 70 % ethanol or RNaseZap®. Similar reagents can be used to reduce RNase contamination from surfaces. If possible, maintain a region of the lab or the bench dedicated to RNA work. Always use aerosol-barrier tips and ultrapure water. Diethylpyrocarbonate or DEPC-treated water to remove nucleases is not necessary for these protocols.

5. Nanodrop spectrophotometers are very easy to use and require only 1 μl of undiluted RNA for analysis. The absorbance ratio (260 nm/280 nm) for RNA should be 1.8–2.0. The RNA concentration is determined (automatically) by the following: μg/ml RNA = absorbance at 260 nm × dilution × 40 μg/ml.

6. Generating complementary DNA can be accomplished in several ways. Total RNA can be reverse transcribed in the presence of random hexamer and nonamer or using oligonucleotide d(T)

primers that preferentially bind to polyadenylated RNA species. An example of an RT reaction of 25 μl consists of the following: RNA template (0.1 to 2 μg), 1.25 μl of RNase inhibitor, 10 mM of primer, dNTP mix (10 mM each of dGTP, dATP, dCTP, dTTP), reverse transcriptase, 2.5 μl of 0.1 M DTT and 2.5 μl of 10× PCR buffer, and water.

7. Incubation of the cDNA reaction mix can be accomplished using a thermocycler, heated chamber, hybridization oven, or water bath. Use the established temperature and time (including activation and inactivation steps) according to the specifications for the enzyme. For example, 37 °C for 50 min is optimal for M-MLV reverse transcriptase, while SuperscriptIII reverse transcriptase conditions specify 50 °C for 50 min.
8. Since the sequences of most genomes and genes have been identified, there are many commercial sources for primers, with Applied Biosystems® at Life Technologies being a primary source. The online database of reagents can be searched using several criteria, including species, gene ID, name, or even sequence. Bioinformatics tools to obtain target sequences include Basic Local Alignment Search Tool (BLAST) from NCBI, Ensembl Genome Browser, and UCSC Genome Browser. However, primers can be designed de novo and examples of primer design algorithms include http://www.ncbi.nlm.nih.gov/tools/primer-blast/, Primer design, and Primer Express. In general, primer and probe sets should have the following features: the oligonucleotide primers should bind across exon junctions to insure that RNA-derived cDNA is amplified over contaminating genomic DNA; the melting temperature of the probe should be the highest, with the optimal differences being 10 °C greater than the forward and reverse primers that have T_m of 55–65 °C; the amplified product should be 60–150 bp long; and the length of the primers should be similar (~20 bp) with no guanosines located at the 5′ terminus of the probe, which would prevent the addition of the fluorescent label.
9. qPCR reaction setup is directed according to the reagents used. In general, it is critical to assay multiple biological replicates and technical replicates (i.e., three reactions for each condition and each template) in addition to non-template and internal reference controls (*see* **Note 12**). A TaqMan®-based detection method uses two primers plus probe labeled with a 5′ fluorescent reporter tag and a 3′ quencher in a prepared reaction mix to assess amplification of a specific PCR product. For example, a 15 μl total volume reaction would contain 7.5 μl of 2× PCR master mix, 0.6 μl of each of primer (10 μM), 0.15 μl of probe (10 μM), template, and water. A SYBR® Green-based detection method uses two primers with a dye

that binds to double-stranded DNA to detect accumulating PCR products. In this case, a 10 μl reaction mix would contain the following: 5 μl of 2× SYBR® Green reaction mix, 0.4 μl of each of primer (10 μM), template, and water. Always prepare master mixes, just before loading onto a PCR plate following the addition of the diluted template. Always include an excess amount of master mix to compensate for any pipetting-induced errors.

10. PCR profiling arrays offer an alternative multiplex profiling approach that supports disease-specific or pathway-focused gene expression studies. PCR profiling arrays simultaneously determine the expression levels of about 80 genes. These pre-plated commercial PCR arrays are typically accompanied with ready-to-use master mixes. Likewise, these arrays provide expression profiling gene primers, housekeeping primers, and RNA quality control targets. Essentially, cDNA that is synthesized from 25 ng to 5 μg of total RNA is mixed with the prepared PCR master mix, aliquoted to wells in a 96-well plate, and then subjected to PCR amplification and analysis, following the manufacturers' protocols.

11. To estimate an absolute quantity of transcript, linear regression based on a known quantity of input molecules must be generated. One approach is to use a plasmid DNA-based standard that contains the PCR amplicon of interest cloned into a vector. The TOPO® TA cloning vector (Invitrogen/Life Technologies) has been specifically designed for subcloning PCR products that contain a single AT base overhang. The plasmid DNA is then harvested from bacteria and molecular amounts are quantified by spectral assessment at 260 nm. The number of molecules is determined based on the following: μg/μl (based on $OD_{260\ nm}$) × (1×10^{-6} g/μg) × (1×10^{18} attomol)/(650 g/bp) × (bp of plasmid) = attomol/μl, where 1 attomol is 602,500 molecules. Prepare dilutions of 500 attomol/μl and then 15 attomol/μl using 0.1 mg/ml of glycogen, an inert carrier, dissolved in water. Subsequently four to five serial 5 to 15-fold dilution aliquots of the plasmid standard are prepared and analyzed to generate standard linear regression statistics. The most efficient PCR amplification will give a line with a slope of −3.3 and correlation coefficient R^2 of 0.99.

12. An internal control used as a normalization reference should be assessed for each sample. These typically consist of gene(s) that should be ubiquitously expressed in many cell types and for which expression does not vary with changes in conditions. These housekeeping genes (i.e., β-actin, tubulin, β2 microglobulin, hypoxanthine phosphoribosyltransferase, glyceraldehyde-3-phosphate dehydrogenase, and ribosomal protein genes) should be analyzed for each cell type as their utility as internal

references is controversial [10–12]. Additionally, the 18S rRNA gene is also used as an internal reference even though this gene is transcribed in greater abundance by RNA polymerase III in contrast to RNA polymerase II-transcribed genes.

13. C_T (or threshold cycle) is a relative measure of PCR product generation and is determined where the amplification curve crosses the threshold of product detection. The comparative C_T method may be employed to determine relative changes in expression compared to an internal reference from the control with a change in condition [13, 14]. The relative amount of target is calculated to be $2^{-(\Delta\Delta C_T)}$ or the fold change in gene expression normalized to an endogenous reference gene and relative to the untreated control. In other words, first normalize gene expression of the target to a reference using the difference in C_T ($\Delta C_T = C_T$ target − C_T reference). Next, determine the change with treatment or tissue type using the difference in ΔC_T ($\Delta\Delta C_T = \Delta C_T$ condition/tissue of interest − ΔC_T untreated control/base tissue).

Acknowledgments

This work was supported by National Institute of Allergy and Infectious Disease grant U19-AI077437 and Radiation Countermeasures Center of Research Excellence (RadCCORE) subcontract U19-AI067798. The technical expertise of Michael Thompson and Karen McKinnon is gratefully acknowledged.

References

1. Alexis NE, Brickey WJ, Lay JC, Wang Y, Roubey RA, Ting JP, Peden DB (2002) Development of an inhaled endotoxin challenge protocol for characterizing evoked cell surface phenotype and genomic responses of airway cells in allergic individuals. Ann N Y Acad Sci 975:148–159
2. Bogaert P, Naessens T, De Koker S, Hennuy B, Hacha J, Smet M, Cataldo D, Di Valentin E, Piette J, Tournoy KG, Grooten J (2011) Inflammatory signatures for eosinophilic vs. neutrophilic allergic pulmonary inflammation reveal critical regulatory checkpoints. Am J Physiol Lung Cell Mol Physiol 300: L679–L690
3. Brickey WJ, Alexis NE, Hernandez ML, Reed W, Ting JP, Peden DB (2011) Sputum inflammatory cells from patients with allergic rhinitis and asthma have decreased inflammasome gene expression. J Allergy Clin Immunol 128:900–903
4. Daheshia M, Tian N, Connolly T, Drawid A, Wu Q, Bienvenu JG, Cavallo J, Jupp R, De Sanctis GT, Minnich A (2008) Molecular characterization of antigen-induced lung inflammation in a murine model of asthma. Ann Allergy Asthma Immunol 100:206–215
5. Di Valentin E, Crahay C, Garbacki N, Hennuy B, Guéders M, Noël A, Foidart JM, Grooten J, Colige A, Piette J, Cataldo D (2009) New asthma biomarkers: lessons from murine models of acute and chronic asthma. Am J Physiol Lung Cell Mol Physiol 296:L185–L197
6. Follettie MT, Ellis DK, Donaldson DD, Hill AA, Diesl V, DeClercq C, Sypek JP, Dorner AJ, Wills-Karp M (2006) Gene expression analysis in a murine model of allergic asthma reveals overlapping disease and therapy dependent

pathways in the lung. Pharmacogenomics J 6:141–152

7. Hernandez M, Brickey WJ, Alexis NE, Fry RC, Rager JE, Zhou B, Ting JP, Zhou H, Peden DB (2012) Airway cells from atopic asthmatic patients exposed to ozone display an enhanced innate immune gene profile. J Allergy Clin Immunol 129(259–261):e1–e2
8. Yu M, Eckart MR, Morgan AA, Mukai K, Butte AJ, Tsai M, Galli SJ (2011) Identification of an IFN-γ/mast cell axis in a mouse model of chronic asthma. J Clin Invest 121:3133–3143
9. Chomczynski P, Sacchi N (2006) The single-step method of RNA isolation by acid guanidinium thiocyanate-phenol-chloroform extraction. Nat Protoc 1:581–585
10. Bustin SA (2000) Absolute quantification of mRNA using real-time reverse transcription polymerase chain reaction assays. J Mol Endocrinol 25:169–193
11. Schmittgen TD, Zakrajsek BA (2000) Effect of experimental treatment on housekeeping gene expression: validation by real-time, quantitative RT-PCR. J Biochem Biophys Methods 46:69–81
12. Suzuki T, Higgins PJ, Crawford DR (2000) Control selection for RNA quantitation. Biotechniques 29:332–337
13. Livak KJ, Schmittgen TD (2001) Analysis of relative gene expression data using real-time quantitative PCR and the 2(-Delta Delta C(T)) Method. Methods 25: 402–408
14. Schmittgen TD, Livak KJ (2008) Analyzing real-time PCR data by the comparative C(T) method. Nat Protoc 3:1101–1108

Chapter 23

Flow Cytometric Methods for the Assessment of Allergic Disease

Adeeb H. Rahman

Abstract

Multiparametric flow cytometry is a powerful technique that allows the quantification and characterization of heterogeneous populations of cells. Advances in flow cytometric instrumentation, software, and reagents are occurring at a rapid pace, and flow cytometric methods are increasingly being applied to better understand cellular responses associated with a diverse array of disease conditions. This chapter provides an overview of some common applications of flow cytometry in characterizing mouse models of allergic airway disease.

Key words Allergy, Lung, Flow cytometry, FACS

1 Introduction

Allergic airway inflammation can involve multiple immune cell subsets including macrophages, dendritic cells, eosinophils, neutrophils, B lymphocytes, T lymphocytes, and natural killer cells. Accurately characterizing the cellular infiltration of the lungs is therefore an important component of investigating the immunological mechanisms responsible for the initiation and progression of allergic airway disease. This has historically been accomplished by cytocentrifugation and differential staining of cells recovered from a bronchoalveolar lavage (BAL), which allows identification of neutrophils, eosinophils, monocytes, and lymphocytes based on morphology and nuclear characteristics. However, this approach is limited in its ability to identify rare cells or accurately distinguish between biologically distinct populations of cells that do not dramatically differ in cellular morphology.

Flow cytometry employs fluorescently conjugated antibodies to identify the phenotypes of individual cells within a heterogeneous population. Multiparametric flow cytometry thereby allows extensive quantitative identification and characterization of a much

Irving C. Allen (ed.), *Mouse Models of Allergic Disease: Methods and Protocols*, Methods in Molecular Biology, vol. 1032, DOI 10.1007/978-1-62703-496-8_23, © Springer Science+Business Media, LLC 2013

broader range of cell populations than traditional differential staining. Recent advances in flow cytometry instrumentation, software, and reagents have greatly enhanced our ability to simultaneously assess the expression of multiple cell markers, which has led to an improved appreciation of the complexity and heterogeneity of the immune response in multiple inflammatory conditions. This chapter discusses some of the common applications of flow cytometry in assessing allergic airway disease.

1.1 Selecting Markers to Phenotypically Characterize Heterogeneous Populations of Cells

While multiparametric flow cytometric methods are increasingly being applied to mouse models of allergic disease, the field is still developing and has yet to reach consensus on the best markers and phenotyping schemes with which to characterize specific models. Thus, marker selection largely depends on the specific experimental objective. For example, an investigator may wish to simply determine the frequency of CD4+ T lymphocytes infiltrating the lungs, which will require a very different set of markers than those used to assess the activation status of lung dendritic cells.

A universal consideration in developing accurate phenotyping schemes is to examine a sufficient number of markers to accurately identify the population of interest. This is easy to accomplish when a population is identifiable by a highly specific marker, but can be challenging when attempting to discriminate between populations with shared or overlapping marker expression. As a general principle, the greater the number of markers that are simultaneously examined, the better the ability to resolve distinct subsets and accurately capture the overall heterogeneity of a population. However, increasing the number of markers requires careful validation of fluorochrome combinations and is ultimately limited by the detectors on the available instrument and the number of fluorochromes that can be simultaneously resolved based on their emission spectra.

The choice of fluorochromes that can be used in an experiment is largely determined by the instrument available to analyze the samples. For example, a BD LSRII with multiple spatially separated lasers will allow the simultaneous analysis of a much broader range of fluorochromes than a BD Calibur. It is therefore important to first determine the lasers and detectors that are available on the cytometer that is to be used for analysis before designing panels of compatible fluorochromes (*see* **Note 1**).

1.2 Fluorescence-Activated Cell Sorting

Fluorescence-activated cell sorting (FACS) is a natural extension of flow cytometric analysis and allows subsets identified in a heterogeneous mixture to be isolated and collected as highly purified viable populations. These sorted cells can then be used for a range of downstream applications, including in vitro experiments, gene expression profiling, and adoptive transfer. The protocols for preparing cells for FACS are largely identical to those used for general flow cytometric analysis, but may need to be scaled up in order to recover adequate number of cells for downstream applications. FACS also requires more complex and expensive cytometric instrumentation than normal flow cytometric analysis, and access to cell sorters is often more limited than to analyzers. Therefore, experiments involving FACS generally warrant more careful advance planning and scheduling, and it is generally advisable to first validate flow cytometry protocols on a normal analyzer before progressing to cell sorting.

1.3 Intracellular Cytokine Detection

In addition to identifying markers expressed on the surface of cells, flow cytometry can also be used to detect intracellular markers. This technique can be used to identify phosphorylated signaling proteins or cytokine production in individual cells, thereby allowing a detailed assessment of functional responses in a heterogeneous population. Given that lung inflammation is thought to be mediated by Th2-polarized CD4+ T cells, intracellular cytokine staining has historically been applied to allergy models to determine the proportion of Th1 and Th2 cells infiltrating the lungs [1, 2]. With the advent of more complex multiparametric flow cytometry, this analysis can be expanded to also simultaneously identify Th9 and Th17 subsets, which have also recently been implicated in the pathology of airway inflammation [3, 4]. While this type of analysis can be accomplished by individually examining the expression of canonical cytokines associated with each of these Th subsets, examining them simultaneously allows the identification of cells that coexpress various combinations of cytokines, thereby providing a more accurate representation of the functional and phenotypic heterogeneity within a population.

2 Materials

2.1 Cell Isolation

1. Experimental mice sensitized and challenged with ovalbumin and appropriately matched control mice.
2. Equipment: Dissecting scissors; fine-tipped forceps; tracheal cannula; 30-G needles; 1 ml syringes; 10 ml syringes and surgical thread (4–0 silk); 30 mm culture dishes; 70 μm nylon cell strainers; 50 ml polypropylene conical centrifuge tubes; and a refrigerated centrifuge.
3. Stock solution of Hank's buffered salt solution (HBSS) without calcium or magnesium.
4. Stock solution of 0.5 M EDTA, pH 8.0.
5. Stock solution of RPMI 1640 medium.
6. Stock solution of penicillin–streptomycin (10,000 I.U. penicillin and 10 mg/ml streptomycin).

7. 100 % bovine serum albumin (BSA).
8. 100 % fetal bovine serum (FBS), standard grade, heat inactivated.
9. DNase I.
10. Collagenase type I.
11. BAL buffer: HBSS with 0.5 % BSA and 0.5 mM EDTA.
12. Digestion buffer (prepare on the day of the experiment): RPMI supplemented with 10 % FBS, 50 I.U./50 μg/ml of penicillin–streptomycin, 1.5 mg/ml of collagenase, and 150 μg/ml of DNase I.
13. ACK lysis buffer: 8.024 mg/l of NH_4Cl, 1.001 mg/l of $KHCO_3$, 3.722 mg/l of Na_2EDTA, pH 7.4.

2.2 Antibody Staining and Flow Cytometric Analysis

1. Equipment: 12 × 75 mm polystyrene round-bottom tubes; a refrigerated centrifuge; and a flow cytometer.
2. Fc block: Purified anti-mouse CD16/CD32 monoclonal antibody, clone 2.4G2 (*see* **Note 2**).
3. FACS buffer: HBSS with 1 % FCS and 0.3 mM EDTA.
4. FACS blocking buffer: FACS buffer with 5 μg/ml of Fc block.
5. Monoclonal antibodies (*see* **Note 3**).
6. Viability dye (e.g., LIVE/DEAD® Fixable Dead Cell Stains, *see* **Note 4**).
7. BD CompBeads (*see* **Note 5**).

2.3 Cellular Activation for Intracellular Cytokine Detection

1. Sterile round-bottom 96-well culture plate.
2. Culture medium: RPMI 1640 supplemented with 10 % FCS, 50 μg/ml of penicillin–streptomycin, and 2 mM L-glutamine.
3. Dimethyl sulfoxide (DMSO, ACS reagent grade).
4. Brefeldin A (BFA): Prepare a stock solution at a concentration of 10 mg/ml in DMSO and store at 4 °C.
5. DNase I: Prepare a stock solution at a concentration of 2 mg/ml in sterile PBS and store in small aliquots at −20 °C.
6. Ovalbumin: Prepare a stock of 50 mg/ml in sterile deionized water and store in small aliquots at −20 °C.
7. Phorbol 12-myristate 13-acetate (PMA): Prepare a stock solution at a concentration of 1 mg/ml in DMSO and store in small aliquots at −20 °C.
8. Ionomycin: Prepare a stock solution at a concentration of 1 mg/ml in DMSO and store in small aliquots at −20 °C.
9. Cell culture-grade monoclonal anti-CD28 antibody (clone 37.51).
10. Cytofix/Cytoperm Fixation/Permeabilization kit (BD Biosciences).

3 Methods

3.1 Preparing a Single-Cell Suspension of Airway Cells (See Note 6)

1. Obtain experimental mice that have been sensitized and challenged with ovalbumin and appropriately matched control mice.
2. Working with one mouse at a time, euthanize the mouse by CO_2 asphyxiation, but do not perform a cervical dislocation. Proceed immediately with the following steps.
3. Place the mouse in a supine position and wipe down the neck and chest area with 70 % ethanol.
4. Make a vertical incision over the upper thoracic cavity and carefully remove the skin and muscle tissue to expose the trachea.
5. Pull up the trachea with tweezers and insert a length of surgical thread behind the trachea and on top of the esophagus.
6. Make a small horizontal incision between two tracheal rings.
7. Insert a tracheal cannula into the incision and secure it to the trachea using the surgical thread.
8. Fill a 1 ml syringe with 900 ml of BAL buffer and fit it to the tracheal cannula.
9. Slowly inject the buffer to fully inflate the lungs and then slowly withdraw the fluid. Transfer the recovered buffer to a 15 ml conical tube and store on ice (*see* **Note 7**).
10. Repeat **steps 8** and **9** three more times to collect approximately 3 and 4 ml of fluid.
11. Centrifuge cells at 300 × *g* for 5 min at 4 °C.
12. Aspirate the supernatant and resuspend the pellet in 1 ml of ACK lysis buffer. Gently swirl the tube for 30–60 s to lyse any residual red blood cells.
13. Fill the tube with HBSS and centrifuge at 300 × *g* for 5 min at 4 °C.
14. Aspirate the supernatant and resuspend the cells in 1 ml of FACS buffer until ready to proceed with cell stimulation for intracellular cytokine detection (*see* Subheading 3.3) or antibody staining to identify cell surface markers (*see* Subheading 3.4).

3.2 Preparing Single-Cell Suspensions of Total Lung and Lung-Draining Lymph Nodes (See Note 6)

1. Obtain experimental mice that have been sensitized and challenged with ovalbumin and appropriately matched control mice (*see* **Note 8**).
2. Euthanize a single mouse by CO_2 asphyxiation, but do not perform a cervical dislocation.
3. Place the mouse in a supine position and wipe down the neck and chest area with 70 % ethanol.
4. Make a vertical incision over the thoracic cavity and carefully remove the skin and muscle tissue. Retract the rib cage to expose the lungs and heart.

5. Carefully remove the mediastinal lymph nodes found below the thymus under the right side of the heart. These lymph nodes can be challenging to find in a naïve mouse, but are generally enlarged in inflamed mice making them easier to identify. Place the lymph nodes into 1 ml of digestion buffer in a 35 mm culture dish and store on ice until the lungs have been isolated.
6. Fill a 10 ml syringe with HBSS and fit it with a 30 G needle. Insert the needle into the right ventricle and maneuver it towards the pulmonary artery. Make a small incision in the left atrium. Very gently perfuse the HBSS to clear cells from the pulmonary circulation. The lungs should turn white during the perfusion step. An additional 10 ml of HBSS can be perfused if adequate perfusion is not achieved on the first pass.
7. Dissect the lung lobes and place them in 5 ml of digestion buffer in a 35-mm culture dish.
8. Use two 30 G needles to break open the lymph nodes. Use a scalpel or a scissors to mince the lung into small pieces. Incubate the dishes at 37 °C for 30 min to allow enzymatic digestion of the tissue.
9. Transfer the lung and lymph node suspensions to separate 50 ml conical tubes passing them through a 70 μm nylon cell strainer. Use the plunger of a syringe to gently mash the residual tissue on the filter. Wash the filter two times with 10 ml of FACS buffer and keep the cell suspensions on ice until the tissues have been harvested from all the animals.
10. Repeat **steps 2–11** for each individual mouse.
11. Centrifuge the cells at 300 × *g* for 5 min at 4 °C.
12. Aspirate the supernatant and resuspend the pellets in 1 ml of ACK lysis buffer. Swirl the tubes for 30–60 s to lyse any residual red blood cells. Add 15 ml of HBSS and centrifuge the cells at 300 × *g* for 5 min at 4 °C.
13. Aspirate the supernatant and resuspend the cells in 1 ml of FACS buffer until ready to proceed with cell stimulation for intracellular cytokine detection (*see* Subheading 3.3) or antibody staining to identify cell surface markers (*see* Subheading 3.4).

3.3 Ex Vivo Restimulation to Induce Cytokine Production (See Note 9)

1. Count the cells and resuspend them in culture medium at a density of 0.2–2 × 10^6 cells/100 μl (*see* **Note 10**).
2. Label a 96-well U-bottom plate to identify samples and stimulation conditions. Pipet 100 μl of the cell suspensions into each of the appropriate wells.
3. Prepare an appropriate volume of 2× restimulation media using culture media supplemented with the components indicated in Table 1 (*see* **Note 11**).

Table 1
Composition of restimulation media

DNase I	40 μg/ml (1:50 dilution of stock)
Brefeldin A	20 μg/ml (1:500 dilution of stock)
(1) Ovalbumin or	1 mg/ml (1:50 dilution of stock)
(2) PMA and	100 ng/ml (1:10,000 dilution of stock)
Ionomycin or	1 μg/ml (1:1,000 dilution of stock)
(3) DMSO	1:1,000 dilution

The components listed in the above table should be added to the culture media for ex vivo cell restimulation to induce cytokine production

4. Add 100 μl of the appropriate 2× restimulation medium to the 100 μl of cells in the wells and mix well.
5. Incubate for 5 h in an incubator at 37 °C with 5 % CO_2.
6. After incubation, proceed to centrifugation of the plate at 300 × *g* for 4 min at room temperature.
7. Rapidly invert the plate to discard the supernatant into a waste container and gently blot the plate onto a paper towel.
8. Resuspend the cells in 200 ml of FACS buffer and proceed to **step 2** of the antibody staining protocol (Subheading 3.4) (*see* **Note 12**).

3.4 Antibody Staining to Phenotype Heterogeneous Cell Populations

1. Divide the cells into an appropriate number of wells on a 96-well round-bottomed plate (*see* **Note 12**) based on the number of available cells and the number of separate staining panels that are to be used.
2. Centrifuge the plate at 300 × *g* for 4 min at 4 °C.
3. Rapidly invert the plate to discard the supernatant into a waste container and gently blot the plate onto a paper towel.
4. Resuspend cells in 100 μl of FACS blocking buffer and leave on ice for at least 10 min.
5. Prepare antibody master mixes in FACS blocking buffer for each staining panel. The specific combination of antibodies in the master mix will depend on the experimental objectives and the available cytometer (*see* **Note 4**). Master mixes should allow for a final staining volume of 100 μl/sample and should include each of the antibodies at a concentration predetermined by titration. This will typically be in the range of 0.2–2 μl/100 μl of buffer.
6. Add 100 μl of FACS buffer to each of the wells.

7. Centrifuge at 300 × *g* for 4 min at 4 °C.
8. Rapidly invert the plate to discard the supernatant into a waste container and gently blot the plate onto a paper towel.
9. Add 100 μl of the appropriate antibody master mix to each well.
10. Incubate for 30 min at 4 °C in the dark.
11. Add 100 μl of FACS buffer to each of the wells.
12. Centrifuge at 300 × *g* for 4 min at 4 °C.
13. Rapidly invert the plate to discard the supernatant into a waste container and gently blot the plate onto a paper towel.
14. Resuspend the cells in 200 μl of FACS buffer.
15. Centrifuge at 300 × *g* for 4 min at 4 °C.
16. Rapidly invert the plate to discard the supernatant into a waste container and gently blot the plate onto a paper towel.
17. If staining for intracellular cytokines, proceed to Subheading 3.5. Alternatively, if the analysis only involves cell surface markers, then resuspend the samples in 250 μl of FACS buffer and transfer them to tubes that are compatible with the available cytometer (e.g., 12 × 75 mm polystyrene round-bottom tubes). Store the samples at 4 °C in the dark until analysis (*see* **Note 13**).
18. Use CompBeads to prepare an unstained and single-stained compensation controls individually stained with each of the antibodies used in the master mix (*see* **Notes 5** and **14**).

3.5 Antibody Staining to Identify Intracellular Cytokines

1. Resuspend the cells in 100 μl of Cytofix–Cytoperm buffer and mix well (*see* **Note 15**).
2. Incubate for 20 min at room temperature in the dark (*see* **Note 16**).
3. Add 100 μl of 1× perm/wash buffer to each of the wells.
4. Centrifuge at 300 × *g* for 4 min at 4 °C.
5. Rapidly invert the plate to discard the supernatant into a waste container and gently blot the plate onto a paper towel.
6. Resuspend the cells in 200 μl of 1× perm/wash buffer.
7. Prepare an intracellular staining antibody master mix in 1× perm/wash buffer allowing for a final staining volume of 100 μl/sample. The specific combination of antibodies in the master mix will depend on the experimental objectives and the available cytometer (*see* **Note 17**).
8. Centrifuge at 300 × *g* for 4 min at 4 °C.
9. Rapidly invert the plate to discard the supernatant into a waste container and gently blot the plate onto a paper towel.
10. Resuspend the cells in 100 μl of the appropriate antibody master mix.

11. Incubate for 20 min at 4 °C in the dark.
12. Add 100 μl of 1× perm/wash buffer to each of the wells.
13. Centrifuge at 300 × *g* for 4 min at 4 °C.
14. Rapidly invert the plate to discard the supernatant into a waste container and gently blot the plate onto a paper towel.
15. Resuspend the cells in 200 μl of 1× perm/wash buffer.
16. Centrifuge at 300 × *g* for 4 min at 4 °C.
17. Rapidly invert the plate to discard the supernatant into a waste container and gently blot the plate onto a paper towel.
18. Resuspend the cells in 250 μl of FACS buffer, transfer them to tubes that are compatible with the available cytometer (e.g., 12 × 75 mm polystyrene round-bottom tubes), and store at 4 °C in the dark until analysis (*see* **Note 13**).

3.6 Flow Cytometric Acquisition

1. Turn on the cytometer and allow sufficient time for the lasers to warm up.
2. Select appropriate lasers and parameters to match the fluorochromes used in the experiment.
3. Load a tube of unstained cells onto the cytometer and begin to acquire events.
4. Adjust the PMT voltages so that the majority of the cells of interest are in the lower left quadrant of a linear FSS and SSC plot and within the first two logarithmic decades for each of the fluorescence parameters (*see* **Note 18**).
5. Briefly acquire an experimental sample and adjust PMT voltages to ensure that none of the fluorescence parameters are off the scale.
6. Acquire the single-color and unstained CompBeads and calculate fluorescence compensation (*see* **Note 14**).
7. Create histograms and cytograms and draw gates to allow the identification of the target populations of interest.
8. Begin acquisition of experimental samples and aim to collect a sufficient number of events to allow statistically justified conclusions to be drawn (*see* **Note 19**).
9. For data analysis and anticipated results, *see* **Notes 20–22**.

4 Notes

1. Having identified the fluorochromes that can be detected using a given instrument, the choice of specific fluorochrome combinations is largely dependent on the markers that are to be assessed. Ideal combinations will include fluorochromes

with maximal fluorescence intensities that have minimal spectral overlap with each other. Identifying appropriate combinations of fluorochromes with these characteristics becomes increasingly challenging with increasing number of markers. Generally, the brightest fluorochromes, such as phycoerythrin (PE) and allophycocyanin (APC), are best reserved for markers that are only expressed on rare cells or at a low density on the cells. Conversely, dimmer fluorochromes, such as Alexa Fluor 700, can be used with markers that are highly expressed on distinct populations. There are a number of useful Web-based tools that have been designed to facilitate the design of complementary fluorochrome panels, including the BD Biosciences Fluorescence Spectrum Viewer, Flourish from Treestar, and CytoGenie from Woodside Logic.

2. Clone 2.4G2 is a rat IgG2b κ antibody and therefore cannot be used with staining panels involving an anti-rat secondary antibody. In this situation, the 2.4G2 Fc blocking antibody can be substituted with 10 % normal mouse serum.
3. It is generally most convenient if all the antibodies used in a panel are directly conjugated to fluorochromes that are compatible with the detectors on the available cytometer. If directly conjugated antibodies are not available, an indirect labeling protocol can be employed using a biotin-conjugated primary antibody followed by streptavidin-conjugated fluorochrome, or an unlabeled primary antibody and a fluorochrome-conjugated anti-isotype secondary antibody. Indirect labeling protocols can result in signal amplification, allowing greater sensitivity than direct labeling; however, they introduce additional complexity to experiments because of the need to identify compatible combinations of primary and secondary antibodies, and because of the potential of secondary antibody cross-reactivity and high background staining. Addressing these issues becomes increasingly more challenging when attempting to combine larger number of antibodies in a panel. All of the antibodies used in a panel should be titrated to determine optimal staining concentrations.
4. As discussed earlier, the specific choice of markers and fluorochromes will depend on the specific experimental objectives. Table 2 presents an example of two phenotyping schemes that could potentially be used with a 4-laser cytometer to accurately identify several major immune subsets in the lung that have been reported to be involved in allergic airway disease [5–8]. These schemes can be modified to focus on particular populations of interest, and the choice of complementary fluorochrome combinations can be optimized to accommodate the capabilities of the available cytometer. Note that these phenotyping schemes include a viability dye (e.g., 7AAD, DAPI,

Table 2
Phenotyping schemes for use with a 4-laser cytometer

A. Antibody panel	Identifiable cell populations and key defining markers
AmCyan anti-CD45 (30-F11)	*NK cells*: $CD3^-$, $NK1.1^+$
Pacific Blue anti-CD3 (17A2)	*NKT cells*: $CD3^+$, $NK1.1^+$
PE-Cy7 anti-NK1.1 (PK136)	*γδ T cells*: $CD3^+$, $TCR\gamma\delta^+$
FITC anti-TCRγδ (UC7-13D5)	*CD4+ αβ T cells*: $CD3^+$, $TCR\gamma\delta^-$, $NK1.1^-$, $CD4^+$, $CD8^{low}$
APC-Cy7 anti-CD4 (RM4-5)	Naïve subset: $CD44^{low}$, $CD62L^{hi}$
Pac. Blue anti-CD8 (53-6.7)	Effector/effector memory subset: $CD44^{hi}$, $CD62L^{low}$
PE anti-CD62L (MEL-14)	Central memory subset: $CD44^{hi}$, $CD62L^{hi}$
APC anti-CD44 (IM7)	*$CD8^+$ αβ T cells*: $CD3^+$, $TCR\gamma\delta^-$, $NK1.1^-$, $CD4^{low}$, $CD8^+$
DAPI (viability stain)	Naïve subset: $CD44^{low}$, $CD62L^{hi}$ Effector/effector memory subset: $CD44^{hi}$, $CD62L^{low}$ Central memory subset: $CD44^{hi}$, $CD62L^{hi}$
B. Antibody panel	**Identifiable cell populations and key defining markers (*see* Fig. 1)**
AmCyan anti-CD45 (30-F11)	*Alveolar macrophages*: $Autofluorescence^{hi}$, $F4/80^{hi}$, $CD11c^{hi}$, $MHCII^{int}$, $CD11b^{low}$
FITC anti-F4/80 (BM8)	*Interstitial macrophages*: $Autofluorescence^{hi}$, $F4/80^{hi}$, $CD11c^{low}$, $MHCII^{low}$, $CD11b^{hi}$
APC-Cy7 anti-Gr-1 (RB6-8C5)	*Inflammatory dendritic cells*: $CD11c^{hi}$, $CD11b^{hi}$, $Gr\text{-}1^{hi}$
Pac. Blue anti-MHCII (M5/114.15.2)	*$CD11b^{hi}$ dendritic cells*: $CD11c^{hi}$, $MHCII^{hi}$, $CD11b^{hi}$, $CD103^{low}$
PE-Cy7 anti-CD11c (N418)	*$CD103^{hi}$ dendritic cells*: $CD11c^{hi}$, $MHCII^{hi}$, $CD11b^{low}$, $CD103^{hi}$
APC-Cy7 anti-CD11b (M1/70)	*Plasmacytoid dendritic cells*: $CD11c^{med}$, $MHCII^{med}$, $mPDCA1^{hi}$
APC anti-CD103 (M290)	*Neutrophils*: $MHCII^{low}$, $CD11c^{low}$, $CD11b^{hi}$, $Ly6G^{hi}$, $F4/80^{low}$
PE anti-mPDCA1	*Eosinophils*: SSC^{hi}, $MHCII^{low}$, $CD11c^{low}$, $CD11b^{hi}$, $F4/80^{int}$
DAPI (viability stain)	*Monocytes*: SSC^{int}, $MHCII^{low}$, $CD11c^{low}$, $CD11b^{hi}$, $F4/80^{int}$, $Gr\text{-}1^{hi}$ & $Gr\text{-}1^{low}$ subsets

The above table lists antibody panels that can accurately identify several major immune subsets in the lung that have been reported to be involved in allergic airway disease

or LIVE/DEAD® Fixable Dead Cell Stain, Invitrogen) to facilitate the exclusion of dead cells, which are often autofluorescent and exhibit nonspecific antibody binding. Certain cell types, such as alveolar macrophages, are also highly autofluorescent and it can be difficult to distinguish this from 488 nm excited fluorochromes, which can present a challenge during data analysis. One useful strategy to deal with this is to keep the 530/50 "FITC" channel open to specifically allow for the detection of cellular autofluorescence, which can be very useful in distinguishing highly autofluorescent macrophages from other cell types [9]. Another strategy, employed in Table 2 and in Fig. 1, is to use FITC-conjugated F4/80, a marker expressed by alveolar macrophages, allowing alveolar macrophages to be identified by any positive signal in the FITC channel.

5. Multiparametric phenotyping schemes generally use combinations of fluorochromes that exhibit some degree of spectral overlap. To address this issue, fluorescence compensation using single-color-stained controls is employed to more accurately represent the true signal in a given detector by subtracting spillover from other detectors. Ideally, compensation should be performed using suspensions of cells or antibody capture beads (e.g., BD CompBeads) individually stained with the same antibodies used in the experimental panel. It should be noted that antibody capture beads provide a number of advantages over cells and are generally preferable for more accurate and consistent compensation. A limitation of antibody capture beads is that they can only capture specific antibody isotypes, and cells must be used in instances where the antibody isotype does not match the beads. In situations where only limited numbers of cells are available, as is often the case with BAL preparations, it can sometimes be challenging to reserve adequate number of cells for single-color compensation controls. However, it should be noted that while the cells used for compensation do need to express the antigen of interest, they do not need to be from the same source as the experimental sample (i.e., splenocytes containing CD4+ T cells can be used to compensate BAL T cell samples stained with an anti-CD4 antibody).

6. The first step in any flow cytometric protocol is to generate a single-cell suspension from the tissue of interest. In the case of allergic airway disease models, inflating the lungs with a physiological saline solution and collecting the resulting BAL fluid offers a way to specifically isolate cells that have infiltrated into the airway space. As a complementary approach, digestion of

Fig. 1 Example of a gating strategy to identify major lung myeloid populations. Whole lungs from a naïve (**a**) and a challenged (**b**) C57BL/6 mouse were digested, processed, and stained with an antibody panel similar to that described in Table 2B. Viable hematopoietic cells are identified as being DAPI^{low} and CD45^{positive}. Lung macrophages (*a*) are identifiable as a distinct F4/80^{high}, CD11b^{intermediate} population. The alveolar macrophages within this population are highly autofluorescent and are CD11c^{high} and MHCII^{intermediate} (not shown). Within the F4/80^{low} population, dendritic cells (*b*) can be identified as being CD11c^{hi} and MHCII^{hi}. These dendritic cells can be further subdivided into Gr-1^{hi}, CD11b^{hi} inflammatory monocyte-derived DCs (*c*), CD103^{+} DCs (*d*), and CD11b^{+} myeloid DCs (*e*). Differences in F4/80 expression and granularity, as assessed by SSC, can be used to identify the MHCII^{low}, CD11b^{hi} cells as neutrophils (*f*), eosinophils (*g*), and monocytes (*h*). The monocyte population can be further subdivided into inflammatory Gr-1^{hi} monocytes (*i*) and resident Gr-1^{low} monocytes (*j*). Data kindly provided by Dr. Daigo Hashimoto

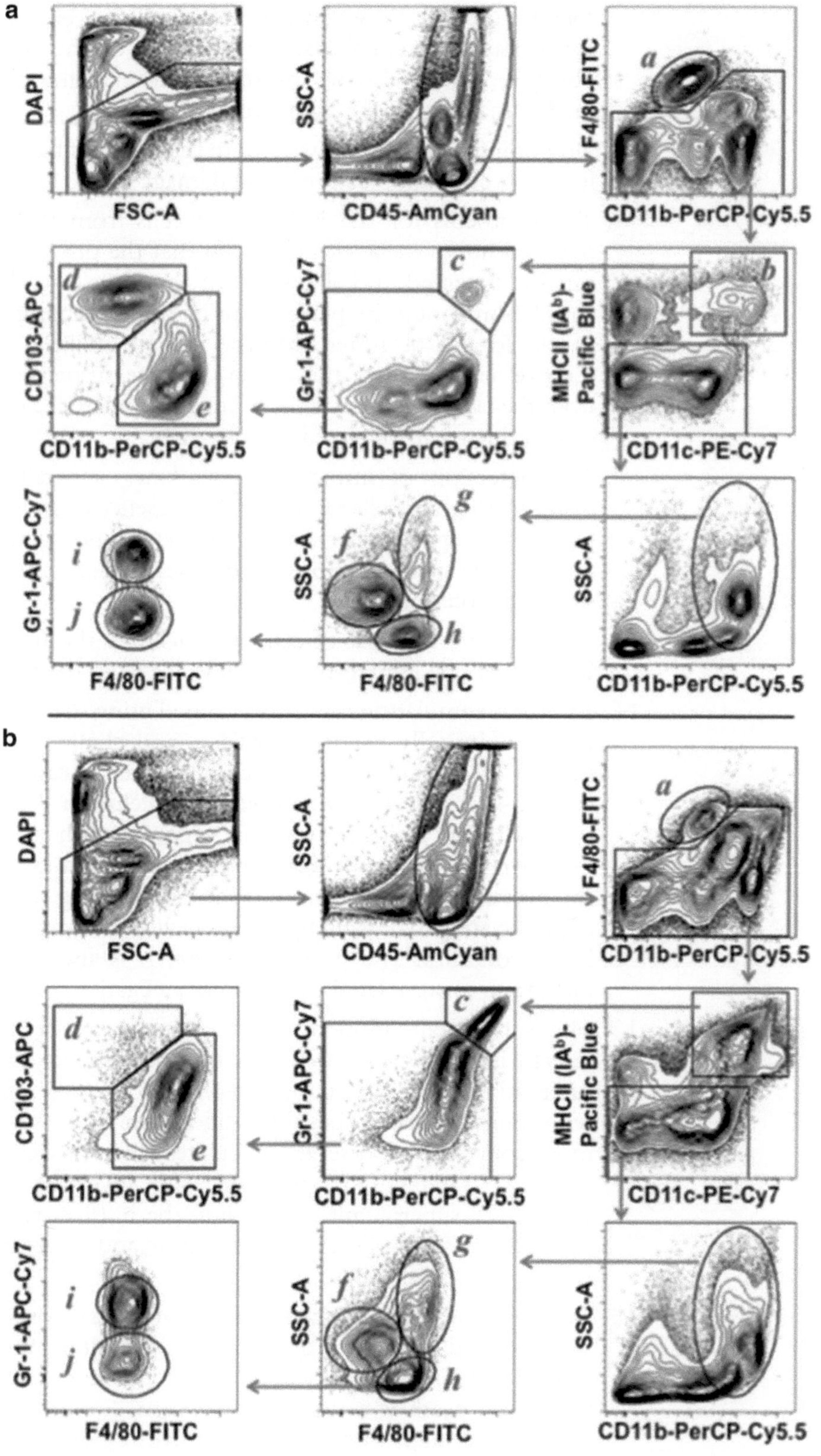
a
DAPI
FSC-A
SSC-A
CD45-AmCyan
F4/80-FITC
CD11b-PerCP-Cy5.5
a
CD103-APC
CD11b-PerCP-Cy5.5
d
e
Gr-1-APC-Cy7
CD11b-PerCP-Cy5.5
c
MHCII (IA^b)-Pacific Blue
CD11c-PE-Cy7
b
Gr-1-APC-Cy7
F4/80-FITC
i
j
SSC-A
F4/80-FITC
f
g
h
SSC-A
CD11b-PerCP-Cy5.5
b
DAPI
FSC-A
SSC-A
CD45-AmCyan
F4/80-FITC
CD11b-PerCP-Cy5.5
a
CD103-APC
CD11b-PerCP-Cy5.5
d
e
Gr-1-APC-Cy7
CD11b-PerCP-Cy5.5
c
MHCII (IA^b)-Pacific Blue
CD11c-PE-Cy7
Gr-1-APC-Cy7
F4/80-FITC
i
j
SSC-A
F4/80-FITC
f
g
h
SSC-A
CD11b-PerCP-Cy5.5

total lung tissue allows an isolation of all the cells in both the alveolar and interstitial spaces. Depending on the experimental objective, it can also be informative to examine cells in the mediastinal lung-draining lymph nodes.

7. Do not inflate the lungs with more than 1 ml of buffer because forced overinflation can result in damage to the lung.
8. The protocols for the isolation of cells from the BAL and digested lung can be combined, in that the pre-lavaged lungs can be dissected and digested. In this case, the pulmonary circulation should be perfused prior to performing the BAL. It should also be noted that the BAL is unlikely to entirely remove all cells from the airways, so the suspension of cells from the lavaged lung will likely contain a mixture of interstitial cells and partially depleted alveolar cells.
9. The detection of intracellular cytokines generally requires restimulating the cells ex vivo in the presence of an inhibitor of protein transport. This section can be skipped if the experimental analysis is only focused on the characterization of cell surface markers.
10. Using higher number of cells will facilitate the final analysis, but this will be limited by the cell yields from the tissues.
11. Ex vivo restimulation can be performed using the same antigen that was initially used to sensitize and challenge the mice (in this case, ovalbumin), which allows an assessment of the antigen-specific cytokine response. The cells can also be stimulated with an antigen-nonspecific agonist, such as PMA and ionomycin, which provides a more generalized assessment of the overall cytokine response. When stimulating the cells with a specific antigen, it is useful to also include a nonspecific stimulation condition as a positive control. It is also important to include an unstimulated condition as a negative control.
12. The subsequent antibody staining steps can be performed directly in the same 96-well plate that was used for stimulation. Alternatively, the cells can be transferred to 12 × 75 mm polystyrene round-bottom tubes for antibody staining. It is generally more convenient to use 96-well plates when processing larger number of samples (>10) because rapidly inverting the plate to discard the supernatant and adding the buffers with a multichannel pipette are faster than aspirating and resuspending the cells in individual tubes.
13. Samples should be analyzed by flow cytometry as soon as possible to avoid potential artifacts that may result from prolonged storage. This is particularly important in the case of unfixed cells where cell death is a significant concern. Formaldehyde-fixed cells that are kept in the dark at 4 °C can generally be stored for longer periods of time but should generally be analyzed within 72 h to minimize loss of fluorescence signal.

14. Accurate compensation controls require single-stained samples for each of the fluorochromes that are being used, and these single-stained samples must be at least as bright as the stained sample. It is also critical to include an unstained sample with identical autofluorescence properties to the single-stained samples. These compensation controls should be acquired on the cytometer on each day of testing using the same photomultiplier tube voltages that are used for the experimental samples. While compensation has historically been performed manually, this process can become very laborious when dealing with large number of fluorescent parameters and can be a significant source of variability. Multiple software platforms that are used for the acquisition and analysis of flow cytometry data now include algorithms for automatic compensation, and the use of these methods is generally preferable to manual compensation. It should also be noted that a number of analysis programs allow compensation to be performed post acquisition. There are a number of resources that provide a more thorough discussion of compensation [10].
15. This section of the protocol uses the BD Cytofix/Cytoperm Fixation/Permeabilization kit and largely follows the manufacturer's instructions. It can be modified to accommodate similar formaldehyde-based fixation and saponin-based permeabilization buffers provided by other manufacturers.
16. Prolonged incubation in formaldehyde-based fixation buffers can result in loss of fluorescent signals and dimmer staining of certain intracellular antigens. Fixed samples can safely be stored for several hours to days prior to proceeding with the permeabilization step. However, it is recommended that after 30 min, the formaldehyde buffer be washed off and the cells resuspended in FACs buffer for prolonged storage.
17. As is the case with cell surface markers, the specific choice of intracellular markers and fluorochromes in a panel will depend on the specific experimental objectives. Table 3 presents an example of an 8-color phenotyping scheme that could be used to subdivide the CD4+ T cell compartment into Th1, Th2, Th9, and Th17 subsets. Depending on the experimental objectives and the capabilities of the available cytometer, this phenotyping scheme could easily be modified to examine alternative combinations of cytokines, for example, simultaneously examining IL-2 and TNFα production by CD4+ and CD8+ T cells.
18. On some instruments, Cytometer Setup and Tracking (CS&T) can be used to automatically determine PMT voltages in the optimal linear response range. In these situations, the CS&T-assigned voltage settings should typically not require drastic adjustments unless experimental samples are off of the scale.

Table 3
8-color phenotyping scheme used to subdivide the CD4+ T cell compartment

Antibody panel	Identifiable cell populations and key defining markers
Surface stain	
AmCyan anti-CD45	*CD4+ αβ T cells*: CD45^{hi}, TCRβ^{hi}, CD4^{hi}, CD8^{low}
Pac. Blue anti-TCRβ (H57-597)	*Th1*: IFNγ^{+}
PerCP-Cy5.5 anti-CD4 (RM4-5)	*Th2*: IL-4^{+}/IL-5^{+}
APC-Cy7 anti-CD8 (53-6.7)	*Th9*: IL-9^{+}
UV LIVE/DEAD stain	*Th17*: IL-17A^{+}
Intracellular stain	
PE-Cy7 anti-IFNγ (XMG1.2)	Note that subsets of CD4+ cells may coexpress combinations of these markers and may not be clearly definable within a single subset
PE anti-IL-4 (11B11) or PE IL-5 (TRFK5)	
FITC anti-IL-17A (TC11-18H10)	
APC anti-IL-9 (RM9A4)	

The above table lists an antibody panel that can accurately subdivide the CD4+ T cell compartment into Th1, Th2, Th9, and Th17 subsets

19. The total number of events collected will depend on background staining levels and the frequency of the population of interest. When dealing with a population that represents a fairly high frequency of the total sample (<10 %), collecting 5,000 events typically results in a coefficient of variation (CV) on the order of 5 %, which is generally acceptable in the field. When dealing with a rarer population, the total number of events collected must be increased. For example, if the population of interest represents only 0.1 % of the total sample, approximately 500,000 total events would need to be collected to ensure a 5 % CV. When acquiring several samples in which the frequency of the population of interest varies, it is generally good practice to gate on the population of interest and set a stopping gate to collect a consistent number of events within this population [11].
20. The acquisition of flow cytometry data results in the generation of a listmode file that can be exported for subsequent analysis. There are a number of free and commercially available programs available for data analysis. While there are significant differences in the interfaces of these programs, the fundamental principles of analysis remain the same. For the applications discussed in this chapter, the analysis largely focuses on determining the frequency of particular subpopulations within the sample, e.g., the percentage of macrophages among lung hematopoietic cells, or the percentage of IFNγ-producing cells among CD4 T cells. This is generally accomplished by sequentially gating populations until the population of interest is adequately identified. Gates are typically drawn based on whether a population is positive or negative for a marker of interest.

This practice is generally straightforward for brightly expressed markers that result in distinct positive and negative populations, but can be more challenging for dim markers or those with a broad distribution. For these challenging markers, additional staining controls should be implemented (*see* **Note 21**).

21. Fluorescently labeled isotype control antibodies have historically been used to help determine background staining levels and thereby identify positively stained cells. While this can be helpful in identifying nonspecific Fc receptor-mediated antibody binding, when conducting multiparameter experiments, it is generally more accurate to employ a "fluorescence-minus-one" (FMO) control [10]. FMO controls are samples stained with all the antibodies in the panel except for the antibody of interest, providing an accurate measure of background staining that can be used to set a threshold for positivity for a given marker.
22. Gating strategies will vary based on the specific markers used in an experiment, and multiple strategies can typically be used to ultimately identify the population of interest. In complex multidimensional experiments it is often wise to attempt to visualize populations using several alternative gating strategies to determine the best way to identify sample heterogeneity. Figure 1 provides an example of a gating strategy used to identify major myeloid populations in total digested lung that was stained using a panel similar to that presented in Table 2B.

References

1. Winterrowd GE, Chin JE (1999) Flow cytometric detection of antigen-specific cytokine responses in lung T cells in a murine model of pulmonary inflammation. J Immunol Methods 226:105–118
2. Randolph DA, Carruthers CJ, Szabo SJ, Murphy KM, Chaplin DD (1999) Modulation of airway inflammation by passive transfer of allergen-specific Th1 and Th2 cells in a mouse model of asthma. J Immunol 162:2375–2383
3. Wilson RH, Whitehead GS, Nakano H, Free ME, Kolls JK, Cook DN (2009) Allergic sensitization through the airway primes Th17-dependent neutrophilia and airway hyperresponsiveness. Am J Respir Crit Care Med 180:720–730
4. Soroosh P, Doherty TA (2009) Th9 and allergic disease. Immunology 127:450–458
5. Hoffmann PR, Gurary A, Hoffmann FW, Saux CJ-L, Teeters K, Hashimoto AC, Tam EK, Berry MJ (2007) A new approach for analyzing cellular infiltration during allergic airway inflammation. J Immunol Methods 328:21–33
6. van Rijt LS, Kuipers H, Vos N, Hijdra D, Hoogsteden HC, Lambrecht BN (2004) A rapid flow cytometric method for determining the cellular composition of bronchoalveolar lavage fluid cells in mouse models of asthma. J Immunol Methods 288:111–121
7. Stevens WW, Kim TS, Pujanauski LM, Hao X, Braciale TJ (2007) Detection and quantitation of eosinophils in the murine respiratory tract by flow cytometry. J Immunol Methods 327: 63–74
8. Pastva AM, Mukherjee S, Giamberardino C, Hsia B, Lo B, Sempowski GD, Wright JR (2011) Lung effector memory and activated CD4+ T cells display enhanced proliferation in surfactant protein A-deficient mice during allergen-mediated inflammation. J Immunol 186(5):2842–2849
9. Vermaelen K, Pauwels R (2004) Accurate and simple discrimination of mouse pulmonary dendritic cell and macrophage populations by flow cytometry: methodology and new insights. Cytometry A 61A:170–177
10. Roederer M (2001) Spectral compensation for flow cytometry: visualization artifacts, limitations, and caveats. Cytometry 45:194–205
11. Roederer M (2008) How many events is enough? Are you positive? Cytometry A 73A: 384–385

Chapter 24

Generation of Bone Marrow and Fetal Liver Chimeric Mice

Eda K. Holl

Abstract

The creation of bone marrow and fetal liver chimeric mice has proven to be a valuable tool in the field of immunology. Chimeric mice are used to study the contribution of various cell types of hematopoietic versus non-hematopoietic origin in the course of an immune response. In this chapter, we describe a detailed method to obtain bone marrow or fetal liver chimeric mice and assess the efficiency of donor cells to repopulate the hematopoietic compartment of recipient mice.

Key words Bone marrow transplant, Fetal liver transplant, Congenically labeled cells, Radiation, Assessment of reconstitution, Antibodies

1 Introduction

Transplantation of congenically labeled bone marrow or fetal liver cells into lethally irradiated mice has significantly improved our ability to study cellular and humoral immune responses. Many studies use this technique to distinguish the contribution of hematopoietic cells versus non-hematopoietic cells during the course of an immune response [1, 2]. A variety of immune responses can be recreated in vitro using cell lines and in vitro-differentiated cells (dendritic cells, macrophages, T and B cells) [3–5]. However, these studies are limited due to the complexity and time-course of many immune reactions that take place in vivo. Bone marrow chimeras have allowed the study of hematopoietic cell development and their participation in long-term immune responses in a physiological setting.

Reconstitution of lethally irradiated mice can be conducted using cells obtained from (a) bone marrow of adult donor mice [6] and (b) fetal liver cells obtained from embryonic day 14 (E14) mouse fetuses [7]. Reconstitution of lethally irradiated mice with fetal liver cells is useful when studying the immune system of embryonic lethal animals. Here, we describe how to prepare

Irving C. Allen (ed.), *Mouse Models of Allergic Disease: Methods and Protocols*, Methods in Molecular Biology, vol. 1032,
DOI 10.1007/978-1-62703-496-8_24, © Springer Science+Business Media, LLC 2013

radiation chimeras using both sources of hematopoietic cells. This protocol utilizes congenic mouse strains that differ at the common leukocyte antigen (CD45) locus. The CD45 antigen is expressed by all nucleated cells and allows donor cells to be easily distinguished from host cells [8]. Expression of the CD45 allele on the surface of nucleated cells has proven to be advantageous not only for detection of donor cells, but also for their isolation and usage in subsequent assays.

Recipient mice are subjected to predetermined lethal or sublethal doses of X-ray or γ radiation and then injected with donor bone marrow- or fetal liver-derived cells. The mice are then screened by flow cytometry for the presence of donor cells 4–6 weeks post adoptive transfer. A detailed study published in 1988 by Spangrude et al. demonstrates the ability of hematopoietic precursor cells to reconstitute all blood cell types [9]. Additionally, the long-term fate of reconstituted hematopoietic cells has been followed and published by Jordan and Lemischka in 1990 [10]. This chapter aims to provide a comprehensive method by which to obtain chimeric mice and notes common measures that can be taken to ensure successful transplantation and mouse survival.

2 Materials

2.1 Preparation of Bone Marrow or Fetal Liver Chimeras

1. Bone marrow recipient animals: C57BL/6 males, 8–10 weeks old (National Cancer Institute).
2. Bone marrow donor animals: C57BL/6 CD45.1 males, 2–5 months old (National Cancer Institute).
3. Fetal liver donor animals: C57BL/6 CD45.1 animals, embryonic day 14.
4. Control bone marrow donor animal: C57BL/6 CD45.2 males, 2–5 months old (National Cancer Institute).
5. X-ray machine or cesium irradiator for γ irradiation.
6. Mouse irradiation chambers (Braintree Scientific, Inc.).
7. Animal CO_2 euthanasia chamber.
8. Antibiotic water: 2 mg/ml of neomycin sulfate prepared in autoclaved water, pH = 2 with 2 N HCl.
9. Cold phosphate-buffered saline (1× PBS).
10. PBS with 3 % fetal bovine serum (FBS).
11. Straight surgical forceps and scissors.
12. Non-tissue culture-treated sterile petri dishes (100 × 20 mm).
13. 70 % Ethanol.
14. 1 ml syringes with 27-guage needles.
15. Cell strainers (70 μm).

16. Mouse restraining chamber (Braintree Scientific, Inc.).
17. Infrared heating lamp.

2.2 Assessment of Reconstitution

1. Irradiated and reconstituted mice.
2. Heparin tubes for blood collection (Becton Dickinson).
3. Submandibular bleeding lancets.
4. PBS.
5. Red cell lysis buffer (Beckman Coulter).
6. PBS containing 3 % FBS.
7. FACS buffer: PBS, 3 % FBS, 0.04 % Sodium Azide. Mix, filter sterilize, and store at 4 °C.
8. Monoclonal antibodies to detect recipient and donor hematopoietic cells (CD45.1 and CD45.2 alleles), as well as B cells and T cells (CD19, CD3, CD4, and CD8) (Beckman Coulter).
9. 5 ml centrifuge tubes or 96-well plate.
10. Centrifuge.
11. Flow cytometer.

3 Methods

3.1 Preparation of Bone Marrow Chimeras

1. Irradiate bone marrow-recipient animals using the X-ray machine or the cesium irradiator at the appropriate dose as detailed below.
2. The animals are placed in a pie chamber (holds up to 11 mice). This method allows for even delivery of the radiation dose by ensuring that all animals are placed at the same distance from the radiation source. It is important to reduce the amount of time the animals will spend in the pie chamber to maintain sufficient oxygen flow and reduce overheating of the animals.
3. The irradiation dose will vary by mouse strain. The laboratory should determine the appropriate dose of irradiation for their mouse strain. This protocol will outline the doses used for C57BL/6 wild-type animals.
4. Animals are exposed to a lethal dose of irradiation (900–1,100 rad) to prevent recovery of endogenous hematopoietic cells. Radiation can be delivered in one single dose the day before bone marrow transplant or in two equal doses 6 h apart to minimize damage of gut and lung cells. If the radiation dose is split into two equal doses the animals should be exposed to the highest dose of irradiation (1,100 rad) to achieve elimination of endogenous progenitor cells (*see* **Note 1**).

5. Euthanize the donor mice: C57BL/6 CD45.1 males and one control C57BL/6 male as approved by the institution's animal protocol.
6. Isolate bone marrow cells using the following protocol: Spray the mice with 70 % ethanol and cut the abdominal skin. Cut the skin all the way to the hind legs and remove it using forceps and scissors. Remove the feet and place the legs in 70 % ethanol for 2 min. Transfer the legs to cold PBS for 2 min, two times. Remove excess flesh from the leg bone and cut off the ends of the bones. Place the bones in media while flushing the bone marrow. Flush the bones using a 27-guage needle.
7. Once finished, make a single-cell suspension of all the marrow and passage the cells through a strainer.
8. Pool cells from all mice and adjust the density to 5×10^6 cells/ml of PBS. One mouse yields about 70×10^6 bone marrow cells. In the author's laboratory, cells are usually pooled from three different mice to ensure sufficient number of cells to perform bone marrow transplants into a large number of animals.
9. Inject 200 μl of bone marrow cell suspension intravenously into irradiated recipient and control animals (*see* **Note 2**). One can inject anywhere from 1 to 5×10^6 cells/recipient.
10. Maintain animals on neomycin sulfate water (2 mg/ml) for 2 weeks following transplantation to prevent infection. Fill a 2 L glass bottle with water and adjust the pH using HCl. Autoclave sterilize water and allow cooling to room temperature. Water is autoclave sterilized to ensure removal of *Pseudomonas aeruginosa*, a common waterborne pathogen. Add 4 g of neomycin sulfate and allow it to dissolve. Wrap the bottle with aluminum foil to protect the water from light. Water can be stored at 4 °C for up to a week. We replace the water in the mouse cages two times a week.
11. Six to eight weeks post transplantation, recipient mice can be analyzed for the presence of donor-derived cells via flow cytometry.

3.2 Preparation of Fetal Liver Chimeras

1. Irradiate the fetal liver-recipient animals using the X-ray machine or the cesium irradiator at the appropriate dose as detailed in Subheading 3.1.
2. Euthanize the donor mice: C57BL/6 CD45.1 pregnant female mice at gestation day 14 (*see* **Note 3**).
3. Isolate fetal livers using the following protocol: Spray the mice with 70 % ethanol and cut the abdominal skin. Expose the embryonic sac. Using forceps and scissors remove the embryos and place in a petri dish with media (the embryos will look like pearls on a string). Remove individual embryos from embryonic sac and remove the surrounding tissue. Cut the abdominal skin

of the embryos and expose the fetal liver. The fetal liver is very fragile and should be carefully removed using two forceps.

4. Once finished, make a single-cell suspension of the fetal liver cells by passing the liver through a 1 ml pipette tip. Passage the cells through a strainer.
5. Pool cells from all mice and adjust the density to 5×10^6 cells/ml of PBS. One mouse yields about 5×10^6 fetal liver cells.
6. Inject 200 μl of the fetal liver cell suspension intravenously into irradiated recipient and control animals. One can inject anywhere from 1 to 5×10^6 cells/recipient.
7. Maintain animals on neomycin sulfate water (2 mg/ml) for 2 weeks following transplantation to prevent infection.
8. Six to eight weeks post transplantation, recipient mice can be analyzed for the presence of donor-derived cells via flow cytometry.

3.3 Screening Animals for Donor-Derived Cells

1. Collect 200 μl of peripheral blood from irradiated and reconstituted animals into heparinated tubes to prevent clotting. Resuspend the blood in heparin by inverting the tubes 2–3 times.
2. Add 100 μl of blood into 2 ml of red blood cell lysis buffer and resuspend by vortexing. The solution will go from turbid to clear red as the cells lyse (2–3 min). Add 2 ml of 3 % FBS/PBS to all tubes and spin down to pellet cells. Wash all cells one more time and aspirate the solution.
3. Resuspend the cell pellet in FACS buffer (*see* **Note 4**). Transfer cells into several 5-ml centrifuge tubes or a 96-well plate depending on the number of stains that will be evaluated.
4. Prepare the antibody cocktail for staining. Make a master mix for all of the stains (*see* **Note 5**).
5. The cells will be stained with anti-CD45.1 and CD45.2 antibodies to determine the donor vs. host cell composition. Often T cell markers, such as CD3, CD4, and CD8, are added to the staining cocktail to determine the percentage of donor T cells. T lymphocytes are the most radiation-resistant cell type and usually take the longest to be reconstituted [11].

4 Notes

1. T cells are the most radiation-resistant cell type. Therefore, if the irradiation dose will be split into two separate doses it is recommended that at least a combined dose of 1,100 rad be given to the animals. Irradiate the mice the day before bone marrow transplant.

2. We find that it is easier to perform tail vain injections with mice whose body temperature is brought closer to 38 °C. We usually use an infrared heat lamp to increase the body temperature of the animals. The increase in temperature exposes the veins to the surface for injections.
3. In order to obtain E14 embryos, female and male mice are bred overnight. Male mice are taken out of the cage the following morning and females are checked for the presence of plugs. Fourteen days post breeding, pregnant mice are euthanized and the E14 pups are harvested. Fetal livers are harvested from the embryos and resuspended into single cells. If genotyping of the embryos is required at the time of harvest, the fetal livers can be placed on ice for several hours. An expedited genotyping protocol is recommended in order to minimize the number of dying cells.
4. Resuspend cells at 20×10^6 cells per mL of FACS buffer. We use 50 μl for each stain that will be transplanted. If screening a large number of mice, a 96-well plate is recommended for staining as it saves time during staining and washing.
5. Titrations should be performed for all antibodies prior to use to identify the proper concentration for optimal staining. A master mix for all stains is also recommended to limit sample-to-sample variability.

Acknowledgment

This work was supported by the NIH grant F32DK094543-01.

References

1. Yang D, Postnikov YV, Tewary P, de la Rosa G, Wei F, Klinman D, Gioannini T, Weiss JP (2012) High-mobility group nucleosome-binding protein 1 acts as an alarmin and is critical for lipopolysaccharide-induced immune responses. J Exp Med 209(1):157–171
2. Vatakis DN, Koya RC, Nixon CC, Wei L, Kim SG, Avancena P, Bristol G, Baltimore D, Kohn DB, Ribas A, Radu CG, Galic Z, Zack JA (2011) Antitumor activity from antigen-specific CD8 T cells generated in vivo from genetically engineered human hematopoietic stem cells. Proc Natl Acad Sci USA 108(51):E1408–E1416
3. Wong AW, Birckey WJ, Taxman DJ, van Deventer HW, Reed W, Gao JX, Zheng P, Liu Y, Li P, Blum JS, McKinnon KP, Ting JP (2003) CIITA-regulated plexin-A1 affects T-cell-dendritic cell interactions. Nat Immunol 4(9):891–898
4. Kuraoka M, Holl TM, Liao D, Womble M, Cain DW, Reynolds AE, Kelsoe G (2011) Activation-induced cytidine deaminase mediates central tolerance in B cells. Proc Natl Acad Sci USA 108(28):11560–11565
5. Holl TM, Haynes BF, Kelsoe G (2010) Stromal cell independent B cell development in vitro: generation and recovery of autoreactive clones. J Immunol Methods 354(1–2):53–67
6. Allen IC, Tekippe EM, Woodford RM, Uronis JM, Holl EK, Rogers AB, Herfarth HH, Jobin C, Ting JPY (2010) The NLRP3 inflammasome functions as a negative regulator of tumorigenesis during colitis-associated cancer. J Exp Med 207(5):1045–1056
7. Choi YI, Duke-Cohan JS, Ahmed WB, Handley MA, Mann F, Epstein JA, Clayton LK, Reinherz EL (2008) PlexinD1 glycoprotein controls migration of positively selected

thymocytes into the medulla. Immunity 29(6): 888–898
8. Shen FW, Saga Y, Litman G, Freeman G, Tung JS, Cantor H, Boyse EA (1985) Cloning of Ly-5 cDNA. Proc Natl Acad Sci USA 82(21): 7360–7363
9. Spangrude GJ, Heimfeld S, Weissman IL (1988) Purification and characterization of mouse hematopoietic stem cells. Science 241(4861):58–62
10. Jordan CT, Lemischka IR (1990) Clonal and systemic analysis of long-term hematopoiesis in the mouse. Genes Dev 4(2):220–232
11. Goldschneider I, Komschlies KL, Greiner DL (1986) Studies of thymocytopoiesis in rats and mice. I. Kinetics of appearance of thymocytes using a direct intrathymic adoptive transfer assay for thymocyte precursors. J Exp Med 163(1):1–17

INDEX

Irving C. Allen (ed.), *Mouse Models of Allergic Disease: Methods and Protocols*, Methods in Molecular Biology, vol. 1032, DOI 10.1007/978-1-62703-496-8, © Springer Science+Business Media, LLC 2013

I

L

M

N

O

P

If you have any concerns about our products,
you can contact us on
ProductSafety@springernature.com

In case Publisher is established outside the EU,
the EU authorized representative is:
Springer Nature Customer Service Center GmbH
Europaplatz 3, 69115 Heidelberg, Germany

Printed by Libri Plureos GmbH
in Hamburg, Germany

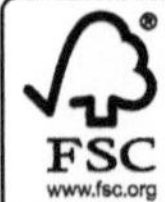

MIX
Papier aus verantwortungsvollen Quellen
Paper from responsible sources
FSC® C105338

If you have any concerns about our products,
you can contact us on
ProductSafety@springernature.com

In case Publisher is established outside the EU,
the EU authorized representative is:
Springer Nature Customer Service Center GmbH
Europaplatz 3, 69115 Heidelberg, Germany

Printed by Libri Plureos GmbH
in Hamburg, Germany